PHARMACEUTICAL PRESS
Essential Knowledge

Management, Leadership and Entrepreneurship in Pharmacy

Zubin Austin
BScPhm MBA MISc PhD FCAHS

Published by the Pharmaceutical Press

66-68 East Smithfield, London E1W 1AW
© Pharmaceutical Press 2023

**PHARMACEUTICAL
PRESS**
Essential Knowledge

is a trade mark of Pharmaceutical Press. Pharmaceutical Press is the publishing
division of the Royal Pharmaceutical Society

First published 2023

Printed in Great Britain by TJ Books Limited
ISBN 978-0-85711-483-9

Disclaimer
The views expressed in this book are solely those of the author and do not necessarily
reflect the views or policies of the Royal Pharmaceutical Society.

For Serena – my sweet gazelle with the sharply arched eyebrow.
For Annalise – so continental, so vexed, so clever, so talented.
For Rosie – editor of the Whig-Standard, rover-clover, and ever-adorable mad-head.
For Paul – y'all right?
And most of all...for Devina.

Table of Contents

SECTION 1: CORE KNOWLEDGE AND SKILLS

SECTION 2: MANAGEMENT IN PHARMACY

SECTION 3: LEADERSHIP IN PHARMACY

SECTION 4: ENTREPRENEURSHIP IN PHARMACY

Preface

Why read a book about management, leadership and entrepreneurship in pharmacy? As a profession, we have been talking about being at a crossroads for over 40 years. Concerns about the ongoing viability of pharmacy as a profession have been part of our culture and have made many of us question our own career choices and trajectory. Can pharmacy survive the evolution of the role of the regulated pharmacy technician? How will pharmacists manage new scopes of practice related to prescribing, physical assessment and public health? How can pharmacies remain economically viable when governments keep cutting back on dispensing fees? With each year, another existential challenge seems to emerge that threatens to destabilise and destroy the profession... yet each year – somehow – pharmacy as a profession continues to survive. And perhaps even thrive. One of the exciting things about this profession is its endless ability to evolve and adapt as the environment around it changes. 40 years ago, the idea that pharmacists would administer vaccinations, independently prescribe medications, or be embedded in GP practices might have seemed absurd...yet here we are today. As a profession, this endless hand-wringing about our future may reflect a more fundamental challenge facing us as individuals: we seem to be perfectly content to allow non-pharmacists to define who we are, direct our work and ultimately decide our future. Across the globe, there have been warnings raised about the 'leadership crisis' in pharmacy – the observation that not enough of us seem interested enough to take on difficult but important roles within our own profession to safeguard its future. When non-pharmacists control our profession they do not understand our history, our culture, our promise, our potential and who we are and want to become. No matter how competent and interested they may be, non-pharmacists simply do not have the same investment in the future of our profession as those who invested time and energy to train as pharmacists or regulated pharmacy technicians. Professional autonomy requires members of our profession to step up and take on difficult roles in order to ensure pharmacy continues to meet the needs of an evolving health care system and its patients. Management, leadership and entrepreneurship by pharmacists and regulated pharmacy technicians will help us to ensure pharmacy continues to grow and thrive in the years ahead.

Why write a book about management, leadership and entrepreneurship in pharmacy? I have been a pharmacist for over 35 years, initially in hospital practice and then as an academic. I have had the good fortune of working at the University of Toronto in Canada. It has provided me with a unique perch to observe and research pharmacy, midway between the United Kingdom and the United States, and with reference to other great health care systems of the world including Australia, New Zealand and Western Europe. I have had the opportunity to teach thousands of students over the years and lecture thousands more pharmacists around the world. I am constantly struck by the immense talent and dedication within our profession. No matter where in the world I may be, pharmacists have an incredible amount of compassion for patients, a high level of knowledge and skills, and an ethical orientation towards care, collaboration and cooperation. Yet world-wide, so many pharmacists and regulated pharmacy technicians seem to eschew management, leadership and entrepreneurship. They may say, 'it's not for me' or 'why would anyone want that headache?' or 'nothing ever changes, so why bother?'. Whatever the reason, the end result is the same: others step into the void and have greater control over our destiny than we do. I believe that every pharmacist and every regulated pharmacy technician is a manager, a leader and an entrepreneur – whether they know it or not, or whether they believe it about themselves or not. Self-confidence may not be our strongest trait in this profession...but we can learn the knowledge and skills needed to be great managers, leaders and entrepreneurs in our own profession. Pharmacy needs to unleash this talent pool now more than ever; our health care systems and our patients need pharmacists to step up and take on these roles in ways that we can't even imagine.

There are so many important topics to cover in a book such as this, and of course not all of them can fit within a single volume. The book is divided into four broad sections. The first section covers general topics of relevance to managers, leaders and entrepreneurs, including emotional intelligence, conflict management and financial literacy. No matter what you do, or where you end up, these topics will be relevant. The second section is focused on management and the specific knowledge and skills needed for success in pharmacy. Topics like workflow and workplace design, nurturing high-performance teams, and hiring and feedback practices will help uncertain managers build their confidence and skills. In the third section, the focus shifts to leadership topics. Chapters include strategic thinking and planning, communication skills, dealing with 'wicked problems' like climate breakdown, and leadership to address misinformation, disinformation and lies. In the final section of the book, the focus is on entrepreneurs and entrepreneurship. Topics such as risk management/mitigation, networking, and understanding the psychology of innovation will help nascent entrepreneurs focus their thinking and energy in more productive ways. Many more topics and concepts should have been included in this book, but of course couldn't be. References in each chapter can help signpost further reading so you can continue your own learning and development.

It is my hope that whoever you are – a pharmacist, a technician, a student, a practitioner, a mid-career professional, or a novice – you will find something to inspire you in this book. Something that makes you reconsider a long-held belief that somehow you aren't made of the right stuff to be a manager or a leader or an entrepreneur. Somewhere in this book you will learn something about yourself and realise that if not you, now...then who, when?

Zubin Austin

About the author

Zubin Austin BScPhm MBA MISc PhD FCAHS is Professor and Murray Koffler Research Chair at the Leslie Dan Faculty of Pharmacy, University of Toronto, Canada. His research focuses on the professional and personal development of the health workforce. He has published over 250 peer reviewed manuscripts and has authored four textbooks including 'Human Resource Management in Pharmacy', 'Communication in Interprofessional Care: Theory and Applications' and 'Research Methods in Pharmacy Practice'. In 2017, in recognition for the global impact of his work, he was installed as a Fellow of the Canadian Academy of Health Sciences, the highest honour for health services researchers in Canada. He is also the only University of Toronto professor ever to have received both the President's Teaching Award for sustained excellence as an educator, and the President's Research Impact Award for the societal significance of his work. He has been named Professor of the Year by students on 20 separate occasions.

CHAPTER 1

Why study management, leadership and entrepreneurship in pharmacy?

Upon completion of this chapter you should be able to:

- define the terms management, leadership and entrepreneurship
- identify key elements of the roles of managers, leaders and entrepreneurs
- understand the differences in the roles of managers, leaders and entrepreneurs
- demonstrate an understanding of the importance of managers, leaders and entrepreneurs.

Why study management, leadership and entrepreneurship in pharmacy?

For many, a profession like pharmacy may seem like a destination or an end-point, rather than simply a step along a pathway. In many ways, there has never been a better time to be a pharmacist, with expanding scope of practice, increased recognition of the invaluable role of pharmacists in primary care, recognition of unique expertise by other health care professionals, and greater integration in health care teams than ever before. Simply being a pharmacist involved in day to day care of patients can be a fulfilling and rewarding career over a lifetime.

Yet 'simply' being a pharmacist may not be enough for many of us: while the rewards of patient care are many, over time these can begin to become overwhelming, or perhaps routine. In other cases, a few years of front-line clinical work can highlight significant opportunities for change and improvement in the practice or the broader health system – changes or improvement that individuals themselves want to make, rather than rely on others to institute. In yet other cases, the highly regulated and formally structured nature of pharmacy practice may inhibit an individual's creativity and ability to innovate – leading to a strong desire to 'break-out' and try something new, daring, and different. All of these situations highlight one of the greatest strengths and most unique feature of a pharmacy degree and background: the diversity of career options and opportunities that await a BPharm, MPharm, or Pharm D graduate over a thirty- or forty-year career.

Management, leadership and entrepreneurship all describe important, possible – but sometimes overlooked – career trajectories for pharmacists. Few pharmacists receive formal education or structured exposure to these areas of the profession during their academic degree or even in the early years of practice. While we are all familiar with 'managers' and 'leaders', we may view them as distant authority figures to be feared rather than pharmacists just like us who have leveraged their personal strengths and interests to assume new roles, responsibilities and opportunities. Those who may quietly think about what else may be possible in their career may quickly dismiss their own potential by believing 'I'm not like those people, I could never do that!'.

It is all-too-common to believe that managers, leaders and entrepreneurs are 'different' than 'normal' people. We may think that they are made of sterner or magical stuff, or are simply better human beings than the rest of us, and so therefore deserve impressive titles, high salaries, and the status conferred on people with big jobs. In other cases, we may cynically believe that management, leadership and entrepreneurship simply aren't worth the pain, aggravation and headaches: 'they might make more money, but I'll be happy with my little job and being able to sleep at night, thank you very much'. At the core of both these observations is the false belief that somehow those people are qualitatively and meaningfully different from us.

Most researchers believe there are real and meaningful differences that exist between human beings[1,2] – and these are often described in terms of emotional intelligence[3]– but equally agree that almost all individuals have the same potential to be managers, leaders and entrepreneurs.[4,5] The specific kind of manager, leader or entrepreneur you can become will of course be a function of your own emotional intelligence (amongst other factors), and the kinds of environments or roles that are best suited to allow you to flourish will differ based on factors including temperament and motivation. Importantly, most researchers note that many of the core skills that appear to differentiate those people from us can, in fact, be learned.[6,7] The things that many of us dread about managerial roles – such as conflict management (see Chapter 5) or dealing with a dysfunctional team (see Chapter 12) – are topics that researchers have focused on to provide specific tools and strategies for better managing.[8,9] The things that leaders do that sometimes seem so magical or super-human – such as leveraging power (see Chapter 20) or advocating effectively (see Chapter 25) – are available to everyone who takes the time to read and learn.[10,11] While it may appear that entrepreneurs are strangely creative and completely carefree individuals who take enormous risks, the reality is that innovation (see Chapter 27) and informed risk-balancing (see Chapter 31) are skills we already use even if we don't think of ourselves as entrepreneurs.[12,13]

This book is written with the philosophy that management, leadership and entrepreneurship are skills available to everyone, not entitlements for a privileged few. As with most skills, they take time to learn, require focused opportunities to rehearse and practice, and benefit from feedback and mentoring.[14] Like most skills, there is a 'muscle-memory' component to consider: the first time you have to lead an organisation through a stressful and complex change process (see Chapter 22) it can be daunting and difficult, but the next time it gets easier;[15,16] the first time you plan for your own business (see Chapter 29) or have to market yourself and your idea publicly (see Chapter 28) it can be challenging to portray confidence and competence – but it gets easier.[17] This is not simply mindless cheerleading or rah-rah boosterism; it is based on managerial sciences and business-focused research that highlights the learnability of skills (including self-confidence)[18,19,20] that makes many of us hesitate in thinking of oneself as anything more or different than simply a pharmacist.

Terminology

The idea of actually taking on some kind of leadership role in an organisation may strike some people as folly or utter madness: why rock the boat, why volunteer for headaches and heartaches if it can be avoided? In part, such opinions may be based on a fundamental misunderstanding of the term 'leadership role': it is frequently used to describe a very diverse array of different jobs, responsibilities, and opportunities. Admittedly not all jobs, responsibilities, and opportunities actually suit or are the best fit for all of us: the kind of self-understanding associated with emotional intelligence (*see* Chapter 2) and personal authenticity (*see* Chapter 26) can help us more accurately reflect on alignment between our personal strengths and interests and professional opportunities.

Part of the misunderstanding relates to vagueness in the way terms are used, particularly for those who are not in leadership roles. While no universal definitions or consensus exist, management researchers are identifying separate though connected understandings of the terms 'management', 'leadership', and 'entrepreneurship'.[21]

What is management?

A dictionary definition of the word management may emphasise the process of 'dealing with or controlling things or people', suggesting that without management, chaos and catastrophe in organisations or society would result.[22,23] Increasingly, management is seen as the coordination and direction of resources needed to allow an organisation, business or practice to operate efficiently and effectively in pursuit of a specific goal.[23] From this perspective, management has an organisational and operational element at its core: managers generally must work with people but also have responsibilities for activities such as budgets, resources, and timelines. Managers will often need to balance a variety of different primary functions including:

- *Setting objectives:* Managers are often central to the process of strategic and business planning (*see* Chapter 19) which will involve articulation of objectives for the organisation or the practice as-a-whole. The manager has the responsibility to share these objectives with the rest of their team and create a workplace culture (*see* Chapter 12) that supports all team members in working collectively towards common goals. Part of the process will involve ensuring the team is, in fact, ready and able to do what is necessary to succeed, and this can involve recruitment, hiring and onboarding of new team members (*see* Chapter 9), and providing performance management and feedback (*see* Chapter 10).
- *Organising the workplace:* A critical role for managers is to organise people, resources, process and workflows to create a harmonious, effective and efficient workplace. This is most frequently accomplished by taking large organisational objectives and goals and subdividing them into smaller, specific tasks and duties that can be accomplished by individual team members. To do so, managers require knowledge and skills related to operations management (*see* Chapter 15 and Chapter 16), financial literacy (*see* Chapter 6) and understanding of the regulatory context within which a profession like pharmacy functions (*see* Chapter 17).
- *Motivating, engaging, and empowering others:* Line managers are the first point of contact in an organisation between an individual pharmacist/employee and the administrative

structure; as a result, managers have unique opportunities to support the psychological positivity necessary to ensure high functioning, high performing teams (*see* Chapter 11). The psychological positivity associated with success in organisations and business requires a sophisticated understanding of organisational structure and culture (*see* Chapter 14).

- *Measuring and monitoring for success:* The fourth role of management is to create and use appropriate measurement systems to ensure organisations and the individuals working within them are actually making progress towards meeting pre-defined goals. Measurement (qualitative or quantitative metrics such as targets) are part of operations management (*see* Chapter 16 and Chapter 17) and organisational structure and culture (*see* Chapter 12 and Chapter 15). In a profession like pharmacy, there are unique measurement and monitoring issues with respect to pharmacy services and delivery of safe and effective care to patients (*see* Chapter 18). Performance management and feedback (*see* Chapter 10) is the crucial vehicle by which measuring and monitoring are translated into management action to support organisational attainment of organisational goals.

- *Developing and nourishing the workforce:* The final, but perhaps most important, function of managers is to help the workforce group and flourish. This management function begins with recruitment, hiring and onboarding (*see* Chapter 9), continues with the creation of high performance teams (*see* Chapter 11), is challenged by conflict and disagreement (*see* Chapter 3, Chapter 5 and Chapter 13) and is enhanced through attentiveness to and embracing of diversity, equity and inclusion in the workforce (*see* Chapter 8). Increasingly, there has been greater attention paid to the managerial role of providing support for a resilient workforce: managing occupational stress and preventing burnout (*see* Chapter 15, Chapter 16 and Chapter 26).[23,24]

Depending on the nature and size of an organisation or practice, there can be various levels or strata of management as depicted in an organisational chart. Front-line or line-managers (e.g. people with titles such as supervisor, team leader or department head) often deal directly and most frequently with employees whom they oversee. They will often do similar work to those they supervise and are thus well acquainted with the day to day realities of the work. Middle managers are generally those in the centre of an organisational chart and may have titles such as 'Chief Pharmacist' or 'Regional Manager'. They usually act as intermediaries between senior management and line managers and work to ensure they appropriately communicate the direction from above to those below. Their focus is generally on supporting front-line managers in achieving better performance within their units. Senior management is the top-tier of an organisational chart and generally holds titles such as 'Chief Executive Officer' or 'President' or 'Director'. These managers typically are responsible for high-level strategic planning and resource allocation decisions for the entire organisation, as well as helping to set the tone for organisational culture and ethics. In for-profit organisations, these individuals are also accountable to company owners and shareholders. Regardless of managerial level within an organisation, all managers must emphasise three key priorities:

- *Communication:* clear, consistent and transparent interactions with all members of an organisation (not simply those to whom a person reports) is essential for success as a manager;
- *Collaboration:* health care is a team sport, and that organisational success is built on the ability to work cooperatively and supportively with others; and

- *Positivity:* managers are by definition, individuals to whom others look to, to set the tone and culture of an organisation...leading by example, being ethical in all interactions, and remaining positive (even when at times it may be difficult) is essential.

What is leadership?

While everyone has a different vision of an ideal leader, the concept of leadership itself is generally connected to notions of influence, persuasive power, and strongly held convictions.[25,26,27] Leaders are sometimes described as those who are able to influence and inspire others to do better, or who are able to convince people to do something they'd rather not do.[25,26] Unlike managers, leaders need not necessarily have a formal job title or a position in an organisational chart: leadership is thus often seen as more of a characteristic of an individual rather than a role.[26,27] Leadership can be exerted through a formal job title, status or role, or through informal means without need for a specific job description.[25,26,27]

The fact that many people struggle to define the word 'leader' and may struggle even more to come to a consensus in terms of who is in fact a good leader highlights one of the reasons why thinking of oneself as a leader can be challenging. For some, leadership involves a unique and valuable skill (like communication, or technical prowess) that is in high demand or need. For others, a leader is an individual capable of leveraging various human qualities like empathy or humility. For yet others, leadership is connected to an idea held with great conviction that can be inspiring or motivating to others.

One common element of leadership in most settings (including pharmacy) is a desire to improve on the status quo and some capacity to rally people towards that better vision.[26] Simply having a vision of a better tomorrow – by itself – generally does not make someone a leader. Similarly, simply rallying people to a cause – by itself – doesn't define leadership; there needs to be something unique, inspirational, and meaningful about the cause that constitutes leadership.

For some, management as a discipline is more practical in its orientation, focused on specific tasks and responsibilities with commensurate skills that can be honed and developed to improve the quality of the manager's work.[28] In contrast, leadership may have more of a psychological and social element as it is more directly connected to the thinking and beliefs of other people.[29] Managers are interested in changing behaviours while leaders are interested in changing minds and hearts.[28,29]

Davis has described leadership as '...the ability to persuade others to seek defined objectives – enthusiastically. It is the human factor which binds a group together and motivates it towards a goal'.[30] From this perspective there are important characteristics of leaders that complement but are different from managers, including:

- It is a group process – leadership cannot exist in a social vacuum, but instead involves others directly and indirectly in the process. A manager may or may not have specific individuals reporting to them, but leaders must have a social context within which leadership is expressed as ultimately it involves inter-personal processes.
- Managers may have specific powers (for example, the power to issue rewards or punishments to incentivise specific behaviours) but leaders generally only have influence (*see* Chapter 20). The ability to influence without formal power is one of the most important – and magical – elements of successful leadership.

- Leaders generally take a longer, strategic view rather than a short-term tactical perspective (*see* Chapter 19). This ability to cast to the horizon and beyond is often what makes leaders inspirational as they are thinking about tomorrow, not just today.
- Leaders have convictions, strong and positive beliefs about their work and its importance. This positive emotional state can be difficult to sustain in an authentic or believable manner but is often one of the most compelling attributes of a leader. Ambivalence or indifference towards the work itself, colleagues, or clients can be problematic in leadership, given the important role leaders have in establishing organisational climate, culture, and tone (*see* Chapter 26).
- Leadership is ultimately an interpersonal activity involving sophisticated use of diverse communication strategies and techniques. While each leader may have a unique leadership style (*see* Chapter 26), the interpersonal demands of leadership are significant and frequently define successful and less-successful leaders. A key communicative competency for most leaders involves difficult or challenging conversations with others (*see* Chapter 3, Chapter 5 and Chapter 13) that are simultaneously affirming and instructive whilst also being clear and principled.
- Within pharmacy, the pace and rapidity of professional evolution has been a struggle for many pharmacists (*see* Chapter 4). Successfully navigating change management (*see* Chapter 22) and understanding the negotiation and advocacy process (*see* Chapter 25) are both crucial skills for leaders.[28,29,30]

Admittedly, the term leadership may have a pejorative or negative connotation given high-profile cases of abuse of authority demonstrated by leaders in fields such as politics and business. Cynicism about leadership – and more specifically, leaders themselves – is commonplace. Ideas such as 'leaders are in it for themselves', or that 'leaders have to always lie to be successful' are corrosive because they bias promising individuals away from thinking about formal or informal leadership roles. Especially in the political sphere or in other high-profile positions, social media abuse and hostility (which is more frequently turned upon women and members of historically disadvantaged groups) can be a significant problem. Particularly where leaders espouse unpopular or polarising ideas that threaten the status quo or privileged position of some members of society, threats can become unbearable. Still, a hallmark of effective leadership is social responsibility (*see* Chapter 24) and enduring in the face of hostility and abuse because it is the right thing to do.

Within leadership there are many different – sometimes competing – visions or models for what leaders do and who they are (*see* Chapter 26). For example, the concept of 'servant leadership' emphasises social interactions, role modelling and mentoring to achieve authority rather than power. In other contexts, hierarchical leadership might be appropriate – situations where leaders make, enact, and enforce decisions in a unilateral manner. In yet other situations, 'leading from behind' describes a leadership philosophy akin to a shepherd tending to a flock. A core responsibility of leaders is to reflect, articulate, and authentically enact their personal philosophy of leadership in ways that resonate with others and are appropriate for the context (*see* Chapter 26).

The challenges faced by leaders today are myriad and the complexity of navigating leadership amongst the noise, confusion, misinformation, hostility and lies is difficult. For those who (understandably) believe it is simply all too much, and certainly too much to personally bear...the question arises if not you, now...then who, when?

What is entrepreneurship?

It is often tempting to believe that entrepreneurs are simply a different species of human being than the rest of us – especially the rest of us who happen to be pharmacists. The very idea of forgoing a stable and predictable job, with a pension and benefits, for the uncertainty and stress of starting one's own business may seem completely other-worldly. The creative genius required to come up with an innovative new idea, plus the breathtaking self-confidence necessary to believe others will find it compelling...these might seem to be psychological traits that can never be learned, leaving entrepreneurship as an impossible dream. Examples of high-profile entrepreneurs like Elon Musk or Richard Branson further compound the issue by suggesting that entrepreneurship is something that is only available to cis-gendered, heterosexual, able-bodied, height-weight proportionate white men, and all others should not even bother to try.

Of course, in reality, entrepreneurs are everywhere and are as diverse as the society in which they thrive. The business definition of an entrepreneur is simply a person who creates and/or extracts value, most frequently involving the process of designing, launching, then successfully running a new business. Entrepreneurship typically involves the ability to translate knowledge, skill, invention, or technology into a concrete product or service for which a market is created that eventually is sustainable and profitable. Not all entrepreneurs are small-business owners, but the principles of small-business ownership are generally applicable to most entrepreneurs.

Historically, the profession of pharmacy has been closely associated with entrepreneurship: in the not-too-distant past, many (if not most) pharmacists owned, operated, and profited from running their own shops. While pharmacists had unique clinical and scientific skills of value to the community, these were channelled through a for-profit business that required discipline and organisation to run successfully. The entrepreneurial roots of the pharmacy profession have in recent years been somewhat attenuated, with a shifting emphasis away from business towards more clinically oriented roles, and today the vast majority of pharmacists work as employees, not as entrepreneurs. Despite this contemporary reality, the core elements of entrepreneurship – identifying an unmet need, generating an innovation or an idea to address it, assuming informed risk to implement it, marketing and advocating for oneself, etc. – are still important in the pharmacy profession today. Arguably, the profession of pharmacy requires more entrepreneurs now than in the past, and the opportunities for pharmacy entrepreneurs today stretch well beyond simply owning a shop.

When contemplating entrepreneurship, many pharmacists will immediately self-handicap by truly believing they lack the psychological temperament for this role. One element of this involves the psychology of innovation (*see* Chapter 27), the process by which ideas are generated and refined by individuals prior to disclosure to others for reality-testing. Another important component of entrepreneurship involves risk balancing and risk tolerance (also called risk management and mitigation) (*see* Chapter 31). While most entrepreneurs assume some degree of personal, professional, and financial vulnerability as part of the process, such vulnerability need not be random or excessive. Self-awareness of one's risk-taking profile and behaviours, coupled with specific techniques to manage and mitigate risks can help even the most cautious of individuals recognise that entrepreneurship is available for everyone. Other core competencies for successful entrepreneurship include general skills necessary for success in everyday life – for example time management, interpersonal communication and conflict management, and networking skills. Perhaps most important of all is the nebulous but essential concept of 'execution', the ability to bring an idea to life in the real world (*see* Chapter 33).

While high profile entrepreneurs typically emphasise their personal dynamism and devil-may-care attitudes, the reality is that all successful entrepreneurs are also individuals who are ruthlessly pragmatic and sufficiently analytical to undertake robust business planning in (*see* Chapter 29). The process of business planning is central to entrepreneurship and can help individuals manage concerns regarding personal risks and vulnerabilities, as well as help to identify opportunities to leverage skills in entrepreneurial marketing (*see* Chapter 30).

The study of successful entrepreneurs highlights the reality that there is no single mould from which entrepreneurs are formed: entrepreneurs are people of all backgrounds and ethnicities, all genders and orientations, and of all types. Increasingly, one's personal background and diversity has been identified as a significant source of strength, ideas, and networks for entrepreneurs. Further, many of aspects of entrepreneurship that pharmacists may fear most – self-promotion, idea generation, risk balancing – are actually skills that can be learned, rehearsed and improved to enhance self-confidence and likelihood of success.

Of course, not all entrepreneurs will always succeed, and a key element of entrepreneurship is the ability to learn from failure (*see* Chapter 34). Equally, not every entrepreneur goes on to become an international superstar and house-hold name. Between failure and stardom...most entrepreneurs are fairly average individuals who have learned important skills, to trust themselves, and to do their best to manage and mitigate predictable risks. The dividends of entrepreneurship are many and varied, and not simply financial. Entrepreneurs frequently report the satisfaction they feel in building something new or innovative, of having their work taken up by others, and of having the freedom and flexibility to explore new opportunities that may not be available to traditional employees. In some cases, entrepreneurs simply prefer not having to report to others or work within an overly structured bureaucratic organisation. Whatever the reason and motivation, entrepreneurship can be an important option for pharmacists to consider, and the skills for success can be learned, rehearsed, and improved.

Summary

A pharmacist graduating today can reasonably expect to work for 30, 35, 40 or more years. While front-line clinical work in traditional hospital, community, or primary care settings can be rewarding, the reality is that over a career lifetime, pharmacists will assume new and different responsibilities, and will have opportunities for career trajectory they may never have imagined. The skills of management, leadership and entrepreneurship are all essential, and complement the scientific and clinical knowledge that pharmacists already have. Do not pre-judge yourself and your abilities and interests; do not write-off certain potential professional opportunities by thinking 'I'm just not that kind of person'; and do not invent stories justifying resistance to take on new roles by shrugging and saying 'who'd want that headache?' or 'you'd have to be crazy to want that kind of big job'. The confidence to assume management, leadership and entrepreneurship roles in pharmacy involves knowledge and skills that can be learned. Expanding your horizons and personal possibilities for enhanced satisfaction and impact can be daunting and will require work and dedication. The benefit in terms of new doors to open, and new opportunities to explore will be well worth it in the long-term.

References

1. Ruble M *et al*. The relationship between pharmacist emotional intelligence, occupational stress, job performance and psychological affective well-being. *J Am Pharm Assoc* 2022; 62: 120–124. https://doi.org/10.1016/j.japh.2021.09.004

2. Sencanski D *et al*. Emotional intelligence and pharmaceutical care: a systematic review. *J Am Pharm Assoc* 2022; 62(4): 11331141. https://doi.org/10.1016/j.japh.2022.02.019

3. Butler L *et al*. Evidence and strategies for inclusion of emotional intelligence in pharmacy education. *Am J Pharm Educ* 2021; Article 8674. https://doi.org/10.5688/ajpe8674

4. Law K *et al*. The construct and criterion validity of emotional intelligence and its potential utility for management studies. *J Applied Psych* 2004; 89(3): 483–486. https://doi.org/10.1037/0021-9010.89.3.483

5. Dries N, Pepermans R. Using emotional intelligence to identify high potential: a metacompetency perspective. *Leadership and Organization Devel J* 2007; 28(8): 749–770. https://doi.org/10.1108/01437730710835470

6. Dulewicz V, Higgs M. Can emotional intelligence be developed? *Int J Human Resource Management* 2004; 15(1): 95–111. https://doi.org/10.1080/0958519032000157366

7. Basu A, Mermillod M. Emotional intelligence and social-emotional learning: an overview. *Psychology Research* 2011; 1(3): 182–185. https://doi.org/10.17265/2159-5542/2011.03.004

8. Bachunsky J, Tindall W. It's time for more pharmacy leadership from within. *Can Pharm J* 2018; 151(6): 388–394. https://doi.org/10.1177/1715163518803875

9. Shikaze D *et al*. Community pharmacists' attitudes, opinions, and beliefs and leadership in the profession. An exploratory study. *Can Pharm J* 2018; 151(3): 44–49. https://doi.org/10.1177/1715163518790984

10. Boechler L *et al*. Advocacy in pharmacy. *Can Pharm J* 2015; 148(3): 138–141. https://doi.org/10.1177/1715163515577693

11. Gregory P *et al*. Community pharmacists' perceptions of leadership. *Res Social Adm Pharm* 2020; 16(12): 1737–1745. https://doi.org/10.1016/jsapharm.2020.02.001

12. Delmar F. The risk management of the entrepreneur: an economic-psychological perspective. *J Enterprising Culture* 1994; 2(2): 735–751. https://doi.org/10.1142/S0218495894000239

13. Li M *et al*. Impact of innovation and entrepreneurship education in a university under personal psychology education concept on talent training and cultural diversity of new entrepreneurs. *Front Psychol* 2021. https://doi.org/10.3389/fpsyg.2021.696987

14. Augustine J *et al*. Identification of key business and management skills needed for pharmacy graduates. *Am J Pharm Educ* 2018; 82(8): Article 6364. https://doi.org/10.5688/ajpe6364

15. Tsuyuki R, Schindel T. Changing pharmacy practice: the leadership challenge. *Can Pharm J* 2008; 141(3): 174–180. https://journals.sagepub.com/doi/abs/10.3821/1913701X2008141174CPPTLC2oCO2

16. Sorensen T *et al*. A pharmacy course on leadership and leading change. *Am J Pharm Educ* 2009; 73(2): Article 23. https://doi.org/10.5688/aj730223

17. Brazeau G. Entrepreneurial spirit in pharmacy. *Am J Pharm Educ* 2013; 77(5): Article 88. https://doi.org/10.5688/ajpe77588

18. Azad N *et al*. Leadership and Management Are One and the Same. *Am J Pharm Educ* 2017; 81(6): Article 102. https://doi.org/10.5688/ajpe816102

19. Park H, Faerman S. Becoming a manager: learning the importance of emotional and social competence in managerial transitions. *Am Review Public Administration* 2019; 49(1): 98–115. https://doi.org/10.1177/0275074018785448

20. Elmuti D. Can management be taught? *Management Decision* 2004; 42(3/4): 439–453. https://doi.org/10.1108/00251740410523240

21. Algahtani A. Are leadership and management different? A review. *J Management Policies and Practices* 2014; 2(3): 71–82. https://dx.doi.org/10.15640/jmpp.v2n3a4

22. Nayar V. Three differences between managers and leaders. *Harvard Business Review* [online] 2013. https://hbr.org/2013/08/tests-of-a-leadership-transiti

23. Tovmasyan G. The role of managers in organizations: psychological aspects. *Business Ethics and Leadership* 2017; 1(3): 20–26. https://doi.org/10.21272/bel.1(3).20-26.2017

24. Buckingham M. What great managers do. *Harvard Business Review* [online] 2005. https://hbr.org/2005/03/what-great-managers-do

25. Winston B, Patterson K. An integrative definition of leadership. 2006; 1(2): 6–66.

26. Carroll B, Levy L. Defaulting to management: leadership defined by what it is not. *Organization* 2008; 15(1): 75–96. https://journals.sagepub.com/doi/10.1177/1350508407084486

27. Reed B *et al*. A systematic review of leadership definitions, competencies, and assessment methods in pharmacy education. *Am J Pharm Educ* 2019; 83(9): Article 7520. https://doi.org/10.5688/ajpe7520

28. Bertocci D. *Leadership in Organizations*. Maryland: University Press of America, 2009.

29. Kotterman J. Leadership vs Management: what's the difference? *J Quality and Participation* 2006; 29(2): 13–17.

30. Davis K. *Organizational behavior: a book of readings*. New York: McGraw-Hill, 1977.

CHAPTER 2

Emotional intelligence

Upon completion of this chapter you should be able to:

- define the term emotional intelligence
- describe the differences between the four typologies of emotional intelligence
- detail the benefits of being aware of and utilising emotional intelligence in pharmacy as a manager, leader or entrepreneur.

What constitutes 'success' as a pharmacist – or as a manager, a leader or an entrepreneur? How do we know if we are being 'effective' in our professional lives? In our personal lives, what is the basis for knowing if we are valued by others? Human life is complicated because human beings are complex and rooted in social interactions and situations that may not always follow clear and logical protocols. The work of managers, leaders and entrepreneurs is inherently social and interactive, and brings us into interpersonal situations on a regular basis.

The term 'emotional intelligence' has been coined to describe the constellation of skills and attributes an individual possesses to allow them to navigate the social and interpersonal world.[1] While traditionally the word 'intelligence' has been associated with facts and logical problem-solving grounded in evidence, the term emotional intelligence highlights the unique and vitally important role of propensities such as empathy, self-assessment, reflection, intuition, and communication skills.[2,3,4] The ability to accurately decipher the meaning-behind-the words spoken by others, or to interpret non-verbal cues transmitted consciously or unconsciously by people in social situations are both examples of how emotional intelligence influences our day to day lives.[7] The work of managers, leaders and entrepreneurs brings them into frequent and routine contact with other human beings, sometimes in less-than-friendly or even outright hostile or challenging situations.[5] Emotional intelligence (EI) is an important vehicle human beings use to help navigate social complexity to achieve positive outcomes in ways that preserve or even build stronger relationships for the future.[6] As such, an understanding of EI is crucial for success and effectiveness in both our professional and personal lives.

What is EI?

No specific definition of EI exists, but it is most often described in terms of an individual's ability to accurately perceive, interpret, use, understand and control/manage one's own and other people's emotions.[3,4] Those with 'high' levels of emotional intelligence recognise the central role that emotions play in all parts of daily life, and in particular with our interactions with other human beings in both professional and personal settings.[7] Emotional intelligence emphasises both an individual's capacity to recognise and self-manage their own emotional state, as well as the capacity to accurately assess and categorise other's emotional states and work effectively through interpersonal situations.[3,6] The concept gained popularity in the 1990s with some of the pioneering work of Daniel Goleman who described the ways in which EI supports management, leadership and entrepreneurship in diverse settings.[8] Since that time, studies have highlighted that those who have greater emotional intelligence self-awareness are more likely to demonstrate better mental health, superior job performance, enhanced career outcomes, and ultimately greater personal and professional satisfaction and happiness.[9,10,11]

Many variations and interpretations of this concept exist; the term 'Emotional Strength' was coined by the famed psychologist Abraham Maslow in the 1950s,[12] while Howard Gardner used the term 'multiple intelligences' to describe similar concepts.[13] More recently, 'strength finders' has been used as a way of helping individuals understand their own propensities, needs, and gifts to better align professional work and personal satisfaction.[14]

The psychology of EI

In the history of business and management sciences, the evolution of EI has been relatively recent and rapid. In large part, this reflects a significant societal bias that has historically existed favouring 'evidence' and 'logic'.[3,8] For millenia, philosophers and average people alike have known that human beings are a complex amalgam of thoughts and feelings, of logic and emotion, of reason and passion. Historically this has been seen as two distinct parts of the self, always in conflict but clearly separated.[8] Much of human history has focused on quelling emotion or suppressing one's feelings and passions, emphasising the primacy of logic, thoughts and reason. The 'stiff upper lip' of the British people represents this notion that feelings can and should be controlled regardless of the consequences.

Today, psychologists recognise that logic and emotion are not separate and distinct but actually entwined within us.[15,16] Further, neurobiologists have highlighted the ways in which emotion, not reason, is actually the primary default state for most human perception.[15] Human beings interact with their environment through their five senses (sight, sound, taste, touch, and smell). Examination of the ways in which information from these senses is communicated neurologically through the central nervous system shows us that the first 'filter' for external stimulus we experience as human beings is the amygdala, sometimes referred to as 'the reptilian brain'.[16] This is the part of our brains where emotional responsiveness resides. From this perspective, we are literally hard-wired to 'feel' before we 'think', respond emotionally to situations before we think about them. We are hard-wired to shoot first, ask questions later.

This neurological hardwiring illustrates how emotion is not a separate and distinct part of who we are, something that can be contained and controlled, but actually integral to the way we perceive sensory information and interact with our world.[17,18] Emotion is the filter through which we see, hear, feel, touch and taste. It colours our understanding and interpretation of our environment and social world, preceding our ability to actually think and apply logic and reasoning. For example, if you are attending a class and you have a particularly dour or mean professor, someone who scares or intimidates you, this emotional response will interfere with your ability to learn and remember the content being taught. In contrast a person whom you like, who makes you laugh and helps you feel comfortable will create a positive emotional filter that will enhance learning and recall. While it may be possible to convince yourself to say 'oh get over it – just because I don't like this person doesn't mean I can't learn from them', this convincing consumes substantial cognitive and emotional bandwidth that actually further reduces the capacity to learn and recall.

Developmental psychologists have highlighted the six core emotions that are both universal and hard-wired as filters to help us understand and interpret our world: joy, sadness, disgust, anger, fear, and surprise.[17,19] It is believed that all human beings – from the time they are born – have these emotional states preprogrammed.[19] The environment and specific social interactions will trigger these emotional responses, and forms the primary filter through which we interpret the world and our interactions with others. You may notice that at least four of these hard-wired emotional states (sadness, disgust, anger, and fear – and perhaps even surprise) are generally thought of as negative emotions to be avoided. Why would human beings be preprogrammed with so many negative emotional filters and only one positive filter (joy)? Evolutionary biologists suggest this is because these negative filters have a survival value, alerting us to potential environmental dangers associated with situations or specific people. The negative emotional filters cause us to withdraw from potentially dangerous situations or people, thereby increasing our chances of survival.[19] For example, the emotion of disgust means that strong tastes or foul smells automatically and subconsciously trigger aversion, so we are less likely to expose ourselves to potentially toxic substances. Over time we may learn that certain strong cheeses are particularly pungent and are an 'acquired taste' – we can (with conscious effort) overcome the initial emotional filter-based response, but it comes at a cost and consequence.

Emotional and cognitive load

A key consideration in understanding human behaviour – and the potential power and value of EI – relates to the concepts of emotional and cognitive load. We are familiar with the experience of feeling overwhelmed by our professional and personal lives; we describe this in various ways, including saying 'I'm burned out', or 'I have no bandwidth'. The experience that there is a maximum capacity in terms of what we are able to manage effectively is rooted in the notion of 'load'. The act of perceiving and interpreting sensory input – whether that is processed cognitively or emotionally – consumes mental resources and energy and there is a finite capacity available. Importantly – and perhaps counterintuitively – our cognitive and emotional capacity for processing are integrated; despite our best intentions and wishes, we can rarely separate cognitive from emotional capacity.[20] Thus, personal and emotional problems we are experiencing that cause us distress or require us to continuously replay or revisit events detracts from our ability to perform mathematical calculations accurately. It is difficult to be emotionally overloaded yet still function effectively in cognitive activities involving logic and reasoning.

Each individual has a different threshold or maximum load they can manage – but every individual does have some maximum bandwidth beyond which additional cognitive or emotional processing becomes difficult or impossible. Unfortunately, few of us are able to accurately define what that threshold is, and as a result we may become overloaded. Cognitive emotional overload can result in poor decision making, diminishment of empathy, lack of caring, and feelings of unhappiness. Worse, over time, chronic overload can result in mental health and well-being issues, including an ability to actually help oneself out of the overload situation.[21]

EI has been described as a 'life preserver' in such situations: those with certain EI competencies related to self-assessment and reflection are better able to self-identify overload situations, more capable of articulating their need for assistance from others, and more effective at preventing overload issues from escalating dangerously to the point of danger.[8] Further, EI can help us to better prioritise environmental stimuli to prevent cognitive and emotional overload from occurring in the first place, thereby allowing us to actually do more and be more effective and productive.[8,9]

Understanding personal EI

It is clear that EI is a crucial concept for managers, leaders and entrepreneurs to not simply understand, but a skill to develop in themselves and others. As noted previously, there is no universally accepted definition or model of EI, nor is there a single or best version of EI that can be used by individuals who are interested in learning more about themselves. Different theories, approaches, models, and tools have been developed, some of which may work more effectively or be more resonant for some people than for others.

Within the pharmacy profession, one model of EI that has been used is built upon learning styles theory first described by David Kolb.[22] As the name implies, learning styles theory was initially formulated in the context of understanding the different preferences of different kinds of students for different modes of instruction and forms of assessment. Kolb's model was built on the observation that learning involves interactions in one's environment, many of them social and interpersonal in nature. The process of learning involves two distinct phases: first, taking in information from the outside world, then second, processing and integrating that information to demonstrate learning has occurred. The intersection of these two different processes produces four distinct 'learning styles'. These learning styles are typologies or idealised models of a specific kind of learner; while few, if any, of us are true and pure representations of these typologies, they serve as a useful way of describing substantive differences in the ways people interact with and learn from their environments. Within pharmacy, Austin and others have adapted the learning styles model within the context of EI, using the same typologies as ways of thinking about different emotional intelligences.[22]

Typologies

A typology is simply a classification system or way of describing a general type of person or situation. It's purpose is to help simplify complex concepts and make them more meaningful and more easily understood. At their worst, typologies can sometimes lead to stereotyping, reductionist thinking, and oversimplification; at their best typologies can provide a common vocabulary and a way to make important and complex concepts more widely understood and discussed.

Typologies have been used to describe different emotional intelligences, and a variety of models have been proposed. Austin's model for emotional intelligence typologies in pharmacy uses the vocabulary and concepts first described by Kolb in learning styles theory, but extends these beyond education settings, with specific relevance and application to pharmacy practice and pharmacists.[22,23] This typology consists of 4 different 'kinds' of emotional intelligence. Importantly, no hierarchy or preference is implied: all emotional intelligences are equally valid and valuable, though in some circumstances, certain emotional intelligences may simply be more efficient or effective in achieving specific objectives than others. The four typologies are:

1. Divergers;
2. Assimilators;
3. Convergers; and
4. Accommodators.

Divergers

The EI of Divergers frequently emphasises interpersonal interactions with a strong need for social harmony. If there were a single sentence summarising this EI, it may be 'let's just all get along, okay?'. Divergers value and draw strength from positive interpersonal interactions and tend to be their most energised and best in highly verbal, interactive, cooperative, and fun environments. To others, Divergers may appear pleasant, conversationalists (to the point of too talkative), empathetic, concerned about others, but less concerned about accomplishments, staying on time, or awards. They place a strong premium on being liked by others, rather than being right. As a result, interpersonal stress and conflict is difficult for them to manage, and they may actively avoid it or (worse) simply agree to things rather than risk a fight. Divergers are generally well attuned to the emotional state of others, and are able to accurately discern non-verbal cues, but at times, this can be overwhelming and can result in Divergers always trying to please and placate others. As the label suggests, Divergers often have multiple interests and fancy themselves to be 'big picture thinkers': at their worst, facts and specifics may bore them and operational/logistical details may be forgotten or overlooked. Divergers place a strong premium on interpersonal harmony and fun, which tends to make them popular and well-liked. Managers and leaders who are Divergers may struggle with their desire to be well-liked and their responsibilities to discipline, supervise, and monitor others. They tend towards being inspirational figures who motivate others by personality, and get others to do difficult things because of interpersonal connection. Divergers can be quite fragile with respect to negative feedback or criticism for others and as a result may have difficulty disciplining or criticising others. Instead they have an infectious optimism that can at times be unrealistic and problematic if not well managed. Divergers can be easily overwhelmed in terms of cognitive emotional load since they place such a premium on liking and being liked. Emotional reassurance and support are essential in helping them manage in such situations; logic and reason may have limited roles in rescuing an overwhelmed Diverger. Occupational studies suggest about 10–15% of pharmacists are Divergers;[22] they mainly work in areas focused on education/teaching, research, or in creative areas of the profession where social interaction and autonomy are valued.

Assimilators

If there were a single sentence that summarised Assimilators, it may be 'lack of organisation on your part should be no reason for an emergency on my part'. Assimilators value planning, details, and operational issues; it is perhaps no surprise that occupational surveys suggest this is the most frequent emotional intelligence style for pharmacists, with approximately 60–65% of pharmacists (especially in community practice) likely being Assimilators.[22] Assimilators have a tendency to subdivide and compartmentalise complexity as a way of managing it more effectively; as a result, they may have the capacity to complete large amounts of work effectively and efficiently. However, this tendency to compartmentalise also extends to cognitive and emotional load, and leads many Assimilators to the erroneous belief that thoughts and feelings can be segregated and independently managed. On the one hand, this provides them with the capacity to focus on details and manage large workloads, but can come at the expense of personal happiness, and accurate self-appraisal. At their worst, Assimilators may appear unempathetic and detached, more interested in things rather than people. At their best, Assimilators get things done, are not blinded by empty promises, and recognise mastery of details and logistics is what produces successful outcomes. Assimilators need and strongly value pre-planning, organisation, and efficient systems, but may have difficulty thinking on their feet or dealing with unexpected situations. They do not necessarily need the limelight, attention, or awards to motivate them. At times, they may appear rigid and rule bound, but they may argue they are merely being conscientious and well-organised. Assimilators are often their own worst critics and can be unreasonably harsh judges of themselves (and sometimes others). They can sometimes confuse 'competence' and 'confidence', mistaking other people's glib fast-talking as evidence of superior intellect or ability. When in a cognitive emotional overload situation, Assimilators typically respond best when they can find something in their immediate environment they can actually manage, plan, and control: rather than emphasise emotional support (as with Divergers), Assimilators need to feel mastery of something, no matter how small or inconsequential, as a way of re-establishing their own self-confidence.

Convergers

If there were a single sentence summarising the Convergers, it may be 'relax everyone – I'm here to help!'. Of all the EI typologies, Convergers frequently come across as the most self-confident, the most relaxed, and the most competitive. At their worst, Convergers may confuse their own confidence with competence and come across as somewhat cocky. Convergers are not detail oriented and prefer not to be dictated to in terms of processes: they generally want to be judged on outcomes, and they are self-confident enough to take direct feedback. Occupational surveys suggest that 10–15% of pharmacists are Convergers, while 50–60% of family physicians are likely this type.[22] Those pharmacists who are Convergers generally view themselves as 'natural leaders' and may gravitate to managerial, leadership and entrepreneurial roles. They tend to be direct communicators who have little difficulty dealing with conflict or directing the work of others; unlike Divergers, they have a stronger need to be right, rather than a need to be liked. At their worst, this may result in insufficient attention to the quality of relationships with others, but at their best Convergers can keep their cool in complex or difficult situations and actually make decisions. Convergers can sometimes bristle when they are not in charge, and may have the tendency to believe they really do know what's best for others; learning to be more attentive to the verbal and non-verbal cues of others and taking the time to actually listen to and hear what others are saying can be difficult. Convergers like fast-paced environments where there is little stability or predictability; they respond well in competitive situations where there are prizes to win, people to help, and an audience to impress. Despite their tendency to agree to do many things, Convergers may be less likely to experience cognitive emotional overload since they are generally confident enough to stop doing things they no longer value, thereby reducing their load. Where Convergers are able to work effectively and harmoniously with Divergers, Assimilators, and Accommodators, they may be at their very best and complement one another.

Accommodators

If there were a sentence summarising Accommodators it may be 'are we there yet?'. Occupational surveys suggest Accommodators represent 5–10% of pharmacists, but may represent closer to 40–50% of pharmacy technicians (or other technological fields).[22] Accommodators pride themselves on being 'doers', not 'thinkers' and have a strong bias towards action, rather than contemplation or reflection. They learn best by doing, not by reading or watching others. Accommodators may be less attentive to details – and quality outcomes – than others, believing 'good enough is good enough' (and frankly, usually they are right). At their best, Accommodators do not obsess about logistics or overemphasise process and quality indicators, and instead simply like to get things done. At their worst, Accommodators may overemphasise efficiency at the cost of interpersonal relationships. Accommodators typically have little interest in management or leadership, and perhaps even less interest in being managed or lead by others: they like to have a clear and well defined job and objectives, then simply be left alone to get it done. As a result, high intensity team settings with significant interpersonal demands can sometimes be challenging for them to manage. Accommodators may be at risk of cognitive emotional burnout because of their tendency to cope by simply doing more work, rather than actively reflect and identify sources of stress that are leading to overload. They may become bored easily and have difficulty spending time on their own or doing more cerebral activities such as reading. An overemphasis on policy and procedure, or a constant need for interpersonal interaction may be challenging for Accommodators to manage and they may therefore avoid environments such as these. Accommodators are not motivated by competition or awards, and generally have a need to be right rather than liked. They may at times come across as less-than-conscientious rule-benders (or breakers) because of their emphasis on efficiency. They may also come across as somewhat resistant to new ideas or changes for the sake of change, unless a clear rationale is presented and is believable.

It is important to remember that the model of EI presented above is simply one conceptualisation of this topic; many other models of EI have been proposed, and may be more relevant to you in different situations.

Applying EI to professional life

The concept of emotional intelligence is a rich terrain of important ideas and has been the subject of countless books and articles. Within a profession like pharmacy there are specific areas that may benefit from a focused application of EI principles, including:

- *Management:* For human resource managers, EI can be an essential tool for both self-betterment and for organisational improvement. Those who manage other people need to recognise their built in blind-spots – biases, assumptions, or emotional filters that prevent them from accurately and fully understanding the nuanced realities of a situation. EI encourages a kind of social perspective taking – understanding how the same words, events, and situations can be interpreted by different people in different ways based on their emotional filters. EI can also provide a powerful tool for organisational development, helping members of a team better understand themselves, and use a common vocabulary to discuss strengths, areas for improvements, and reasons for conflict. The 'difficult conversations' that are part of management can be helped through mindful applications of EI and understanding of one's own – and the other person's – unique EI profile.

- *Leadership:* Leadership is by definition a social activity involving and requiring others. Leaders need to have the capacity to connect with and energise diverse audiences, and this requires not just self-awareness and understanding but equally insights into the needs, wants, and motivations of the audience. The greatest leaders create an intangible but real chemistry with others, one that is rooted in EI principles such as empathy, effective communication, and the ability to accurately read, interpret, and reflect verbal and non-verbal cues. The most effective leaders are those who are able to authentically present their own emotional intelligence in a way that is compelling and inspiring, while simultaneously tune into the EI of others to create mutually satisfactory and lasting relationships built on trust and reciprocity. Leaders do not shy away from emotion, and in fact recognise that facts, evidence, and logic alone are insufficient for the complex tasks of leadership. Instead, creating emotional engagement, investment, and chemistry in authentic and ethical ways provides a kind of psychological fuel that helps good organisations become great, and powers high-performance teams to excel.

- *Entrepreneurship:* The myth of the 'lone wolf' entrepreneur toiling tireless in a cellar to come up with the next great idea overlooks the reality of the social reality of most entrepreneurs. Beyond salesmanship and effusive marketing, what makes entrepreneurs successful is their ability to authentically connect with other people, including bankers/financiers, clients, and even competitors. This notion of 'connection' is central to entrepreneurship: to convince others to believe in you requires that they trust you, and this requires a type of interpersonal connectedness and chemistry that is built on emotional intelligence. Successful entrepreneurs recognise and build on their own strengths and do not try to morph themselves or change based on what they feel an audience wants from them; this is both unethical and unsustainable and in most cases is entirely transparent and ineffective. Instead, successful entrepreneurs play to their EI strengths, work to develop new strengths, and commit to the act of connecting with others through empathy, communication, and interpersonal chemistry.

Applying EI to personal life

Perhaps more important than professional success, the model of EI can provide an important roadmap to a more successful and happy personal life. At its root, EI is all about personal self-awareness and building a vocabulary to support better communication designed to build stronger, sustainable relationships. Rather than respond randomly and unreflectively to difficult situations, self-understanding of EI can help us to step back and better understand our responses and motivations, with the hope of finding common ground with others to prevent small problems from escalating into bigger ones. Recognising that our emotional filters affect the way we interpret everyday events – and that the same events will be interpreted by different people because of this reality – helps us to be more empathetic and less self-righteous in our dealings with others. EI can also give us tools to be more mindful and intentional in our conversations and communication, taking the time to truly listen and hear both what people are thinking and what they are feeling, knowing that the amalgam of both is what defines behaviour.

Summary

Human – and professional – life is inherently social and interactional, and as a result we spend our lifetimes trying to understand ourselves and others. It is all too easy and tempting to assume we are right and others aren't, yet we also know that such thinking is reductive and counterproductive. Emotional intelligence is a powerful tool and model that encourages us to reflect more deeply on ourselves and accept that emotion is integral to cognition, that feeling and thinking are conjoined twins that cannot (and should not) be separated. Instead, learning to be more attentive to our emotional selves – rather than suppressing and denying – can help us to build better, stronger, and more sustainable relationships with others, which is the core of success in professional and personal life.

Table 1: *A summary of emotional intelligence typologies*

	Divergers	Assimilators	Convergers	Accommodators
Summarising statement	'Let's just all get along, okay?	'Lack of planning on your part is no reason for an emergency on my part'	'Relax everyone, I'm here to help'	'Are we there yet?'
Openness to new ideas/experiences	Values innovation and creativity	Prefers predictability and stability	Likes to be in control of change May become bored easily	Likes to be in control of own work; may resist change unless clearly explained
Conscientiousness and attentiveness to detail	Less focused on details, more big-picture thinker Respects rules but may have difficulty following them	Strongly values clear rules and policies Functions best in high-rule environment with clear enforcement	Rule-flexible Does not respond well to strict enforcement Believes other people will manage the details	Prefer to not be burdened with procedures Want to be judged on outcomes, not processes
Degree of extraversion	Socially affiliative and relationship oriented	More introverted, prefers boundaries and separation of personal/professional	Enjoys social interaction but sometimes gets bored with others	Neither wants nor needs a high degree of social interactions with others
Degree of agreeableness	Prefers being liked to being right	Can confuse other's confidence with competence	Prefers being right to being liked	Somewhat indifferent to being liked or opinions of others
Feedback	Needs positive affirmation and gentle corrective nudges	Values clarity and feedback based on pre-defined criteria, not just general statements	Emphasise what needs to be improved; don't waste time in idle praise	Believes self-assessment is accurate enough so doesn't necessary value external feedback
Motivational factors	Harmony Fun Relationships	Organisation Structure Predictability	Recognition (titles, awards) Decisiveness Completion of work Efficiency	Completion of work Efficiency

References

1. Birks Y, Watt I. Emotional intelligence and patient-centred care. *J Royal Society of Medicine* 2007; 100(8): 368–374. https://journals.sagepub.com/doi/10.1177/014107680710000813

2. Romanelli F *et al*. Emotional intelligence as a predictor of academic and/or professional success. *Am J Pharm Educ* 2006; 70(3): Article 69. https://doi.org/10.5688/aj700369

3. Sa B *et al*. The relationship between self-esteem, emotional intelligence, and empathy among students from six health professional programs. *Teach Learn Med* 2019; 31(5): 536–543. https://doi.org/10.1080/10401334.2019.1607741

4. Arnone R *et al*. The role of emotional intelligence in health care professionals burnout. *European J Public Health* 2019; 29: 588–589. https://doi.org/10.1093/eurpub/ckz186.553

5. Landry L. Why emotional intelligence is important in leadership. *Harvard Business Review Online Business Insights* [online] 2019. https://online.hbs.edu/blog/post/emotional-intelligence-in-leadership

6. Mayer J. Leading by feel. *Harvard Business Review* [online] 2004; 1. https://hbr.org/2004/01/leading-by-feel

7. Srivastava K. Emotional intelligence and organizational effectiveness. *Ind Psychiatry J* 2013; 22(2): 97–99. https://doi.org/10.4103/0972-6748.132912

8. Drigas A, Papoutsi C. A new layered model on emotional intelligence. *Behav Sci* 2018; 8(5): Article 45. https://doi.org/10.3390/bs8050045

9. Rosete D, Ciarrochi J. Emotional intelligence and its relationship to workplace performance outcomes of leadership effectiveness. *Leadership and Organization Development J* 2005; 26(5): 388–399. https://doi.org/10.1108/01437730510607871

10. Prati L *et al*. Emotional intelligence, leadership effectiveness, and team outcomes. *Int J Organizational Analysis* 2003; 11(1): 21–40. https://doi.org/10.1108/eb028961

11. Carmeli A. The relationship between emotional intelligence and work attitudes, behaviour, and outcomes. *J Managerial Psychology* 2003; 18(8): 788–813. https://dx.doi.org/10.1103/02683940310511881

12. Taormina R, Gao J. Maslow and the motivation hierarchy: measuring satisfaction of the needs. *Am J Psychology* 2013; 126(2): 155–177. https://doi.org/10.5406/amerjpsyc.126.2.0155

13. Gardner H, Hatch T. Multiple intelligences go to school: educational implications of the theory of multiple intelligences. *Educational Researcher* 1989; 18(8): 4–10.

14. Comer R *et al*. Impact of students' strengths, critical thinking skills, and disposition on academic success in the first year of a Pharm D program. *Am J Pharm Educ* 2019; 83(1): Article 6499. https://doi.org/10.5688/ajpe6499

15. Jung N *et al*. How emotions affect logical reasoning: evidence from experiments with mood-manipulated participants, spider phobics, and people with exam anxiety. *Front Psychol* 2014; 5: 570. https://doi.org/10.3389/fpsyg.2014.00570

16. Solomon R. The logic of emotion. *Nous* 1977; 11(1): 44–49. https://doi.org/10.2307/2214329

17. Lerner J *et al*. Emotion and decision making. *Annu Rev Psychol* 2015; 66: 799–823. https://doi.org/10.1146/annurev-psych-010213-115043

18. Dane E, Pratt M. Exploring intuition and its role in managerial decision making. *Academy of Management Review* 2007; 32(1): 1. https://doi.org/10.5465/amr.2007.23463682

19. Bailey R, Barnes S (2015). *Brain science – inside out*. Harvard Graduate School of Education. https://www.gse.harvard.edu/news/uk/15/09/brain-science-inside-out

20. Plass J, Kalyuga S. Four ways of considering emotion in cognitive load theory. *Educational Psychology Rev* 2019; 31(13): 5. https://doi.org/10.1007/s10648-019-09473-5

21. Heer S *et al*. Shaken and stirred: emotional state, cognitive load, and performance of junior residents in simulated resuscitation. *Can Med Educ J* 2021; 12(5): 24–33. https://doi.org/10.36834/cmej.71760

22. Austin Z. Learning styles of pharmacists: impact on career decisions, practice patterns and teaching method preferences. *Pharmacy Education* 2004; 4(1): Article 59. https://pharmacyeducation.fip.org/pharmacyeducation/article/view/59

23. House R, Aditya R. The social scientific study of leadership – Quo Vadis? *J Management* 1997; 23(3): 409–473. https://doi.org/10.1177/014920639702300306

CHAPTER 3

Communication skills

Upon completion of this chapter you should be able to:

- define the term communication
- explain why communication is important for managers, leaders and entrepreneurs in pharmacy
- list the attributes of good and effective communication
- detail the differences between summarising, paraphrasing and empathising statements
- understand the importance of non-verbal cues.

Introduction

Management, leadership and entrepreneurship are all inherently social activities,[1] with a high degree of interpersonal interaction with diverse audiences in different contexts.[2,3] At times, these interactions can be challenging – for example, in situations of conflict, or negotiation, or trying to persuade individuals to do something they would rather avoid. A common and critical skill that is required is the ability to communicate effectively.[4] Most individuals in such roles already have a high natural degree of communicative competency,[5] but the unique demands of management, leadership and entrepreneurship can sometimes exhaust even the best of us – and lead us to want to avoid such roles in the first place.[6]

What is communication?

Some people believe that managers, leaders and entrepreneurs have it easy: they don't need to 'communicate', they simply need to 'tell' and everyone will listen to what is said. The notion that simply having a title somehow confers great power and unique skills is false: if anything, the communication burden increases and the challenges are amplified.[7]

We all intuitively know what communication is, even if we may have different ideas about what constitutes good or effective communication skills. At its core, communication can be described as 'a reciprocal dynamic between receivers and senders involving verbal and non-verbal cues'.[8] This description highlights some important elements:

Communication is not simply information download or a one-way transmission of facts.[9] The reciprocal nature of communication means that both parties involved in communication are engaged in an ongoing interaction and information flows in both directions.

The notion that receivers and senders of communication are engaged in a dynamic that roles will constantly shift during an interaction: at times, one person will be the primary sender of information while the other is the receiver, but that changes moment to moment. Indeed, if it does NOT change moment to moment ... that can be an indication that true communication is not occurring and information download is happening instead.[10]

How we send and receive information is intimately connected to factors including emotional intelligence (*see* Chapter 2). The emotional filters that act as the primary way in which human beings screen and interpret information from the external environment will shape how we 'hear' and understand information sent by others.[11] Equally, our emotional intelligence governs how we deliver information.[12] Receivers and senders in communication are not interchangeable and passive agents filling pre-defined roles: their unique emotional intelligence fundamentally shapes the way in which the reciprocal dynamic forms and evolves.[13]

The 'information' that is sent and received is most frequently in the form of verbal and non-verbal cues.[14] We are generally more familiar with the importance of verbal cues – the words we choose to convey the ideas, feelings, and beliefs we have about a situation.[15] While it may seem unambiguous to a sender, a receiver may 'hear' certain words in different ways. For example, consider the difference between the following two sentences: 'Umm...we have a problem' *vs* 'Umm...we have a situation'. In the English language, in this case, the words 'problem' and 'situation' might be considered synonyms – words having substantially the same meaning. However, for many English speakers, there is an intensity to the word 'situation' in this case that perhaps evokes greater concern or even a sense of panic than the word 'problem'. Verbal cues may be transmitted by senders with a certain intention – but if the receiver doesn't hear that intention, problems (or situations) may arise. While verbal cues may generate miscommunication, non-verbal cues can be even harder to interpret even though in many cases the non-verbal cues are actually more important in terms of information communicated. Examples of non-verbal cues include eye-rolls, heavy sighs, tone and intonation, body language, hand gestures and errant verbal interjections that are less than words, such as 'uhhhh' or 'hmmm'. The emphasis or stress a sender places on a specific word in a sentence often cues the receiver to what the sender believes is actually important. For example, 'WE have a situation' will be interpreted differently than 'We have a SITUATION': the first version emphasises personal involvement and attachment, while the second emphasises the situation itself.

As can be seen, communication can be extremely complex even at the best of times – and for managers, leaders and entrepreneurs, sometimes communication is actually happening at the worst of times. Noise is sometimes described as the external interference in this reciprocal dynamic that can further confuse and undermine messaging.[16] Examples of noise can include loud background distraction (music, other people's conversation, traffic) but can also include more subtle things like someone wearing perfume or cologne that is too strong, or a receiver or sender who is dressed inappropriately or in a distracting manner. Messages transmitted where noise interferes with receivers and senders will become garbled and miscommunication can result.

Why is communication so important?

Most of us want to be clear and effective communicators because we recognise the value this brings to our relationships, and because we know it increases likelihood that we will accomplish our objectives. Particularly (though not exclusively) in the context of a health profession like pharmacy, communication is central to most day to day activities. Communication can be thought of as the foundation of a pyramid – or the start of a process – that has the ultimate objective of building stronger and more sustainable interpersonal relationships (*see* Figure 1). In this relational model, relationships between people are central to most human interactions. Few people respond positively and genuinely if they are 'told' something by someone they don't know or actually dislike. They may fake listening or disingenuously agree, but without a relationship between individuals, 'telling' is rarely successful in causing people to change or do something different. Similarly, 'warning', or 'threatening' may provide a superficial sense that someone will listen and hear, but ultimately warnings and threats that are not grounded in a relationship simply won't work as a communication technique.

Figure 1: *The pyramid of building strong and sustainable relationships.*

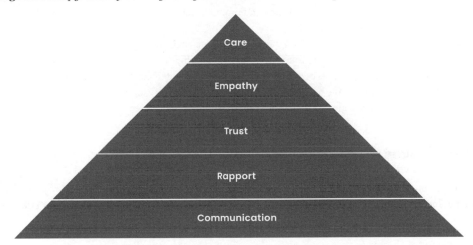

This model suggests that effective communication is the bedrock – or first step – in the process of building rapport between individuals.[8] Rapport is a type of intangible interpersonal chemistry that exists when receivers and senders start to understand and can reliably predict one another's verbal and non-verbal cues within a reciprocal dynamic. Rapport permits certain communication shortcuts – where rapport exists, a knowing smile, or a twinkle in the eyes is immediately understood in an accurate manner, based on previous reliable experiences between sender and receiver. Rapport provides both receiver and sender with a mutual and subjective sense of safety and well-being, a feeling of being heard and understood. Where effective communication exists and rapport builds ... it simply feels good.

As rapport between receiver and sender builds, the next layer to develop is trust. Trust between individuals is one of the most important yet difficult elements of interpersonal life to achieve.[17] The communication shortcuts that can be enabled through rapport are reinforced over time and in this way, trust builds. Hallmarks of trust include reliability and predictability, alignment between expectations and reality, as well as reinforcement of the reciprocal dynamic at the centre of communication. Importantly trust takes time and consistency to build; a single event of good communication does not automatically produce meaningful or deep trust.[18]

With trust and time, true empathy can evolve. Empathy is a particularly powerful part of relationships as it involves individuals figuratively being able to see the world through the other person's eyes. Empathy is one of the most powerful motivators of human behaviour;[19] when it is inauthentic or fake, it is usually quite evident. The connections between communication, rapport, trust and empathy are essential to understand; the benefits of empathy for the strength of a relationship are significant, leading to 'over-and-above-the-call-of-duty' or 'going the extra mile' kinds of activities that simple communication on its own generally cannot generate. From empathy, the deepest forms of human connection can evolve – relationships rooted in care. Health professionals like pharmacists frequently emphasise the importance of developing 'caring' relationships with patients, or the value of 'pharmaceutical care', but the way in which care evolves within an interpersonal dynamic is complex and requires significant time, consistency, and a strong foundation in effective communication.[20]

Managers want to know that their staff care about their work. Leaders attempt to create organisational cultures where everyone cares for one another and for the outcomes of the group. Entrepreneurs rely on others' caring about their innovations sufficiently to invest, buy, or promote. All of these outcomes rely on a solid foundation of effective interpersonal communication and consequently this is a critical skill to develop, nurture, and enhance.

What makes for 'good' communication?

Given the pivotal role of communication in building caring relationships, it is useful to reflect on our personal communication strengths and areas for improvement. Attributes of good or effective communication include:[8]

- *Honesty:* While, in the short-term, white lies or obfuscation might prevent conflict, we generally recognise that this is not a viable long-term strategy. A reputation for dishonest or dissembling communication can be difficult to overcome, and will stunt evolution towards caring relationships because it prevents formation of trust.
- *Proactive:* Good communicators recognise it is valuable to prevent small problems from becoming big problems and they tend to take a pre-emptive role in dealing with issues. Being proactive highlights an important aspect of good communication: it requires us to actually notice the verbal and non-verbal cues we are receiving and make sense of them. There are situations where it is easier to pretend we haven't heard someone sigh heavily, or haven't seen them roll their eyes upward with disdain. Proactive communication means actually noticing,

acknowledging, and respectfully following up on these obvious cues that there are problems rather than simply ignoring them and hoping they magically go away.

- *Asking the right questions … in the right way:* Between receiver and sender, there are many things that require clarification and further detail, and the way this is addressed is generally through the use of questions. Respectful questions asked with genuine interest telegraphs the kind of concern that leads to trust, empathy and care. The use of open-ended questions (i.e. questions that require more than yes/no answers) provides greater opportunities for senders and receivers to share information and connect. Overuse of close-ended questions (i.e. questions that can be answered with a single word like 'yes' or 'no') do not lead to rapport and may stifle evolution of caring relationships.
- *Be clear and concise:* Good communicators do not use jargon and use the minimal number of words necessary to clearly convey the point. Use of unnecessarily complicated terms, excessive use of adjectives, and repetition are boring for receivers and starts to shut down communication, inhibiting formation of rapport.
- *Be reliable:* The transition from good communication to rapport and trust is based on reliability and predictability: consistency in communication and responsiveness conveys a sense of safety which eventually translates into trust. Highly volatile and unpredictable emotional states, guesswork in terms of 'will-he-answer-or-won't-he-answer' or erratic changes of mind all undermine the reliability necessary for trusting relationships to form.
- *Listen … and hear:* Asking questions doesn't automatically produce empathy. A technique sometimes referred to as 'effective listening' has been used for many years to help receivers and senders better understand the important reciprocal dynamics of questions and responses within conversations.

Effective listening: the cornerstone of good communication

Social psychologists sometimes describe conversations between individuals as an ongoing series of choices.[21] In a conversation we receive a diverse and sometimes overwhelming amount of verbal and non-verbal information and have to filter and sort it out before deciding what parts to pay attention to in our response. Often, we pick the path of least resistance … if a heavy sigh indicates lack of agreement, but the person we are speaking with says 'yeah, sure', let's ignore the negative and focus on the affirmative and just keep moving ahead. As noted above, an attribute of good communication is being proactive and actually noticing such cues – and not deliberately avoiding or overlooking them when they appear inconvenient or problematic.

Effective listening describes a series of communication and conversational techniques that help build conversations, enhance the quality of communication, and ultimately bring us closer to the kind of empathy that is essential for caring relationships to form.[8,22] It requires us to engage both our cognitive and emotional selves fully, and filter what we hear and what we say in ways that are meaningful. To illustrate, consider the following example:

Box 1: Example

Fazia is the owner of a mid-sized high street pharmacy. The pharmacy has a staff of six part-time pharmacists, two full-time and one part-time technician, as well as other front-shop staff. Fazia wants to introduce a new clinical program focused on cardiovascular screening and referral. She holds a dispensary staff meeting explaining how workload and workflow may change as a result and highlighting both the benefits for patients and the additional revenue stream for the pharmacy. Fazia noticed that the pharmacists in particular seemed quiet and asked no questions. Four months later, while reviewing the pharmacy's operations, Fazia notes that only a handful of screenings have been completed. She meets with Orville (one of the part time pharmacists) to ask what's happened:

> **Fazia:** 'Orville, thanks for meeting with me. Let me get straight to the point – I've been reviewing the statistics on the CV screening program and they're abysmal. Any explanation?'

> **Orville:** 'Yes it's been really difficult the last few months, we've been chasing down supply chain problems, then Fran was off those three weeks for her surgery, then we had the water main break …'

> **Fazia:** 'Yes, yes. But you'd said at the meeting that you thought it was a good idea and that you'd be able to do at least 7 or 10 screenings each week. You've not been able to do any at all in the last four months.'

> **Orville:** 'Well, yes but like I said it's been really busy and all these …'

> **Fazia:** 'Let's get to nub here. What's the problem you're having with this program?'

It seems quite predictable where the conversation will flow from here. As pharmacy owner, Fazia has a clear interest and reason to pursue expansion of a new clinical service; as pharmacists, both Fazia and Orville should have a clear professional interest and reason as well. This conversation between Fazia and Orville appears to be heading in exactly the wrong direction if Fazia's objective is to motivate Orville to change his behaviour.

Effective listening begins with the understanding that interpersonal conversations are as much about talking as they are about listening. As we analyse this brief interchange between Fazia and Orville a few communication-related issues arise:

Fazia behaves as most direct communicators do: using short sentences, and overusing the word 'you'. To some receivers, the word 'you' will sound accusatory and threatening, even if that is not the sender's intention. It appears to have provoked a defensive response from Orville on several occasions.

Fazia appears to pride herself on 'getting straight to the point'. Rather than assuming an open and questioning stance, she is using many narrowing, close-ended communication methods that are shutting down conversation rather than opening it up to find out more about what is actually happening. Her communication style is pushing Orville into a subversive stance: rather than working collaboratively and openly to try to come to a mutually beneficial resolution, he is perceiving Fazia as a threat and actively undermining by coming up with reasons (excuses?) that don't truly address the underlying issue.

A pharmacy owner is a combination of manager, leader and entrepreneur. Fazia may erroneously assume these titles equate with a certain kind of power which allows her to be very direct and directive in telling Orville what to do. Further, she may even believe she is supposed to be this direct and directive, even if it doesn't come naturally or easily to her – because that's just how leaders are supposed to behave and what those who are being lead expect. In opting for such a communication style, she is harming her relationship with Orville: she is not building rapport and consequently will not be able to establish trust or empathy.

If Fazia were to reflect on this conversation, she may find opportunities for improvement. First, reducing the direct and directive tone (e.g. stop over-using 'you') would be helpful. It would also be useful to actively and effectively listen rather than tell. At several points in the conversation, Fazia has an opportunity to apply a basic principle of effective listening: appropriate use of summarising, paraphrasing and empathising statements.

At the point where Orville says 'Yes it's been really difficult the last few months, we've been chasing down supply chain problems, then Fran was off those three weeks for her surgery, then we had the water main break …' Fazia now has a choice as a receiver of this information. What is the next message that she can send?

A *summarising statement* provides the sender with an opportunity to reflect back on the facts of a situation and to clarify factual inconsistencies or misunderstandings.[8] A summarising statement does not emphasise or reflect the emotion or tone with which these facts were initially sent or received. In response to Orville's statement about supply chain issues, etc. an example of a summarising statement from Fazia might be, 'I see, so all of these issues meant you didn't have enough time to start the new service – do you think we should look at increasing the other pharmacists' hours slightly to get over the short-term problems to get the program off the ground?' In this summarising statement, Fazia is drawing inferences from Orville's statement about causes of the problem and is trying to put forward practical solutions. At its best, summarising statements are solution focused and attempt to clarify the root cause of problems. At their worst, summarising statements can give the impression of jumping to conclusions, without paying sufficient attention to the actual emotional needs of the other person. In overlooking or ignoring Orville's emotional needs, this can stunt evolution of the relationship and inhibit formation of rapport, even if it gives the impression that a solution has been found for this particular issue. A summarising statement generally sends a signal to the receiver that the sender has taken the time to listen to what has been said and is now working to solve a problem. Importantly, the summarising statement does not attempt to blame Orville (as in the original conversation), simply to understand the situation for the purpose of problem-solving.

In contrast, a *paraphrasing statement* attempts to clarify both the factual statements and the emotional tone of what the other person has just said.[8] In attempting to integrate both thoughts and emotions, facts and feelings, the paraphrasing statement represents a higher and more impactful form of effective listening, but it can be somewhat more challenging to deliver given its additional complexity. An example of a paraphrasing statement in this case may be, 'wow I hadn't realised how much everyone has been juggling right now and how exhausting that must be, right when we were hoping to start a new clinical program'. Note, that in the paraphrasing statement, there is no immediate jumping to a conclusion or attempt to solve the problem; by using a word like 'exhausting', Fazia has shown her willingness to hear more about Orville's personal and emotional state and that she has not overlooked or ignored its impact. By not using the word 'you' at all in this statement (instead, using 'everyone'), she is emphasising collective action rather than subtly blaming Orville. By not jumping to a solution right away, she is giving Orville a further invitation to continue to share his experiences, thoughts and feelings. The power of a paraphrasing statement is that it sends a signal to receivers that not only have they been listened to, but they have actually been heard. This is a crucial distinction: while the words 'listen' and 'hear' may appear synonymous, being heard is a much more impactful experience for most of us … it means the other person is truly interested and more fully engaged with our concerns and needs. Paraphrasing statements are the foundation for building trust and empathy; by reflecting and truly hearing another person (not simply listening to them), a more full, frank, and honest conversation becomes possible.

An *empathising statement* provides Fazia with the opportunity to not only listen and hear, but also to indicate she understands and acknowledges what is happening.[8] An example of an empathising statement in this situation might be: 'I'm sorry I hadn't noticed or thought about the impact of all of this on you and everyone else. Of course, I can see now why there's been such a struggle to get this new program up and running. Tell me more so we can figure out what's the best path forward for all of us'. In this statement, Fazia acknowledges and accepts responsibility for not noticing what was happening in the pharmacy, and the resultant impact not just on Orville but on everyone else. In doing so, she is implicitly demonstrating trust in Orville's assessment: she is not questioning his facts or his interpretation. By indicating she is sorry, she is demonstrating empathy towards Orville, which should increase substantially Orville's willingness to demonstrate trust and empathy in return. By inviting Orville to discuss the situation further, and highlighting the collaborative nature of problem-solving (rather than leaping to a solution herself, without him), she is also indicating she needs to rely on Orville for his expertise and skills, which further amplifies the relationship-building nature of this conversation. Some may feel Fazia is being weak or not leader-ly enough in this statement, and that she may be compromising her future status and power in being apologetic for problems not within her control. This is a misreading of leadership; saying 'I'm sorry' does not imply responsibility for supply chain shortages or Fran's surgery, or even for pushing the clinical program forward. Instead it is simply an acknowledgement of a difficult period of time that has taken a personal and professional toll on Orville. In the long run, use of empathising statements builds stronger and more collaborative relationships and ultimately will result in better outcomes for all.

The use of summarising, paraphrasing, and empathising statements may appear formulaic and perhaps even a cynical attempt to manipulate Orville. While there are common features to each kind of effective listening statement, this does not make it a formula. A formulaic approach to communication is immediately apparent to the receiver; a generic statement like 'that must be very frustrating for you' makes the receiver feel unheard and unacknowledged and is delivered with a patterned tone or disinterested attitude. It is insulting to 'fake' empathy and actually will worsen relationships and diminish rapport and trust. Being mindful that the to-and-fro of a conversation means that each time receivers and senders switch roles there are choices to be made, highlights the importance of gaining skills in effective listening. Using summarising, paraphrasing, and empathising statements in a genuine and meaningful way may not come easily or naturally, but it can be learned and it can enhance the quality of communication between individuals.

What not to do

Reflecting upon this chapter and the concept of effective listening may be overwhelming, and may appear like an impossible task. In the event it is neither feasible nor reasonable to apply communication principles discussed in this chapter, it may be useful to consider 'what not to do' strategies with respect to interpersonal interaction. These common communication pitfalls that should be avoided diminish rapport and worsen relationships, and include:[8]

Judging: In response to Orville's statement regarding supply chain shortages and Fran's surgery, Fazia may have said something like: 'it's always busy in a pharmacy, you just have to learn to manage time better'. This is an example of a judging response. It is demeaning to Orville, assigns undeserved blame, and inhibits formation of rapport and trust. Judging statements such as this are regrettably common in everyday life and can be uttered by senders without fully recognising the implications of what's been said. Of course, like all the statements in this section, judging should be avoided.

Advising: Most of us have had the experience of someone providing sincere, well-meaning but unsolicited advice. In many cases, when we are describing a problem to someone, we are not actually asking them to solve our problem: we simply want a sympathetic ear and an empathising response to make us feel better about our situation and to help refill our emotional capacity and bandwidth. When we expect a sympathetic ear and an empathising response, and instead we are given unsolicited advice, it makes us feel unheard, unappreciated, and disconnected from the other person. An example of an advising response to Orville in this situation might be: 'maybe if you blocked off an hour in your calendar each day to implement the new program, you'd ring-fence that time and still manage to get everything done'. Such a statement sounds insulting – Orville might legitimately think, 'what, do you think I'm so stupid that if such an obvious answer to the problem existed, I wouldn't have already thought about it?'. It also cuts off any discussion of feelings and emotions, and leaves Orville feeling unheard and unacknowledged. Advising responses inhibit rapport and cut off evolution of relationships.

Placating: In response to Orville's statement, Fazia might have used a placating statement such as: 'oh my that's a lot going on!'. While the statement may have been intended as empathetic it comes across as dismissive. Without explicitly acknowledging Orville's emotional response, or acknowledging Fazia's role in this, a placating statement can sound perfunctory and inhibit formation of rapport. It casts Orville in the role of a child who needs soothing, rather than in the role of a professional colleague being engaged to collaboratively address an issue.

Generalising: A generalising statement attempts to equate an individual's unique situation and circumstances with a vaguely defined group of others, as a way of suggesting or implying it's not that bad. For example, Fazia might have said, 'yeah every pharmacy I know is dealing with supply chain shortages and staff absences and findings ways of getting on with things'. This statement makes Orville feel like he is personally deficient, and not keeping pace with 'every pharmacy'. It does not open the conversation to specific reasons or circumstances in this particular pharmacy that need to be addressed, and does not make Orville feel listened to, heard, or acknowledged.

Quizzing: One of the most frequently used 'what-not-to-do' responses is quizzing, the rapid deployment of a series of close-ended questions are often invoked when senders and receivers are feeling emotionally disconnected and uncomfortable with one another. In this situation, a quizzing series of statements from Fazia might include: 'What drug shortages did we have? Did we get the medications in? Did they come in good time? Did we miss any prescription refills because of this?'. These questions do not necessarily relate to the reason for the conversation in the first place, and the structure of each question makes it difficult for Orville to say anything other than 'yes' or 'no' in rapid succession. Quizzing responses are exhausting and eventually lead to receivers losing interest and energy in the conversation and thus should be avoided.

Distracting: Particularly in situations where there is clearly an emotional issue at the centre of a discussion, senders may feel uncomfortable acknowledging or even accepting this reality. In such cases, a distracting response may be used as a kind of conversational circuit-breaker designed to move attention off the uncomfortable emotional tone that is building. For example, in this case, Fazia may have said: 'yes it was great how we rallied during Fran's surgical leave – she told me how much she appreciated the card and the present we sent'. Fran's surgical leave may be tangentially relevant to the conversation with Orville, but by shifting to such a glowing testimonial from Fran in the midst of a difficult conversation with Orville, Fazia is using a distracting technique that is both transparently unhelpful and confusing. It will lead Orville to conclude Fazia is unpredictable in her communication and consequently inhibit formation of rapport and trust.

There are many other examples of unhelpful communication techniques that should be avoided, even if application of effective listening is difficult or not realistic. Of course, in real time, conversations and interpersonal communication move quickly and we have little time to reflect and be mindful in all of our responses when senders and receivers shift roles. Our spontaneous and natural responses can sometimes be inadvertently unhelpful and counterproductive and learning to be more intentional in use of effective communication can be challenging. It is however an essential area for skill development for managers, leaders and entrepreneurs.

Non-verbal cues

The communication case study between Fazia and Orville depicted above is glaringly deficient in one key respect: as a written dialogue on a piece of paper, the non-verbal cues sent and received in a typical conversation were not present. We know that non-verbal communication transmits upwards of 80% of the 'information' in a conversation: things like heavy sighs, eye rolling, hand gestures, tone of voice, etc. say much more than words do.[23] Learning to integrate non-verbal cues with the words spoken to have a more nuanced understanding of what is truly meant (and not simply what is said) can be challenging. One element of non-verbal communication can be of particular importance for managers, leaders and entrepreneurs: tone. Tone is an encompassing term that describes different elements including the manner of speaking and carrying oneself, the tenor or quality of voice and the general attitude of the sender. Tone conveys important non-verbal information related to what senders actually truly think and believe about receivers: tone conveys contempt, disrespect, irritation, a sense of superiority and a variety of other emotions that words alone rarely capture. Mindfulness regarding one's tone is imperative: every attempt to use effective listening or other verbal strategies to enhance communication will fail miserably if tone is not appropriate. It can be challenging to accurately self-assess one's tone, and most often we rely on feedback from trusted others, or our ability to accurately assess how receivers are reflecting our comments. While we may not be entirely conscious of the tone we are projecting, if we begin to notice discomfort from receivers, it may be useful to think about whether we are projecting something negatively through tone in a less-than-conscious manner.

Summary

No single chapter can possibly summarise the complexity and convey the importance of effective communication in building strong relationships that underpin everything managers, leaders and entrepreneurs do and hope to accomplish. Reflecting upon one's own communication styles, and honestly self-appraising one's strengths and areas for improvement are life-long tasks that enrich not only our professional work but our personal lives. Mindfulness and intentionality in our communication can be challenging to enact, but choosing our words carefully and setting the right tone in conversations is central to effectiveness in all areas of life.

References

1. Nutall J. Modes of interpersonal relationship in management organizations. *J Change Management* 2004; 4(1): 15–29. https://doi.org/10.1080/1469701032000154944

2. Schlenker B, Weigold M. Interpersonal processes involving impression regulation and management. *Ann Rev Psychology* 1992; 43: 133–168. https://doi.org/10.1146/annurev.ps.43.020192.001025

3. Schrader M *et al*. The functions of management as mechanisms for fostering interpersonal trust. *Advances in Business Res* 2014; 5: 50–62.

4. Jankelova N, Joniakova Z. Communication skills and transformational leadership style of first-line nurse managers in relation to job satisfaction of nurses and moderators of this relationship. *Healthcare* 2021; 9(3): 346. https://doi.org/10.3390/healthcare9030346

5. Arendt J *et al*. Mindfulness and leadership: communication as a behavioural correlate of leader mindfulness and its effect on follower satisfaction. *Front Psychol* 2019; 10: 667. https://doi.org/10.3389/fpsyg.g.2019.00667

6. Shikaze D *et al*. Community pharmacists' attitudes, opinions, and beliefs about leadership in the profession: an exploratory study. *Can Pharm J* 2018; 151(3). https://doi.org/10.1177/1715163518790984

7. Day D *et al*. Assessing the burdens of leadership: effects of formal leadership roles on individual performance over time. *Personnel Psychology* 2004; 57: 573–605. https://doi.org/10.1111/j.1744-6570.2004.00001.x

8. Austin Z. *Communication in interprofessional care: theory and applications*. Washington DC: American Pharmacists' Association, 2020.

9. Gonzales M. Hear what employees are not saying: a review of literature. *J Education and Training Studies* 2014; 2: 119–126. https://dx.doi.org/10.11114/jets.v2i4.520

10. Thomas F *et al*. How to capture reciprocal communication dynamics. *J Communication* 2021; 71(2): 187–219. https://doi.org/10.1093/joc/jqab003

11. Petrovici A, Dobrescu T. The role of emotional intelligence in building interpersonal communication skills. *Procedia – Social and Behavioural Sciences* 2014; 16: 1405–1410. https://doi.org/10.1016/j.sbspro.2014.01.406

12. Sigmar L *et al*. Strategies for teaching social and emotional intelligence in business communications. *Business Communication Quarterly* 2012; 75(3): 301–317. https://doi.org/10.1177/1080569912450312

13. Codier E, Codier D. Could emotional intelligence make patients safer? *Am J Nursing* 2017; 117(7): 58–62. https://doi.org/10.1097/01.NAJ.0000520946.39224.db

14. Fichten C *et al*. Verbal and non-verbal communication cues in daily conversation and dating. *J Social Psychology* 2014; 132(6): 751–769. https://doi.org/10.1080/00224545.1992.9712105

15. Hull R. The art of non-verbal communication in practice. *Hearing Journal* 2016; 69(5): 22–24. https://doi.org/01.HJ.0000483270.59643.cc

16. Edmonds J. Overcoming noisy communication *Training Journal* 2016; 10. https://www.trainingjournal.com/articles/feature/overcoming-noisy-communication

17. Gregory P, Austin Z. Understanding the psychology of trust between patients and their community pharmacists. *Can Pharm J* 2021; 154(2): 120–128. https://doi.org/10.1177/1715163521989760

18. Kunyk D, Olson J. Clarification of conceptualizations of empathy. *J Advanced Nursing* 2001; 35(3): 317–325. https://doi.org/10.1046/j.1365-2648.2001.01848.x

19. Fuller M *et al*. Conceptualizing empathy competence: a professional communication perspective. *J Business and Technical Communication* 2021: 35(3): 333–368. https://doi.org/10.1177/10506519211001125

20. Hardee J. An overview of empathy. *Permanente J* 2003; 7(4): 51–54. https://www.thepermanentejournal.org/doi./10.7812/TPP/03-072

21. Yeomans M *et al*. The conversational circumplex: identifying, prioritizing, and pursuing informational and relational motives in conversations. *Current Opinion in Psychology* 2022; 44: 293–302. https://doi.org/10.1016/j.copsyc.2021.10.001

22. Jahormi V *et al*. Active listening: The key of successful communication in hospital managers. *Electron Physician* 2016; 8(3): 2123–2128. https://doi.org/10.19082/2123

23. Hans A, Hans E. Kinesics, hapsics, and proxemics: aspects of non-verbal communication. *IOSR J of Humanities and Social Science* 2015; 20(2): 47–52.

CHAPTER 4

Understanding professional identity

Upon completion of this chapter you should be able to:

- define the term identity
- explain the concept of intersectionality
- detail the importance of considering professional identity in pharmacy
- consider the role of identity in managers, leaders and entrepreneurs.

Ping has been a pharmacist for five years and has generally enjoyed his work. Of course, there are ups and downs – every job has its challenges some days, right? Recently there have been some changes in the workplace, and there is an opening for a new manager. Ping's colleagues believe he would be great for the job but he's not sure if he is 'management material'.

In his years as a pharmacist, Greg has seen so many great things – expanding scope of practice, new respect from primary care colleagues, important new roles. But Greg also knows there are problems – corporatisation of the profession, a fixation on costs, non-pharmacists in leadership roles. He is thinking of putting his name forward for a leadership role in a professional association. He strongly believes pharmacists need to take control of their profession or risk losing it, but his partner William is worried that being in the limelight might expose Greg to more heartache than he deserves.

Beth has enjoyed working as a pharmacist, but recognises now it's not a life-long career. She has always enjoyed dabbling in developing mobile apps, and wonders if she has come up with a real winner of an idea – a tracking system to help pharmacies manage medication shortages that connects them to other pharmacies that may have supplies they can share. Everyone tells her it's a great idea and she should run with it ... she knows the idea is great but she doesn't think she's got a head for business or the stomach to handle the risk of starting a new venture.

What is a pharmacist? Perhaps more specifically – who is a pharmacist? The characteristics and identity of those who select pharmacy as a field of study and a profession have been the endless source of social speculation and more recently of academic interest.[1,2,3,4] The notion that those who select the same profession may have certain common traits has been described in different ways.[5] Chapter 2 introduced the concept of emotional intelligence as a way of understanding the collective group of people known as pharmacists. Occupational studies suggest that while, of course, not all pharmacists are the same, a large proportion (>60%) share a common emotional intelligence learning style (Assimilator) which may highlight a reason why a unique and distinct culture that describes pharmacy has evolved.[6] Recent research has gone further and enumerated common core attributes of many community pharmacists, including: a) lack of self-confidence;

b) avoidance of new responsibility due to high need for perfection; c) paralysis in the face of ambiguity; d) a strong need for approval from others; and e) risk aversion.[5,7] If the brief case vignettes above resonated with you as a reader, it could be because they confirm broad stereotypical traits many of us associate with pharmacists.

What is identity – and why does it matter?

Psychologists have long noted the central role of identity in defining who we are as individuals.[8] There is no precise definition of identity; it is an amalgam of different memories, experiences, relationships, beliefs, and values that creates an individual's sense of self, and understanding of who they are. Identity is not necessarily fixed and unchangeable; for some individuals, identity may continuously and incrementally evolve over a life time, while for others, it may rapidly change.[9,10]

The question of identity is fundamentally existential – we all struggle with the answer to the question 'who am I?' and 'who do I want others to think I am?' or 'who do I want to be in the future'. Identity is frequently rooted in certain characteristics over which an individual has little or no control over, including race, gender, sexual orientation, social class,[11] and even basic biological factors such as height or weight.[12] Layered on top of these characteristics are socialised factors generally coming from the family of origin, including religious beliefs, culture, and dietary preferences and requirements.[8,9] The number of factors that inform a person's identity are enormous, and the combinations and permutations of ways in which they combine in differently-weighted ways results in the enormous diversity of human beings we encounter every day.

Where identity can become an issue is where individuals struggle to express, accept, or come to terms with a core aspect of themselves.[8] For example, for most human beings, sexuality is a critically important component of identity, but one that doesn't always warrant specific attention. Those who have minority sexual orientations (including gay, lesbian, bisexual or asexual individuals) may feel a strong social need to 'hide' their true feelings, thoughts and beliefs from others, and this can consume significant cognitive-emotional load (see Chapter 2). Over time, this can crowd-out other important elements of identity and can lead to serious physical and emotional health issues. Alternatively, individuals who choose not to hide their identity may still suffer from overt and subtle forms of discrimination precisely because of their identity, and this too introduces a cognitive-emotional load that can be exhausting and ultimately debilitating.

In a perfect world, most of us would prefer to live authentic lives in which we are fully at peace with our true identity (warts and all) and are able to express our identity without fear or guilt. Of course – sadly – for many people no such perfect world of authentic identity expression exists, and the existential pain this can cause becomes the foundation for both personal pain and growth, and the beginnings of social movements such as Black Lives Matter, #metoo, and ActUp!. Identity is central to self-understanding and the presentation of oneself to others in social settings. Most human beings intuitively understand this based on their own experiences, yet recently the idea of identity has become increasingly weaponised in political terms. Certain politicians and politically-oriented individuals may decry the idea of 'identity politics', claiming it is a way of dividing and disunifying individuals and society as a whole; they claim that when we focus on a demographic characteristic such as sex, sexual orientation, race, or ethnicity and assume it is of paramount importance to an individual, we reduce them to a stereotype and consequently negate their personhood. They claim that a 'colour-blind' view of individuals – judging them solely on merit rather than on characteristics – is ultimately more fair and just than considering identity at all. This perspective may have appeal, but of course negates the reality that identity is central and is crucial to personhood and personality formation. For example, a gay person who has spent much of life 'hiding' in the closet due to fear of stigma or internalised shame will have had a psychological development process entirely different to a person who could be open about their sexuality and preferences. To pretend that this formative experience does not directly contribute to how a person sees the world is naïve at best, disingenuous at worst. Similarly, a person who has experienced Islamaphobia, sexism, or societal discrimination due to a disability will have had an entirely different view on social relationships and society than others – and this cannot help but become part of their identity, which in turn shapes thoughts, feelings, behaviours, actions, and beliefs.

Intersectionality

To address the claims of those who negate identity and advocate for total colour-blindness in human interactions, there has been an increasing interest in the concept of intersectionality as it relates to identity.[13] For some, the kernel of truth behind the accusation that identity-based policies and politics reduce and stereotype an individual's personhood is the recognition that not all gay people are the same – just as not all women are the same, or all individuals who use a wheelchair. Single-issue focused identities do run the risk of being reductionist and stereotyping. For example, it may be simplistically convenient to assume that all devout Christians are also opposed to same-sex marriage and thus devout Christians are, and are supposed to be, homophobic. The reality, of course, is that there are many Christians who are not only supportive of same-sex marriage – they may also be gay themselves. Individuals have multiple identities, some of which may not conveniently align with stereotyped preconceptions.[14]

The concept of intersectionality helps us to recognise that all human beings have multiple intersecting and overlapping identities that they navigate and negotiate on a regular basis. In a specific time, place, and context, some of these identities may come to the foreground while others are in the background. For the same person in a different time, place and context, identities may shift in their emphasis. When we think about the totality of a person, we think about how their multiple identities intersect with one another to produce a unique and distinct human being. Single-issue identity politics can risk oversimplifying and reducing individuals; intersectionality attempts to build our understanding of the importance of the many different identities we all carry and the ways in which these shape us. Recognising that a single demographic or characteristic is not the sum of a human being, and supporting the notion that not all members of an identifiable group must think and act in the same way, opens us to the possibility that individuals can be individuals in all their complexity and contradictions.

Thinking intersectionally means we see people from different angles: the obvious visible characteristics as well as the less-visible characteristics. Even so-called obvious characteristics (such as age, sex, or race) are not always as obvious as they seem: think of the times we may erroneously make assumptions about a person's gender identity or sexual orientation because they behave in ways that may not be stereotypically conventional of a 'straight' or 'gay' person. When we consider the intersections that shape and define who we are – and who everyone else is – we recognise that people are unique individuals, not bound to one specific identity or characteristic, and free to be who they choose, want, and need to be.

What about professional identity?

As a manger, leader and entrepreneur, it is important to reflect deeply and meaningfully on the central role of identity in human development and human relationships. As pharmacists, it is also valuable to consider how professional identity has emerged as a central concern for the profession of pharmacy in helping us to understand pharmacy practice evolution.

As with personal identity, professional identity is an amalgam of many intersecting factors and characteristics. To begin, professional identity is one of the intersections that shape who we are as human beings. The label 'pharmacist' is often associated with stereotypes and reductionist thinking: a pharmacist is quiet, tidy, efficient, detail oriented, but a bit stand-offish, more bookish, not a people-person. Some go so far as to say that people become pharmacists specifically so they don't have to touch people (like doctors) or interact with them (like nurses).

Pharmacy has struggled to define its professional identity for generations.[1-4] At the core, is the question of whether pharmacists are truly health care professionals or whether they are profit-taking business people.[1-4] On the one hand, the public impression of most pharmacists is rooted in a retail setting where money is exchanged for goods and where profit is expected. For the last 40 years, many in pharmacy have been trying to shift the identity away from corporate and financial interests towards health care, highlighting the clinical role and medication expertise of pharmacists. It has been an uneasy struggle; while arguably many in the profession want to feel more like clinical experts and less like business people, the reality is the majority of pharmacists today work in for-profit business settings. Despite the rhetoric across the profession (and certainly in academic programs) the reality is that in the public eye and in day to day experience of pharmacists – it is a business whether we choose to recognise that or not.

This reality highlights an interesting feature of identity: the struggle to actually define oneself and to project that definition into the world may not be as successful as we like to think. Other people may find it confusing or simply bemusing that pharmacists take themselves so seriously and continuously advocate for an identity for themselves that is either unrealistic, non-existent or not really visible to most of society. Yet this struggle to advocate for this identity is in itself a crucial part of the identity of pharmacists – aspirational, earnest, trying to figure out who we truly are. This evolution of professional identity in pharmacy is particularly relevant as it mirrors the experiences of others with respect to personal identity formation.

The struggle to define pharmacists' identity has been rooted in the changing nature of the field itself.[1-4] A hundred years ago, apothecaries used to have a very unique and defined skill set that was of great importance to society: they were highly trained individuals who understood the art and science of actually making medicines that healed and saved lives. This unique and special skill defined a clear remit for pharmacy and made it a 'profession' on par with other similarly unique and skilled professionals such as physicians or lawyers. Of course, by the mid 20th century, the multi-national pharmaceutical industry co-opted the vast majority of compounding activities: big corporations could make, produce and distribute medications much more safely, cost-effectively, and efficiently than apothecaries working on their own. Suddenly – the major raison d'etre for the profession no longer existed and pharmacy's claim to be a profession with a unique, important, and defined skill no longer existed. It was around this time that the idea of a 'clinical' role for pharmacists first evolved, as a way of offsetting the loss of prestige and power associated with the apothecary role. Shifting away from manufacturing/compounding towards a clinical advisory role to physicians to support appropriate medication use, leveraged the pharmacist's knowledge base and skill but in a new and different way. Importantly, this shift in professional identity away from compounding and towards clinical advice, allowed the pharmacist to maintain self-pride because it was an equally important, albeit different, role.

The limitations of the clinical advisory role for pharmacists became more apparent towards the end of the 20th century as the internet and instantaneous access to information became more available for all.[1-4] Gradually it became apparent that doctors and patients didn't need a pharmacist to provide clinical advice: they could look up information for themselves and by themselves. The unique and important skills associated with a clinical advisory role became less valuable as information became more widely available to all. Again, a crisis of identity in pharmacy became apparent, as pharmacists struggled to identify what they could contribute to ensure value and pride in their own profession. Around this time, a new professional identity began to evolve: pharmaceutical care, the notion that pharmacists weren't simply encyclopedias with feet that provided information, but actually caring professionals who made decisions and took responsibility for patient outcomes. As the pharmaceutical care identity evolved, there were changes in scopes of practice for pharmacists that enabled greater responsibility – for example, prescribing rights or the ability to administer injections. In this way, pharmacists started to resemble other more traditional health care professionals like nurses and doctors.

Both the clinical advisory and the pharmaceutical care identities began to create tensions with the reality that the majority of pharmacists still worked in for-profit businesses. While more and more pharmacists began working within physicians' offices/GP surgeries or within National Health Service (NHS) roles, high street pharmacies continued to be the largest employers and these organisations are traditional retail operations focused on profit optimisation. The ways in which the advisor identity and the carer identity of pharmacists conflicts with a for-profit motivation of businesses is an ongoing source of tension in the profession.

Today, it may be argued, pharmacists suffer from an identity crisis.[1-4] While academics may argue for a purer version of the profession than actually exists, most average pharmacists struggle to reconcile what they actually are, what value they bring, and how to balance business/corporate/ financial interests with patient care/clinical advisory roles. This manifests, for example, in the structure of community pharmacy where products with no proven medicinal value are still sold in a place purported to be a health care centre. The continuing sale of 'junk food' in pharmacies belies the rhetoric that pharmacists are carers or advisors, despite the reality that sales of high-margin items like crisps supports financial viability of pharmacies as businesses.

In personal life, the kind of identity crisis faced by pharmacists typically leads to demoralisation, unhappiness, and a behavioural paralysis based on indecisiveness.[15] Arguably, the identity crisis in the profession of pharmacy is leading to similar behaviours across the profession. Without clear identity – without a clear sense of who we are, why we matter, what we contribute – a type of lackadaisical passivity emerges, one that perhaps helps us better understand the state of pharmacy today.

The identity of managers, leaders and entrepreneurs

An intersectional complexity in professional identity in pharmacy relates to those who find themselves in managerial, leadership or entrepreneurial roles. The identity of these roles is distinct from that of a pharmacist; pharmacists can 'afford' to be ambivalent or negative about their profession, but leaders and managers are expected to be relentlessly positive and optimistic to inspire others. Indeed, many pharmacists deliberately avoid managerial titles and leadership roles specifically because they feel they cannot fake it or pretend to be enthusiastic.[16] Others simply cannot see themselves as managers, leaders or entrepreneurs – that identity label feels uncomfortable or unrealistic. In some cases, individual personal identity characteristics may interfere with one's ability to see oneself as a manager or leader – 'why would anyone listen to someone like me?'. In other cases, personal identity factors prevent us from thinking about taking risks, self-promoting, or advocating.

The identities of managers, leaders and entrepreneurs builds upon personal and professional identity characteristics, and creates new and interesting intersections that may be barriers or facilitators to growth and advancement. The instinct to say no to promotions, leadership roles, or risky ventures may initially feel comfortable, but on reflection, it reveals the ways in which identity fundamentally shapes our thinking, behaviour and choices. Learning to see oneself as a manager, a leader or an entrepreneur means learning a new identity and intersecting it with existing identities. For some, this may be an easy and natural process, but for others, it may be very difficult.

In particular, for those who have pre-existing personal identities rooted in discrimination these new identities can be challenging to visualise. For example, an individual who has historical personal experience of being in the closet, hiding their true self from others due to fear, shame, or stigma, may have identity-driven behaviours that reinforce a notion they should remain hidden, out of sight, quiet, and simply fly under the radar to avoid notice from others. The idea that this person could also be a manager or leader – someone with a voice, who others listen to, who compels others to act – might seem irreconcilable with their personal identity. Learning to overcome the legacy of this personal identity and recognise the possibilities to become a manager, a leader or an entrepreneur can be challenging and difficult work, but it is essential if each person is to realise their fullest potential.

While not all of us have the experience of hiding our true selves from public view, most of us have similar personal identity issues or characteristics that potentially interfere with managerial, leadership, or entrepreneurial aspirations. How can these be reconciled to allow us to achieve our full potential? The first step involves reflection, leading to understanding and self-acceptance. Identities that are not easily hidden from the judgement of others are identities that may interfere with professional aspirations. This means not simply tolerating or accepting but proudly embracing one's personal identities fully in order to be authentic and engaged. It is easy and natural to assume certain identities automatically confer certain privileges on certain individuals: for example, it is tempting to believe that able-bodied, heterosexual, cis-gendered white males have all the luck, all the power, and all the cards dealt in their favour. While historically, and to this day, there are a variety of different powers and privileges associated with certain demographic characteristics, intersectionality also teaches us that we stereotype at our own peril. Self-understanding means recognising that there are many less obvious but equally important privileges all of us have regardless of our personal identities, and finding ways of concentrating our attention and focus on those – rather than lamenting the things we are not – can be (within reason) helpful in supporting leadership aspirations. That is not to say that privilege, discrimination, and asymmetrical opportunities are not important or do not exist – clearly, they are real and impactful. Learning to not simply accept oneself, but actually embrace our multiple personal and professional identities as sources of strength, not weakness, and promote this face to the world may sound naïve and idealistic but it is an important technique for overcoming negativity bias that can inhibit one's professional development and trajectory.

What stops us from wanting to be and do more?

Identity is a complex and fraught concept, and we can be forgiven if most of us would rather ignore or avoid the whole topic as it can lead to emotional and cognitive discomfort. Despite recent anti-woke rhetoric to the contrary, identities are real, important, and fundamentally shape who we are as human beings. Our identities are the foundation of our beliefs, behaviours, thinking, feelings, and actions. Some of our identities are fixed and immutable, while others may evolve over time. All human beings juggle multiple identities and these intersections between identities are the places where human nature and personality form.

While we rarely reflect closely enough on our personal identities, it is rarer still that we consider our professional identities. For pharmacists, our professional identities have evolved over the years and continue to be in flux. Kellar has coined the term 'pile-up' to describe the multiple competing and sometimes contradictory identities that pharmacists today juggle:[1] are we business people or health care professionals? Are we scientists or care-givers? Are we all of these things at once – and if we are, how is that even possible? The consequences of the identity crisis in pharmacy – the 'pile-up' or collision of competing professional identities – is a kind of rootlessness, a lack of commitment, ambition and full engagement in our work. If we can't even accept our professional identity, why would we even bother to try very hard to do the job to the best of our ability?

From this morass of professional identity, the managers, leaders and entrepreneurs of pharmacy must emerge. It can be challenging, and perhaps explains why some people claim there is a 'leadership crisis' in pharmacy today.[17-20] Without clear commitment to a professional identity as a pharmacist, why would anyone want to manage, lead or take risks as an entrepreneur? There may be many good reasons to shrug and say 'no, not me'. Overcoming negativity and inertia in order to take on new professional challenges is not easy but it is essential for the profession to thrive – and for each individual to grow and develop personally. One important first step in overcoming this negativity is honest self-appraisal and reflection on the ways in which existing personal and professional identities may act as barriers or enablers to taking on new roles, responsibilities and opportunities. Where one's instinct is to say 'no, not me', understanding how our identities make this our default position is essential. Recognising that no matter what privileges we may or may not have because of our identities, all of us have the potential to be and do more. What's getting in your way?

Summary

One of the most important challenges in the profession of pharmacy today is trying to mobilise pharmacists to actually want to take on management, leadership and entrepreneurial roles. In other fields, such roles are sometimes viewed as prestigious, an honour, and a recognition of accomplishment, but for many pharmacists, the words 'leader' or 'boss' are sometimes viewed pejoratively or negatively. One perspective on this connects to the intersections of personal and professional identities that, in pharmacy, may have produced a culture of 'no – not me!' as a default posture. This is regrettable, since such negativity may mean many individuals do not live up to their fullest potential and have the most impactful and interesting careers possible. In part, an important driver of this 'no – not me!' posture may be difficulty in actually visioning oneself as a manger, a leader or an entrepreneur, which in turn may connect to professional identity ambivalence and personal identity characteristics.

Pharmacy is a profession filled with intelligent, creative, skilled, and compassionate individuals – yet something seems to hold many people back from considering management, leadership and entrepreneurship as possible career options. It may be too easy to simply blame the system, the profession, or nameless others for this. Considering the ways in which our professional and personal identities are constructed, intersect, and at times 'pile-up', is an important pathway forward towards greater opportunities that allow our diverse profession to truly flourish.

References

1. Kellar J *et al.* A historical discourse analysis of pharmacist identity in pharmacy education. *Am J Pharm Educ* 2020; 84(9): 7864. https://doi.org/10.5688/ajpe7864

2. Elvey R *et al.* Who do you think you are? Pharmacists' perception of their professional identity. *Int J Pharm Pract* 2013; 21(5): 322–332. https://doi.org/10.1111/ijpp.12019

3. Kellar J *et al.* Professional identity in pharmacy: opportunity, crisis, or just another day at work? *Can Pharm J* 2020; 153(3): 137–140. https://doi.org/10.1177/17151635209130902

4. Nelson N *et al.* The pharmacist's professional identity: preventing, identifying, and managing medication therapy problems as the medication specialist. *J Am College Clinical Pharmacy* 2021; 4(12): 1564–1571. https://doi.org/10.1002/jac5.1538

5. Rosenthal M *et al.* Pharmacists' self-perception of their professional roles: insights into community pharmacy culture. *J Am Pharm Assoc* 2011; 51(3): 363–367. https://doi.org/10.1331/JAPhA.2011.10034

6. Austin Z. Learning styles of pharmacists: impact on career decisions, practice patterns, and teaching method preferences. *Pharmacy Education* 2003; 4(1): Article 59.

7. Rosenthal M *et al.* Are pharmacists the ultimate barrier to practice change? *Can Pharm J* 2010; 143(1): 37–43. https://doi.org/10.3821/1913-701X-143.1.37

8. Carter M. Advancing identity theory: examining the relationship between activated identities and behaviour in different social contexts. *Social Psychology Quarterly* 2013; 76(3): 203–223. https://doi.org/10.1177/0190272513493095

9. Simons J. From identity to enaction: identity behaviour theory. *Front Psychol* 2021; 12. https://doi.org/10.3389/fpsyg.2021.679490

10. Leary M, Tagney J, eds. *Handbook of Self and Identity,* 2nd edn. New York: The Guildford Press, 2012.

11. Matthews J *et al.* Professional identity measures for student health professionals – a systematic review of psychometric properties. *BMC Medical Education* 2019; 19: 308. https://doi.org/10.1186/s12909-019-1660-5

12. Verplanken B, Sui J. Habit and identity: behavioural, cognitive, affective, and motivational facets of an integrated self. *Front Psychol* 2019; 10. https://doi.org/10.3389/fpsyg.2019.01504

13. Carbado D *et al.* Intersectionality: mapping the movements of a theory. *DuBois Rev* 2013; 10(2): 303–312. https://doi.org/10.1017/S1742058X13000349

14. Kellar J *et al.* How pharmacists perceive their professional identity: a scoping review and discursive analysis. *Int J Pharm Pract* 2021; 29(4): 299–307. https://doi.org/10.1093/ijpp/riab020

15. Hekman S. Identity crises: identity, identity politics, and beyond. *Crit Rev International Social Political Philosophy* 1999; 2(1): 3–26. https://doi.org/10.1080/1369823990843266

16. Shikaze D *et al*. Community pharmacists' attitudes, opinions, and beliefs about leadership in the profession: an exploratory study. *Can Pharm J* 2018; 151: 3. https://doi.org/10.1177/1715163518790984

17. Tsuyuki R. A leadership crisis in pharmacy. *Can Pharm J* 2019; 152(1): 6–7. https://doi.org/10.1177/1715163518816963

18. White S. Will there be a pharmacy leadership crisis? *AJHP* 2005; 62(8): 845–855. https://doi.org/10.1093/ajhp/62.8.845

19. Ali R *et al*. Developing leadership skills in pharmacy education. *Medical Science Educator* 2022; 32: 533–538. https://doi.org/10.1007/s40670-022-01532-x

20. Schmeltzer B *et al*. Addressing the pharmacy leadership crisis in Canada: a call to action for a unified approach. *Can Pharm J* 2022; 155(3): 140–142. https://doi.org/10.1177/17151635221089293

CHAPTER 5

Conflict management, resolution and negotiation

Upon completion of this chapter you should be able to:

- define the term 'conflict'
- recognise the early warning signs of conflict
- list the strategies for de-escalating conflict
- describe the steps in conflict management
- understand the importance of negotiation and mediation as a manager, leader or entrepreneur.

One of the most commonly stated reasons for avoiding management, leadership and entrepreneurship in pharmacy is a desire to avoid conflict.[1] The reality of modern life in organisations is that conflict is commonplace and that many people feel they lack the skills or temperament to manage it, resolve it, or successfully negotiate an acceptable outcome.[2,3] Conflict management skills may not come naturally, but they can be learned and improved to enhance confidence and to support individuals who may otherwise be interested in managerial roles.[4]

What is conflict?

From a managerial perspective, conflict is most frequently described in interpersonal terms as 'a stated disagreement between two or more parties, based on a situation where the parties believe they have incompatible goals or objectives'.[5] An alternative way of viewing conflict is to describe it as an intellectual disagreement coupled with emotional involvement.[6] From this perspective, conflict involves both a cognitive and an emotional component. Simple intellectual disagreement can be stimulating and enjoyable for some people – sparring in a debate when you don't have any particular investment in the outcome can lead to sparkling conversations and witty exchanges. For many people, conflict becomes troublesome when they have a personal interest in the situation or outcome, or where the result of the conflict could be perceived as emotionally damaging or threatening. The intersection of intellectual disagreement and emotional investment is often why conflict can be difficult to manage.[7]

What makes conflict so challenging for many of us?

Conflict is frequently rooted in threat perception, the belief that the other party can somehow harm or damage us.[8] A common trigger for conflict is the feeling of being disrespected by the other person; our emotional response to being overlooked or diminished by another person is strong and visceral.[9]

Importantly, emotion and cognition are separate but interconnected components of our central nervous systems and this parallel processing can sometimes lead to us feeling overwhelmed during conflict.[10] Human beings are literally hard-wired to experience emotion prior to engaging cognitively with a situation: sensory inputs (from sight, sound, taste, touch and smell) first route through a part of the brain called the amygdala, sometimes referred to as the 'reptilian brain'.[11] The amygdala is thought to be the centre for most primal human emotion. At one point in human evolution, there may have been a strong survival advantage to this wiring: responding emotionally to stimuli engaged a fight-or-flight response, quickly and without cognitive burden, that may have prevented us from harm. Today, this hard-wiring can lead to problems when our stimuli are more interpersonal in nature.[12]

Cognitive processing of external stimuli is slightly time delayed compared to emotional processing, by approximately 0.3 seconds.[10] With these 0.3 seconds, the history of human kind has been written: we are literally hard-wired to 'shoot first, ask questions later', to feel before we think, and consequently may respond in disproportionate, inappropriate, or unhelpful ways before we have an opportunity to actually think through what we are doing.[11] When intellectual disagreement becomes entangled with emotional involvement, it can be difficult to contain strong emotional impulses through rational thought and this can lead to unintentional and rapid escalation.[12]

Threat perception is frequently the driver for conflict escalation, and the emotional element of this can sometimes lead us to inappropriately assess or inaccurately distort the reality of a situation.[13] When the other person involved in a conflict is behaving in a similar manner, this can cause significant difficulty. A key component of effective conflict management involves self-awareness of the emotion–cognition connection, and finding ways of managing the 0.3 second delay between emotional and cognitive processing in order to allow opportunities for thinking to control feeling...a difficult but necessary task indeed!

Managerial challenges in conflict management

Managers, leaders and entrepreneurs often see conflict in diverse ways. They may personally be involved in conflict with others (including employees, competitors, customers, or their supervisors). Alternatively, they may need to mediate conflict between other people in order to restore harmony to their team. They also need to be vigilant to prevent small disagreements from escalating into open conflicts and find ways to diffuse these situations artfully. Finally, they must find ways of ensuring that all of these different sources of conflict do not taint them or bias them away from certain individuals, so they can treat everyone fairly and equitably.

A key principle of conflict management is to embrace the reality that conflict is inevitable.[14] Try though we may to avoid it, conflict is unavoidable and will happen in all workplaces. Accepting this and actively looking for signs, symptoms, and early warning indicators are essential tasks for successful managers. It is not helpful to wilfully overlook signs of brewing conflict: when disagreements are only intellectual in nature and do not involve significant emotional entanglement, they are frequently easier to address and resolve before they escalate. At this stage, gentle humour, compromise, explanations or agreeing to disagree may be sufficient to calm troubled waters and prevent escalation. However, it is also important to not simply assume everything will be fine going forward. Consistent, supportive communication and checking in may be necessary to ensure the situation has not tipped into emotional entanglement.

Early warning signs of conflict

Managers, leaders and entrepreneurs need to be familiar with the early warning signs of brewing conflict and attempt to diffuse the situation before escalation. Such early warning signs include:

- *Changes in body language:* Observe the way in which individuals communicate with you and with each other. Body language is an important non-verbal cue that can help us gain an insight into the way people feel about each other and a situation. 'Closed' body language (e.g. folding of arms, avoidance of direct eye contact, tense or pursed lips, rapid blinking, heavy sighs, etc.) may indicate a brewing heightened emotional state that reflects emotional entanglement. Body language is frequently difficult to fake or hide, so there may be situations where individuals say they are fine and say they agree with you, but if their body language is not consistent with their verbal statements, this can be an important clue that something is amiss – and needs to be dealt with.[15]
- *Changes in behaviour:* Unexplained or unexpected behavioural or affective changes can be another clue that conflict is in the air: formerly relaxed and jovial colleagues who suddenly go quiet, or who surprisingly spend more time than normal isolated at their desk away from others, may be stewing or fuming about something but have not yet reached the point of being able to articulate it. Behavioural changes may presage sudden escalation towards conflict and identifying and addressing this both productively and sensitively can help prevent small problems from becoming big ones.
- *Emergence of new alliances or cliques within a team:* All workplaces are complex social groupings in which individuals with similar interests may form stronger interpersonal bonds and friendships with some people rather than others; this is both to be expected and perfectly natural. During times of intellectual disagreement, typical social interaction patterns may start to shift as individuals seek allies who reinforce their own beliefs; the expression 'adversity makes strange bedfellows' highlights how new cliques and alliances that are situational and opportunistic – but not necessarily healthy or helpful – can be an early warning sign of potential trouble.
- *Verbal cues:* As emotional involvement becomes entangled in intellectual disagreement, individuals start to articulate how these feelings and thoughts are affecting them. It may be reflected through the use of unusually strong words to describe relatively inconsequential events, or through a pattern of studied formalism that illustrates how each word is being carefully selected so the person has control of their feelings. Changes in typically conversational patterns between colleagues and with managers can be reflective of cognitive processing that is anticipating open conflict.
- *Lack of bandwidth to manage slightly unexpected events:* The capacity to 'roll with the punches' and respond effectively to small deviations in expected practices reflects an individual's cognitive and emotional capacity; where small surprises produce outsized or disproportionate responses, it can indicate that an individual is at, or has exceeded, their bandwidth and are at a point of fragility that can quickly escalate into conflict. A lack of tolerance for other's small mistakes can be an important managerial clue of conflict problems ahead. Where people are accustomed to staying a few minutes late to tidy up the day's work, and now suddenly go home on the dot and leave unfinished business, this may indicate bandwidth saturation that can presage open conflict ahead.

- *Unusual sick time or absences:* Lack of attentiveness to these early warning signs can sometimes trigger further problems including unexplained or suspicious sick time and absences, where people simply feel they need to stay away from work for their own mental health and well-being. At this point, workplace productivity and morale will be adversely impacted and open conflict becomes more likely.

There are, of course, other potential early warning signs of conflict that exist, and that may be unique to individuals. Managers, leaders and entrepreneurs need to be mindful of the many different ways in which these early warning signs may manifest – and most importantly not ignore them or simply hope they go away. Proactive identification of conflict warning signals can help us to self-manage our own emotional responses where we are involved in the conflict directly, or provide a trigger to intervene in some way to de-escalate conflict involving other parties.

De-escalating conflict

Rather than managing open conflict, it is often helpful to try to prevent conflict from escalating into the open in the first place. Where early warning signs are noted, one should attempt several strategies to help disentangle the cognitive from the emotional. Strategies that can be considered include:

- *Move to a private area to discuss:* Threat perception is a common trigger for conflict escalation, and is strongly correlated with feelings of shame, embarrassment, or disrespect. Trying to address a problem in public, with others listening or observing, can be interpreted as a sign of disrespect and can further escalate emotional entanglement. Separating parties and providing private spaces for discussion is essential for de-escalation.
- *Respect personal space and boundaries:* The heightened emotional state that is a feature of conflict means that physical presence can become frightening and intimidating. A well-intentioned gesture to place an arm around a shoulder, or to reach out and touch a forearm, can be misinterpreted as threatening. Be conscious of providing those in a conflict mode with the physical space needed to feel safe and respected. There will likely be a time where some form of physical contact is needed and helpful, but it is not likely at the point of escalation.
- *Be mindful of power dynamics transmitted through body language:* When conflict is escalating, small things like height differences can be distorted out of proportion. When conflict is brewing, attempt to bring parties together in a seated position to minimise threat perception and create greater equality in physical positions. Where conflict involves individuals of different physical proportions, ensure one person does not 'loom' over another, further amplifying threat perception. Being seated at a table can provide both physical space and distance, as well as make it easier to establish equitable eye-to-eye contact.
- *Try to engage the cognitive rather than the emotional:* It may be tempting to say things like 'how is everyone feeling right now?' but reinforcing the supremacy of emotion over cognition can be counterproductive to the goal of de-escalation. Instead, trying to emphasise what people are thinking and why they are behaving in a certain way can engage cognitive processes that will actually help tamp down and contain emotional responses.

- *Be mindful of non-verbal cues:* Non-verbal cues generally reflect our internal emotional state and this can result in a ricochet escalation of other's emotional responses. Keeping your tone of voice and body language neutral can help calm others. Be conscious of your personal 'tells', non-verbal cues that one has little control over but that reflect internal feelings vividly to others – what you are actually feeling and thinking despite the words you may be using. This can be particularly important – but difficult – if the other party is being directly hostile, challenging or belligerent. Learning to control non-verbal cues is an indirect but powerful form of learning to control emotional responses. Where anger is met with calmness, anger is more likely to dissipate.
- *Learn to ignore provocation:* Conflict generates many challenging situations, including deliberate provocation through the use of abusive language and slurs. While completely unacceptable and inappropriate, the reality, of course, is that such language and slurs are a part of the emotional response that is generated by conflict. Finding ways of not engaging directly with provocation can be very challenging, particularly where slurs are of a highly personal nature and targeting, for example, an individuals culture, race, religion, sexual orientation, or gender identity. Such slurs are an attempt to wield power by dehumanising the other individual: trying not to succumb to that power by not actually being dehumanised or responding is extraordinarily challenging but an important skill to learn.
- *Use words effectively:* Chapter 3 highlights techniques for effective listening and empathetic responses. Though it may be difficult, using empathy during conflict can be one of the most disarming and effective techniques to quell emotional surges. A combination of summarising, paraphrasing and empathising statements, the use of open-ended questions to encourage dialogue, and attentive engagement in conversation, are all important ways of engaging cognitive problem-solving and supressing emotional responses.

De-escalation techniques such as those listed above, are offered in the spirit of trying to manage conflict productively and constructively. Regrettably, however, it is essential to also note that these should only be attempted where physical and psychological safety are reasonably certain and possible. Societal acceptability of hostility, intimidation, and outright violence has become distressingly commonplace, and in some settings and countries, proliferation of tools of violence (including guns and knives) means that *pro forma* conflict management techniques must always take a back seat to safety concerns. Removing oneself from such dangers must be paramount: conflict management in these situations must be balanced against other priorities and an awareness of procedures around contacting police, security personnel, or others trained to deal with such situations. Be careful and stay safe.

From de-escalation to management and resolution

The objective of conflict de-escalation is to disentangle emotional involvement from intellectual disagreement. Once individuals have greater self-control over their cognitive and emotional selves, it becomes possible to shift towards conflict management and ultimately some form of acceptable resolution.

Conflict management is essentially a cognitive activity that engages problem-solving while monitoring emotional responsiveness. Conflict management is built upon skills such as listening, root cause analysis, effective communication, and prioritising. It requires significant cognitive bandwidth and engagement. Steps in conflict management include:

- *Talking:* Dialogue is essential in conflict management. Attempts to manage conflict through email or pre-recorded phone messages are generally less effective than face to face dialogue. Physical presence sends a strong signal that compromise is possible and that person to person connections will be part of the solution.
- *Emphasise behaviour and events, not personalities:* Conflict management is essentially a problem-solving process – clearly defining and actually asking the question, 'what's the problem we're trying to solve here?' can help focus attention away from personalities and on to concrete issues that are at the heart of the intellectual disagreement. It will often be tempting to answer the question of 'what's the problem?' by responding 'you're a jerk' but of course, that's not helpful. Agreement on the actual problem itself and the reason for intellectual disagreement is an essential first step in managing the conflict.
- *Establish ground rules for discussion that give everyone uninterrupted time and space to speak:* It is critical that individuals involved in conflict are given sufficient time to tell their stories and reflect their perspectives on the problem, without interruption or intimidation. Before even starting this discussion, clearly establish this ground rule and work collaboratively to enforce it. Part of this involves a commitment from everyone to listen and to control emotional responses to statements that are made.
- *Start by finding 'low-hanging-fruit', the points where you already agree:* Searching for points of agreement first can help establish a tone of compromise and collegiality that can make other difficult discussions less fraught. For example, most pharmacists can agree that keeping patients safe is a priority, even if the way this is achieved may be a point of disagreement. Clearly stating points of agreement sets a positive tone for further discussion.
- *Accept and acknowledge that not all disagreements will be addressed in one conversation:* Defining realistic priorities for an initial conversation will be important; not everything will be solved in a single discussion. Shifting from low-hanging-fruit of agreement to the most essential priorities for right now – and sticking with this – is important.
- *Develop a plan to keep talking:* Successful conflict management requires multiple conversations over time, and this requires planning and scheduling. Do not leave it to informal 'you'll sort it all out later, right?' methods; formalise the process of ongoing discussion so parties are clear with respect to the next steps and objectives.
- *Celebrate accomplishments:* Rather than grudgingly and reluctantly engaging with one another through the toil of conflict management, find ways of actually celebrating when even small compromises and successes are achieved. This kind of positive reinforcement can be energising and support further success. Part of this celebration can involve other bystanders who are not actually part of the conflict itself but who may have been peripherally or indirectly affected by it. Highlighting this kind of team-based spirit and collaboration can help build the interpersonal connections that can prevent problems in the future.

While this kind of approach to conflict management may appear overly naïve or idealistic, it is rooted in the concept that thinking and cognition must be engaged to control feeling and emotion in a productive and constructive way. Lists such as those presented in this chapter, engage us cognitively and provide a structure that can be helpful to consider and refer to when our emotions get the better of us.

Conflict resolution

There is some disagreement as to whether conflict resolution is ever truly possible or if simply containing conflict is all that is realistic.[16] The notion that resolutions to conflicts are possible is optimistic and also opens opportunities to heighten self-awareness of one's personal relationship to conflict. Chapter 2 introduces the concept of 'emotional intelligence', and the emotional intelligence styles described in that chapter can provide us with insights into how we behave in a conflict and what conflict resolution might look like. For example, Divergers, who strongly emphasise harmony, may view resolution in mainly interpersonal terms, rather than framing it as a specific quantitative outcome. Convergers, in contrast, may view resolution in more competitive terms, such as winning and losing. Each emotional intelligence style has a different understanding and framework for considering what 'resolution' means and what it may look like.

Another widely used tool to support self-reflection around conflict resolution, is the Thomas–Kilmann Conflict Mode Instrument (TKI). This tool proposes the existence of different conflict management styles and highlights how each individual's style contributes – or does not – to conflict management and resolution.[17] Importantly, the dominant strategies used by each style has unique strengths and benefits as well as potential weaknesses; there is no 'right' or 'best' conflict management style; instead, understanding how, in emotional and fast-changing circumstances, we instinctively and subconsciously respond to conflict can help increase awareness of better options. Furthermore, being aware that others also have their own style can help us to respond more appropriately during conflict. The TKI is a commercially available instrument and training program that can be useful for managers. There are other models and tools available, including the Conflict Management Scale,[18] that are free to use.

The TKI highlights five different, somewhat complementary, conflict management styles:

1. *Collaboration:* Collaborative conflict resolution involves a combination of both assertiveness and cooperation; the goal being to identify solutions that fully satisfy everyone involved, optimising outcomes whilst minimising negative emotional responses. Collaboration is important when the maintenance and nurturing of a long-term relationship with other parties is as important as successful resolution of the conflict itself. Collaboration requires a give-and-take spirit and the ability to see a situation from other people's perspectives.
2. *Competition:* Competitive conflict resolution generally involves an assertive personality type who are somewhat uncooperative and willing to pursue personal objectives at another person's expense. In this situation, the outcome is more important than the maintenance and nurturing of the relationship. It may be a useful conflict resolution style in some cases – for example, when dealing with another organisation where a long-term relationship is not necessary or desired – but should generally not be used by colleagues within an organisation who will likely need to keep working together and have some form of positive relationship. The competing style is high-risk, high-reward: even in the most competitive settings, there may be times in the future where an overly competitive conflict resolution style can result in unanticipated blow-back.

3. *Avoidance:* Avoidance is characterised by both unassertive and uncooperative behaviours, and usually takes the appearance of chronic distancing or sidestepping of difficult situations. There will be times where avoidance is the best conflict resolution style: for example, where threats of violence or intimidation are in place. Where safety is a concern, avoidance is appropriate, so long as it is framed in the context of postponement rather than completely ignoring a situation. In other circumstances, where the actual substance of the conflict is not particularly grave or concerning, such as a colleague who once in a while makes personal phone calls during work hours, avoidance may be a reasonable first pathway for conflict resolution – it's simply not worth engaging at this point. Should 'once in while' become 'all the time', then it may be appropriate to revisit avoidance as an approach.

4. *Accommodation:* The opposite of competition, accommodation involves conflict resolution akin to 'caving in' and simply accepting the other's point of view and demands. While this may take on the appearance of being self-sacrificing and generous of spirit, accommodation runs the risk of looking weak and causing resentment. Accommodation is most likely to occur when the ongoing quality of the relationship between individuals is more important than the actual outcome. Importantly, if accommodation becomes a default conflict resolution approach or style, this can start to breed internalised resentment and anger, which may ultimately explode at an inopportune moment.

5. *Compromise:* Compromises involve quick, reasonable and mutually agreed upon solutions that only partially satisfy both parties, and involves a balance of assertiveness and cooperativeness. Compromise is usually best used when the outcome is not critical and there is a time pressure involved. However, by definition, compromises mean that no one is actually truly satisfied with the outcome, so compromises can sometimes mean the conflict re-emerges later in an amplified manner.

The recognition that conflict resolution can (and should) look different in different situations, is important. Understanding how personal emotional intelligence connects to different conflict resolution styles, and recognising the balance between the importance of the outcome and the importance of a healthy long-term relationship between parties in a conflict, can provide some guidance in understanding how best to proceed in difficult situations.

Negotiation and mediation

Managers, leaders and entrepreneurs may find themselves in difficult situations involving different employees or other stakeholders: while they themselves may not be involved with or part of a conflict, they may be called upon to find ways of managing and resolving conflict involving others, and this can be challenging. It can be difficult to maintain impartiality, openness, and transparency in such situations, but, of course, it is essential to not be seen taking sides or favouring one person/group over another in a biased or unfair manner, and without justifiable cause.

There is an important distinction between the concepts of negotiation and mediation, and there are times and circumstances where one, but not the other, may be more appropriate. Negotiation typically is described as a process where the individuals or groups involved in a conflict or a dispute, find a way of reaching a settlement amongst themselves that both can agree to (or at least live with).[19] In mediation, this process involves a neutral third party that assists the individuals/groups in reaching a solution. Mediation requires strict neutrality in order to be perceived as fair.[20] Managers, leaders and entrepreneurs need to understand advantages and disadvantages of both approaches and what managerial roles exist in both cases.

In negotiation, identified individuals (negotiators) actually represent each party and deal directly with one another to identify areas of common agreement as well as where compromises can occur. Negotiation is often best used in situations where there is general comparability or equality between the parties involved, so that one does not have a particular advantage over the other. Negotiation can be a stormy process at times, but when it works, it often produces a satisfactory outcome as well as helping to strengthen relationships between the parties. Where negotiation is being used, managers may find it most effective to simply step away and provide the negotiators with time and space to find a mutually acceptable solution, without outside interference or involvement. There is, however, a risk with negotiation that the 'mutually acceptable solution' to the parties may in fact not be workable from a managerial perspective; without a third party present to facilitate the process, negotiation can sometimes lead to unexpected and unworkable outcomes.[19]

In contrast, with mediation, an impartial facilitator, with no specific link to either individual/group involved and with no interest in the issue itself, focuses on the process of ensuring respectful, productive, and constructive dialogue as a prelude to identifying and selecting alternatives and solutions. It is quite unusual for the mediator to be the manager themselves, since the manager likely has some interest in the issues that are the source of the disagreement, but the manager can provide an important role in offering an organisation the services of a mediator. In larger organisations, managers from unrelated areas might serve as mediators. The extent to which mediators represent a third party in a conflict – the interests and needs of the organisation as a whole, distinct from the interests and needs of the individuals/groups involved in the conflict itself – is a very difficult subject to navigate. In some cases, mediators can and should provide a valuable 'reality check' to the disputants, but in a way that still preserves impartiality and fairness. Explicitly representing management's views on an issue as part of a mediation is rarely successful, it frequently accelerates or worsens conflict and should be avoided. Crucial to the success of mediation is finding a mediator who can reconcile these many concerns and needs, and present an impartial perspective that is trusted and respected by the disputants. Their focus should be on facilitation, not on content: ensuring parties are heard, voices are respected, and ground rules for conversation are adhered to consistently.[20]

Managers, leaders and entrepreneurs need to recognise when negotiation is useful and when mediation is required, depending on the severity of the conflict and other organisational issues. In both negotiation and mediation, it is essential to clearly define and find common ground on what issues are subject to negotiation or mediation; failure to agree upon a defined parameter for the discussion will likely mean that conversations devolve quickly into personality disputes.[19,20]

Negotiation skills and tips

There is no one-size-fits-all formula for successful negotiation, but there are certain principles that generally apply:

- *Don't be a tough guy:* Negotiation that is rooted in force or intimidation rarely succeeds and does not produce a win–win outcome. Both parties need to enter a negotiation believing (and wanting) a mutually acceptable outcome where everyone gets something of value.
- *Coinage matters:* In negotiation, the term 'coinage' refers to an item that has significant meaning to one party but is not particularly important to the other.[21] Coinage is frequently the most common way in which the give-and-take of negotiation proceeds; one party's willingness to concede or give something that isn't all that important to them can have an enormous value on enhancing the tone and collegiality of the negotiation – increasing the willingness of the other party to find suitable coinage in return. Initial negotiations focusing on coinage rather than the more sticky issues that matter significantly to both parties, can proceed more efficiently and create a positive climate.
- *Clarity around what negotiators can and cannot do:* It is essential that those involved in negotiation actually know what authorities and powers they have, particularly if they are representing a group or other people. Negotiators can sometimes make decisions but in many cases they need to check in with the rest of their group prior to commitments being made – building this into the negotiation process is essential.
- *Tone and environment matter:* Conflicts frequently escalate in stressful, crowded, and disorganised workplaces: negotiation should be removed from these environmental distractions to set a more positive tone, so both parties can truly concentrate, listen, hear, and focus their attention on one another.
- *Impasses will occur:* No negotiation is a smooth, straight-line process: if it were that simple, no conflict would have erupted in the first place. Expecting and planning for an impasse (the point at which neither side has coinage or the ability to compromise) is essential, and most often requires a physical break from discussions for a period of time. Realistically, not all negotiations are successful, and even successful negotiations will leave some elements that are unnegotiated behind.

Mediation skills and tips

Mediators must have sophisticated communication and problem-solving skills in order to be successful. Like negotiation, there is no one-size-fits-all formula for success as a mediator, but certain practices have emerged as being likely to engender a positive outcome:[22]

- *Focus on the problem:* Mediators must use verbal and non-verbal language to emphasise the problem itself, rather than personalities or individuals involved. This can be complex because by the time conflict erupts, personalities and individuals have become part of the problem. Finding ways of decoupling personalities from problems, and framing the mediation as a discussion around issues alone, is one of the most important skills mediators must possess.
- *Encourage the parties to jointly problem solve:* It can be tempting for mediators to think of themselves as the wise judge who has the answer, but successful mediation rarely occurs when the mediator does all the talking. Mediators should refrain from prematurely offering their opinions or their uninformed solutions for fear they will be perceived as impartial or unfair. Instead, mediators need to ask open-ended questions to test the strength of ideas/solutions proposed by the parties themselves.

- *Don't ignore verbal and non-verbal cues:* In mediation, much of the information the mediator will have will come from the communication of the disputants. Being mindful of this information and responding to it (rather than ignoring it) is essential. An eye roll or heavy sigh in response to a statement conveys a wealth of information that the mediator needs to use effectively in deciding what to say next.
- *Ensure ground rules for respectful dialogue are enforced:* Disputants may assume that a mediator is a referee who makes the final decision when the individuals/parties can't agree. This is not the case: mediators are not referees in a decision making sense, but they do have the important role of ensuring respectful conversation and tone are maintained throughout. Each mediator needs to find the language and non-verbal cues that work most effectively to signal – respectfully but clearly – when one of the parties has crossed the line. Most frequently, this involves the use of words like 'we' or 'us' rather than 'you' or 'them'. For example, when conversation becomes heated, rather than saying 'you're out of line', it may be preferable to say 'let's all take a break to catch our breath and start with new energy'. Failure to address disrespectful discourse clearly and effectively will diminish trust in the mediator and may imply a lack of impartiality.
- *Demonstrate confidence that mediation can work:* The mediator has to believe mediation is useful for the disputants to buy-in. Confidence that mediation can work does not imply mediation will solve all problems: instead, mediation can help parties advance their discussions respectfully and perhaps establish a foundation for ongoing discussions to continue to address challenging issues in the future.

Many jurisdictions have mediator certification programs. Mediators come from a variety of different backgrounds; finding a trusted and respected mediator with the skills necessary to facilitate discussions between disputants will take time and energy, but the reward of finding such a mediator can be significant. Word of mouth and referrals from professional colleagues are the most frequently used ways that managers can find good mediators. Human resource departments and lawyers may also have advice regarding mediators that can be effective in particular cases or situations. Mediators can be expensive depending on their background and qualifications so this may be a consideration in many cases; avoid the temptation of being penny-wise but pound-foolish and using less qualified or well-meaning amateurs, when only professional mediators could truly manage the complexity of a situation. The costs of not having a good mediator in terms of productivity, broken relationships, and further stress on the organisation are frequently much higher than the fees charged by an effective and experienced mediator.

Summary

Conflict is a reality in any workplace, and managers need to accept and work with this reality. Managers may themselves be part of a conflict situation or be called upon to find ways of resolving conflict between other parties. In most cases, conflict itself is a function of both intellectual disagreement and emotional involvement, an amalgam of thinking and feeling. Strategies to decouple emotional entanglement to allow for better problem-solving are an important part of conflict de-escalation. Conflict management and resolution are functions of both communication skills and emotional intelligence; self-awareness and self-reflection can support the development of skills with respect to dealing with conflict.

References

1. Shikaze D *et al*. Community pharmacists' attitudes, opinions, and beliefs and leadership in the profession: An exploratory study. *Can Pharm J* 2018; 151(5): 315–321. https://doi.org/10.1177/1715163518790984

2. Sportsman S, Hamilton P. Conflict management styles in the health professions. *J Professional Nursing* 2007; 23(3): 157–166. https://doi.org/10.1016/j.profnurs.2007.01.010

3. Cullati S *et al*. When team conflicts threaten quality of care: a study of health care professionals' experiences and perceptions. *Mayo Clinic Proc Innov Qual Outcomes* 2019; 3(1): 43–51. https://doi.org/10.1016/j.mayocpiqo.2018.11.003

4. Overton A, Lowry A. Conflict management: difficult conversations with difficult people. *Clin Colon Rectal Surg* 2013; 26(4): 259–264. https://doi.org/10.1055/s-0033-1356728

5. Thakore D. Conflict and conflict management. *IOSR J Business and Management* 2013; 8(6): 7–16.

6. Gregory P, Austin Z. Conflict in community pharmacy practice: the experience of pharmacists, technicians, and assistants. *Can Pharm J* 2107; 150(1): 32–41. https://doi.org/10.1177/1715163516679426

7. Haumschild R *et al*. Managing conflict: a guide for the pharmacy manager. *Hosp Pharm* 2015; 50(6): 543–549. https://doi.org/10.1310/hpj5006-543

8. Evans C *et al*. Conflict resolution in retail community pharmacy: Drugmart Pharmacy case. *J Business Studies Quarterly* 2010; 1(3): 53–67.

9. Thomas KW. Conflict and conflict management: reflections and update. *J Organizational Behavior* 1992; 13: 265–274.

10. Kang Y *et al*. Purpose in life and conflict-related neural responses during health decision-making. *Health Psychol* 2019; 38(6): 545–552. https://doi.org/10.1037/hea0000729

11. Freedman BD. Risk factors and causes of interpersonal conflict in nursing workplaces: understandings from neuroscience. *Collegian* 2019; 26(5): 594–604. https://doi.org/10.1016/j.colegn.2019.02.001

12. Westen D, Gabbard GO. Developments in cognitive neuroscience: I. Conflict, compromise, and connectionism. *J Am Psychoanalytic Assoc* 2016; 50(1): 53–98. https://doi.org/10.1177/00030651020500011501

13. Rousseau DL, Garcia-Retamero R. Identity, power, and threat perception: A cross-national experimental study. *J Conflict Resolution* 2007; 51(5): 744–771. https://doi.org/10.1177/0022002707304813

14. Samuel AP, Lucent-Iwhiwhu H. Inevitability of conflict in business organizations. *Int J Innov Social Sciences Humanities Research* 2021; 9(2): 118–130.

15. Austin Z. *Communication in Interprofessional Care: Theory and Applications*. Washington DC: American Pharmacists' Association, 2020. https://doi/org/10.21019/9781582123431

16. Omisore BO, Abiodun AR. Organizational conflicts: causes, effects, and remedies. *Int J Academic Res Economics and Management Sci* 2014; 3(6): 118–137. https://dx.doi.org/10.6007/IJAREMS/v3-i6/1351

17. Womack DF. Assessing the Thomas-Kilmann Conflict Mode Survey. *Management Comm Quarterly* 1988; 1(3): 321–349. https://doi.org/10.1177/0893318988001003004

18. Austin Z *et al*. A conflict management scale for pharmacy. *Am J Pharm Educ* 2009; 73(7): Article 122.

19. Zohar I. The art of negotiation: Leadership skills required for negotiation in times of crisis. *Procedia – Social and Behavioral Sciences* 2015; 209(3): 540–548. https://doi.org/10.1016/j.sbspro.2015.11.285

20. Knickle K *et al*. Beyond winning: mediation, conflict resolution, and non-rational sources of conflict in the ICU. *Crit Care* 2012; 16(3): 308. https://doi.org/10.1186/CC11141

21. Hake S, Shah T. Negotiation skills for clinical research professionals. *Perspect Clin Res* 2011; 2(3): 105–108.

22. Fairchild AJ, McDaniel HL. Best (but oft-forgotten) practices: mediation analysis. *Am J Clinical Nutrition* 2017; 105(6): 1259–1271. https://doi.org/10.3945/ajcn.117.152546

CHAPTER 6

Financial literacy

Upon completion of this chapter you should be able to:

- understand the importance of financial literacy for managers, leaders and entrepreneurs in pharmacy
- explain the three key financial statements that form the core of a business
- list the applications of the three key financial statements in business.

Much of management and leadership training focuses on human resources issues related to conflict management, team-building, and motivation techniques; while these are undeniably important, in reality most roles also require additional knowledge and skills in financial management. All businesses and operations – including not-for-profit and public sector organisations – must have a solid and sustainable financial foundation in order to continue to hire and pay workers and to deliver services and care. In most organisations, managers and leaders have significant operational responsibilities related to the development and monitoring of budgets, accounting for variances, and projecting future revenues and expenditures. Entrepreneurs may have personal financial well-being on the line with their own businesses. While many people have some limited accounting or finance experience, there are crucial 'financial literacy' competencies that are essential for success. Managers, leaders and entrepreneurs are constantly making decisions that fundamentally will influence an organisation's financial position, including scheduling, hiring/firing of personnel, approving invoices for payment, and monitoring of budgets. A lack of basic financial skills can result in poor decisions that may ultimately compromise organisational success and sustainability.

Understanding financial statements

While managers, leaders and entrepreneurs are rarely required to actually produce financial statements (a task best left to professionally qualified accountants), it is important that they have basic familiarity with the terminology and layout of these statements so they can understand how their unit, department, business, or organisation is performing. Financial statements are simply written records that summarise a business' activities and financial performance over a period of time. They are routinely audited by external experts to ensure they are accurate, fair, and truly reflective of reality. Three key financial statements form the core of any business, and can be used by managers, leaders, executives, owners, external parties and shareholders to determine the overall health of an organisation:

- *Balance sheet:* The balance sheet provides an overview of the financial position of an organisation. It is best described as a snapshot-in-time since the balance sheet must be dated. A balance sheet consists of three broad categories: assets, liabilities and equity (or net worth). Assets list items and elements in an organisation that have monetary value; they represent some form of ownership, and include contractual rights to future payments from other organisations. Liabilities represent money that an organisation owes to others, including mortgages, future guaranteed salaries or pensions, and contractual promises to pay others for services or goods already received. The formula, assets − liabilities = net worth, describes the overall financial position of an organisation: a positive net worth means there are more than enough assets to pay for liabilities, and reflects a more sustainable financial foundation for future operations. The magnitude (or amount) of net worth is, of course, a crucial consideration for for-profit organisations, but also of importance for non-profit or governmental organisations.

- *Income statement:* The income statement describes operational profits and losses over a period of time. Typically, income statements are generated quarterly (every three months) but must be produced at least yearly. The formula, revenue − expenses = income, helps managers, leaders and entrepreneurs understand what it costs to generate the returns that are received. Where expenses are higher than revenue, income is negative and the business is losing money. In some cases (for example, a start-up business) income may be negative and tolerable for a short period of time. However, in all cases, businesses must ultimately generate positive income in order to be sustainable.

- *Cash flow statement:* Balance sheets and income statements are intuitively accepted as important by most managers without financial training. The third financial statement − cash flow − is sometimes more difficult to understand and so may be frequently overlooked or ignored due to its complexity. However, cash flow statements provide an important piece of information regarding the financial health of an organisation, answering a crucial question of how much cash an organisation hands over to employees for salaries, creditors for materials purchased, owners, shareholders, etc. versus how much cash is retained by the organisation for its own growth, investment in future operations, and a 'safety cushion' for emergencies. Having sufficient cash on hand to fund these items is essential for sustainability: without sufficient cash flow, routine maintenance for a broken pipe or an equipment malfunction requiring fixing can literally bankrupt an organisation.

Taken together, these three different statements provide managers with the clearest understanding of the financial health of the organisation, and can help them make the most informed decisions regarding (for example) hiring, new equipment purchases, or investments in future growth. A more detailed explanation of these three different statements follows below.

The balance sheet

Figure 1: *An example of a balance sheet.*

123 Pharmacy BALANCE SHEET			
ASSETS		**LIABILITIES**	
Current assets		**Current liabilities**	
Cash on hand	£ 50 000	Accounts payable	£ 110 000
Account receivable	15 000	Accrued expenses	40 000
Inventory	60 000	(including salaries/benefits)	
Prepaid expenses	15 000		
Investments	7 500	**TOTAL CURRENT ASSETS**	**150 000**
TOTAL CURRENT ASSETS	**147 000**		
		Non-current liabilities	
Non-current assets		Bank loan	£ 150 000
Property	£ 250 000	**TOTAL LIABILITIES**	**£ 300 000**
Furnishings and equipment	75 000		
TOTAL NON-CURRENT ASSETS	**147 000**	**Net worth**	
		Shares in company	£ 150 000
		Retained earnings	22 500
Total assets	**£ 472 500**	**Total liabilities + net worth**	**£ 472 500**

Each section of the balance sheet needs to be considered separately before forming a full picture of the financial health of the organisation. Current assets are those that can reasonably be expected to be converted into cash in less than one year. Cash on hand represents the amount of money that is already on hand and can be used to make immediate purchases without negotiating a separate loan or liability agreement. Accounts receivable represents work or services provided by the organisation to another different person/organisation; an invoice for this will have been sent and the company is waiting for payment. For example, in many community pharmacies, billing for prescriptions dispensed happens on a monthly or quarterly basis. The pharmacy delivers goods but must wait a period of time before being reimbursed for this by the National Health Service (NHS) or another payor. Accounts receivable are listed as current assets because there is a high, reasonable probability that within a year, what is owed will be paid and thus converted to cash the organisation can use. Inventory represents tangible products that will eventually be sold and converted to cash; a business like a pharmacy must first purchase and store products for a period of time prior to converting this into sales that will then become cash on hand. Prepaid expenses represent a category of current assets that will help reduce liabilities in the future. For example, some organisations may pay certain operational expenses (such as electricity or heating bills) to a utility company in advance to take advantage of a discount offered to companies. These are future liabilities that would have to be paid eventually, but for the snapshot-in-time of the balance sheet, they are considered an asset as they have not yet been incurred. Investments represent short-term cashable products (usually held in banks) that provide a convenient but readily accessible way of an organisation saving money for a rainy day, or building up its reserves for an upcoming purchase.

Non-current assets represent more long-lasting or enduring investments in the organisation that are expected to be held for more than one year and are not quite as easy to convert to cash on hand. This includes the property or building within which the business operates (if it is owned by the business itself) and the equipment and furniture that allows the business to function. In general, property prices will appreciate (or gain financial value) over time, while equipment and furniture will depreciate (or lose financial value) over that same time period. Complex formulas for calculating appreciation and depreciation exist and must be included in balance sheet calculations in order to accurately portray the health of the organisation. One type of non-current asset, not represented in this sample balance sheet, is the 'intangible asset'. Intangible assets are non-physical assets that still have some monetary value. The most common non-tangible assets include 'goodwill', intellectual property, patents, or copyrights. Goodwill represents the relationships the business has with clients and its community: the more connected and respected an organisation is, the more likely it is to have repeat customers and build new clients, and this can be quantified and expressed in the balance sheet as an asset. Similarly, beloved and respected brand names also have a financial value since customers often demonstrate brand loyalty and seek out specific businesses to buy from simply because of their name. This too can be expressed on the balance sheet as an asset. The traditional formula for calculating goodwill/brand as an asset is the difference between purchase price of a business and the fair value of all net assets (i.e. assets minus liabilities). However, great care must be exercised in interpreting brand and goodwill claims on a balance sheet as fewer rules govern how they are financially calculated and they can be misrepresented or misstated more easily.

The sum of current and non-current assets represents the financial strength of an organisation. In the sample balance sheet presented above, there are a few observations of note. First, there appears to be a large percentage of cash on hand, with relatively little invested. This represents a lost opportunity, since money in the bank at least earns interest and this grows with time, while cash on hand is more inert. It may be prudent to reduce cash on hand and transfer to a high interest savings account at a bank so the money is readily accessible, so if not currently being used it can at least generate some interest. Inventory appears somewhat high, even for a product intensive business like a pharmacy. This may mean poor purchasing decisions are being made. While inventory is an asset, too much inventory means products expire, additional resources are consumed for storage and maintenance, and inefficient use of money is occurring. Finding the right balance of inventory is challenging – if inventory is too tight, shortages will occur and customers will be lost. If inventory is too high, costs are also too high. The non-current asset of furnishings and equipment also appears quite high; more than 15% of this organisation's assets are in a depreciating asset that, over time, will become worthless as they become outdated. Of course, proper equipment and furniture are essential for a business, but understanding why so much of the asset base is dedicated to this would be worth exploring further to see if efficiencies could be found.

Next, let's examine the right hand side of the balance sheet. The liabilities represent money owed by the organisation to others, usually for goods and services already purchased but not yet paid. Accounts payable usually represents purchases made on credit, often linked to inventory. The selling organisation would issue an invoice for payment, stipulating the time frame for receipt of the payment. Failure to pay an invoice on time usually results in some kind of financial penalty; this should be avoided as it is wasteful and depletes cash reserves. Accrued expenses are expenses a company needs to account for, but for which no invoices have been received and no payments have yet been made. Examples of accrued expenses can include interest on bank loans, taxes payable to governments, utilities that will likely be paid, or rent on space. Wages (including salaries and benefits) are also examples of accrued expenses since organisations know what they will owe their workforce in the year ahead and need to account for it. Similar to assets, current liabilities represent those financial obligations that will need to be paid within the next year. Non-current liabilities – in this case, a bank loan – have repayment terms longer than one year. The principal amount of the loan is listed as a non-current liability, while the interest payments for that loan will be listed under accrued expenses.

The liabilities portion of the balance sheet provides some interesting observations for managers. First, accounts payable seems quite high, representing more than 23% of the total of the balance sheet. This could reflect problems or inefficiencies in the way in which invoices are processed. It may also suggest the organisation has been on a 'spending spree' and perhaps is not making the wisest purchasing decisions. Coupled with the seemingly high amount of inventory noticed on the asset side, this could be a cause for concern for the organisation and its long-term sustainability. While of course all businesses must buy in order to sell at a profit, there is a balance that is healthy and in this balance sheet it is not clear that the balance of purchases is healthy. Accrued expenses appear somewhat low which may indicate that understaffing of the organisation is a problem; given the existence of a large bank loan and other utility expenses, it is unclear how sufficient staff is in place to actually run the business well and profitably. Under non-current liabilities, the bank loan represents more than 30% of the balance sheet. This may be reasonable and proportionate for a company that is growing, though of course care must be taken to ensure interest payments on this loan (represented in accrued expenses) are monitored closely, especially should bank interest rates rise quickly.

The final portion of the balance sheet – labelled 'net worth' (or sometimes 'shareholder equity') – represents the difference between assets and liabilities. In some cases, when a business is just starting, or an existing business is undergoing rapid growth or temporary difficulties, it may be reasonable to expect that (for a short period of time) liabilities may exceed assets. Of course, this cannot be sustainable beyond a short period of time without bankruptcy occurring. Shares in a company represents a category of net worth related to investments made by individuals in the business itself. For example, when this business was first starting out, someone may have given the owner a sum of money to get off the ground. This could have been structured as a loan repayable in a specific period of time with a defined interest rate (in which case it would be represented under non-current liabilities). In this case, it appears as though this person gave the owner a sum of money in exchange for 'shares' in the company and its future profitability. A loan is fixed in its duration and does not represent an open-ended claim on future profitability and growth of the company. In contrast, a share represents a percentage of business ownership which translates into a long-term obligation for the company. In some cases, shareholders will receive annual dividends, representing a share of the year's profits, while still maintaining their ongoing claims to future company profits. Retained earnings represents the amount of money the company keeps (or its profits) after all other expenses have been paid. These earnings are traditionally used to reinvest back into the business to ensure its future growth and sustainability. In this case, retained earnings represent less than 5% of the balance sheet, which may be a cause for concern if the company is anticipating growth and will need resources to invest in that growth.

Overall, this balance sheet provides an interesting snapshot of a business that may have some risks ahead and may need to have tighter managerial controls. Inventory may be excessive and draining profitability, while expenditures (as represented by accounts payable) need to be scrutinised more closely to ensure they are necessary and appropriate. Staffing levels may be too low, while purchases of equipment and furniture (both depreciating assets) might be too high. Managers reviewing a company balance sheet should be able to draw similar inferences, and use this data in order to investigate further and ensure financial decisions are made that will ensure the sustainability of the business into the future.

Income statements

Income statements (sometimes called 'profit and loss statements') provide a different lens through which the financial health of the organisation can be understood and complement balance sheets by providing a 'moving picture' view of a business, rather than a snapshot-in-time. The income statement has three main sections: revenues, expenses, and profit/loss. There are several variations of income statements that can be used (e.g. 'single step' versus 'multi-step') but the general purpose will be the same: to help managers understand how much it costs to generate revenue received, which in turn translates into a profit or a loss for the company. *See* Figure 2.

The vertical presentation of financial data in the income statement highlights the ways in which revenues and expenses ultimately determine profit. At the macro level, revenues are simply the dollar amount of sales minus the cost of the goods sold. In this simplified version, all goods sold in pharmacy XYZ (over-the-counter, prescription, front shop, etc.) are collapsed into a single dollar amount; of course, in real life these would be individual line items, allowing the manager to better understand what share of revenues comes from what part of the pharmacy. This can allow for staffing decisions in the future: for example, if the bulk of sales in a pharmacy is coming from cosmetics, not prescriptions, it may be helpful to redeploy non-professional staff to that part of the operation to further maximise profits.

Cost of goods sold (COGS) is a somewhat complex calculation but it must be accurately and carefully reported in order to ensure income statements truly reflect financial realities. Briefly, COGS – beginning inventory + purchases (during the time period) – ending inventory. As a result, one of the primary management functions in pharmacy is ensuring accurate and timely physical inventory counts are undertaken; this is the only way that COGS can accurately be calculated. There may be a temptation to try to shortcut the painful and laborious process of physically counting inventory on an annual basis but failure to do this will result in inaccurate COGS calculations, and inaccurate income statements. COGS does not include overhead or operational costs of doing business, simply the value of products purchased and sold. If COGS exceeds revenue generated by a company during the reporting period, this means there will be no profit. Accountants employ other, more sophisticated methods for calculating COGS, focused on FIFO, LIFO, and ACM. FIFO means 'first in, first out': since prices typically tend to rise over time, FIFO requires companies to sell less expensive products first, translating into a lower COGS. In contrast, LIFO ('last in, first out') means the latest goods added to inventory (which are likely the more expensive ones to purchase) are sold first, leading to a higher COGS value. In the ACM or 'average cost method', it is assumed that the inventory cost is based on the average cost of goods during the time period. Managers will rarely make the decision as to which accounting method is used for COGS calculations, but need to be aware of the differences and implications, and be prepared to contribute to decision making.

Figure 2: *Example XYZ pharmacy income statement for the year ending June 30 2024.*

XYZ Pharmacy Income Statement For the year ending June 30, 2024		
REVENUE		
Sales (including Rx, OTC, front shop)		£ 600 000
Cost of goods sold		
Opening inventory (as at July 01 2023)	£ 80 000	
Add purchases	240 000	
Less closing inventory	70 000	
Less costs of goods sold		£ 250 000
Gross profit		£ 350 000
Add other operating revenue		
Vaccination services	£ 75 000	
Public health services	25 000	
New medicines/medication review services	50 000	
TOTAL REVENUE		**£ 500 000**
LESS OPERATING EXPENSES		
General and administrative expenses		£ 600 000
Wages, salaries, benefits	£ 280 000	
Rent expenses incl. insurance	60 000	
Depreciation	5 000	
Marketing/advertising/public relations	15 000	
Utilities (electricity, heating, water, telecom)	20 000	
Bookkeeping, bank, audit	9 000	
Bad debt	9 000	
TOTAL EXPENSES		**£ 398 000**
Net profit (EBIT)		£ 102 000

Gross profit simply equals: sales – cost of goods sold. The term 'gross' is used because this only refers to actual products, and does not include many other expenses that, of course, are incurred in order to actually sell the products, including staff, rent, utilities, etc.

The nature of pharmacy practice today means that products are not the only revenue generating items that are 'sold' in a pharmacy. As dispensing margins and fees have become diminished over time, pharmacies are increasingly reliant on the clinical services and the care they provide to strengthen the income statement. In this example, three particular clinical services have been highlighted as revenue generating – vaccinations, public health screening, and new medicines/medicines review programming.

No 'goods' are bought or sold, but these services are billed and remuneration is received for care provided, and so this appears on the income statement. A manager reviewing this income statement would note that a fairly significant proportion of the revenues of the pharmacy comes from these services; of course the next question then will be how much does it 'cost' (in terms of salaries, benefits, overhead, rent, utilities, etc.) to generate service based revenue versus how much it costs to generate product based revenue. The income statement alone cannot answer this question, but it does help identify this as an important area for the manager to research further. A simplistic and rough calculation suggests that sales – cost of goods sold = 600 000 – 250 000 = 350 000, meaning there is a 58% profit on products sold without overhead and expenses considered. In contrast, there is a 100% profit on services provided since there are no 'costs of services sold' noted. This is an erroneous calculation however, since services typically have higher wage/salary/benefits expenses, which points to the importance of the next section of the income statement.

Whether goods or services are being sold, there are always expenses involved in running a business. The expenses highlighted in the sample statement above point to the categories of costs incurred in order to generate revenue. In this case, there is no attempt to separate costs associated with sales of 'goods' (e.g. over-the-counter products, prescriptions, etc.) versus 'services' (e.g. vaccinations), mainly because in day to day pharmacy practice, it is difficult to accurately allocate portions of time of staff members to these different activities. The category of 'general and administrative expenses' covers a wide variety of areas, but it is essential for managers to understand the structure of expenses in order to control them. Some 'fixed' expenses will exist regardless of whether one vaccine is given or 1000 are administered: for example, rent paid in order to provide space, or a refrigerator to store vaccines. Other 'variable' expenses will change as the number of activities (sales or services) increases. In between, there are 'step' expenses: for example, a single pharmacist may be able to administer 40 vaccines in a typical shift, but if 50 people require vaccines, another pharmacist will need to be brought on to administer the additional 10. This second pharmacist will be under-worked (relative to the first pharmacist) but will still be paid the same rate. Step expenses can be complex to manage but important to understand.

One category of expenses that is important in pharmacy is 'shrinkage'. An inventory intensive business like a pharmacy must take into account the reality that theft, expired goods, or product spoilage will occur. The term 'shrinkage' is used to describe inventory that simply goes missing, sometimes for no apparent reason. Monitoring shrinkage through the income statement is important as this can help alert managers to other issues in the pharmacy and should be used as a trigger to prevent unnecessary waste that impacts on profitability.

The final profit or loss calculation is simply a function of revenues minus expenses. The term 'EBIT' (earnings before interest and taxes) or 'EBITDA' (earnings before interest, taxes, depreciation, and amortization) will frequently be used in income statements to highlight that the 'profit' calculated is not the end of the story: taxes must be paid on profits and interest may be payable on losses where loans are required to cover them.

Overall, this income statement suggests the pharmacy is doing relatively well – it is making a reasonable profit and the ratio of revenue to expenses appears sustainable. There appears to be healthy diversification in terms of revenue sources, amongst both goods and services. Despite a relatively high proportion of revenues derived from services (which are inherently more labour intensive), employee related expenses appear well managed. Bad debt and shrinkage is an unfortunate reality in any business, and given the size of the operation, the amount does not appear to be out of proportion.

Cash flow statements

The third element of financial statements involves cash flow. Cash flow statements help managers understand where cash is being generated, and where cash is being used across a business. There are different methods that can be used to track the flow of cash in a business, namely the 'direct method' and the 'indirect method'. While managers will rarely make the decision as to which method should be used, they need to understand the implications of this choice and be prepared to contribute to discussions related to this decision. The direct method of cash flow focuses primarily on cash transactions, separating analysis into cash received versus cash paid. In the indirect method, cash flow begins with net income, and non-cash adjustments are subsequently factored into the analysis.

There are three broad categories of cash use in a business: operations, investments, and financing. Operating cash flow refers to day to day business activities: revenues collected and expenses paid during the year are included in this section, but depreciation costs on equipment or mortgages owing on property to house the business are not. Investing cash flow focuses on the non-current assets that support the business, including property, furnishings, and equipment costs, but not inventory or salaries. Finally, financing cash flow focuses on the structure of the business itself, including transactions related to stocks/shares being sold, debt being assumed through bank loans or mortgages, etc.

Cash flow statements rely heavily on honesty and transparency: the full disclosure principle means that accountants or others preparing cash flow statements must accurately and honestly disclose everything and provide notes in order to help readers understand the financial realities of the business. For example, if a pharmacy is in the middle of a law suit for negligence and has put aside extra cash in reserve to pay for legal or other fees, it might be seen on a cash flow statement as a robust cash reserve, and potentially interpreted as a very positive finding of future financial health and opportunities to invest back in the business. The cash flow statement should provide a note indicating the underlying reason why there is so much additional cash; with this note, a reader can understand that perhaps this is a very negative finding since the organisation is at risk of even greater financial liability in the future.

Figure 3: *Example ABC pharmacy cash flow statement, June 2023.*

Cash flow statement
ABC Pharmacy (June 2023)

Beginning cash position		£ 40 000
Cash receipts		
Cash sales	£ 90 000	
A/R (0–30 days)	150 000	
A/R (31–60 days)	10 000	
A/R (>60 days)	100 000	
Total cash receipts		£ 390 000
Cash disbursements		
Costs of good bought	£ 150 000	
Payroll expenses	110 000	
Operating expenses and supplies	60 000	
Rent	25 000	
Interest on bank loan	35 000	
Total cash disbursements		£ 380 000
Net cash flow		£ (+) 10 000
ENDING CASH POSITION		**£ 50 000**

In this sample, it may be tempting to believe that all is fine because at the end of the month there was more money than at the beginning of the month, and the net cash flow is positive. However, there are some red flags of concern that a manager, leader or entrepreneur needs to examine further. A/R (or accounts receivable) represents cash flow from invoices sent by the pharmacy to others, for services delivered or goods already purchased but not yet paid in full. In essence, A/R is a promise of future income, not necessarily money in the bank. One issue of this in pharmacy is the large proportion of A/R that is dated at 60 days or longer: this means the pharmacy has expended cash already and needs to wait several months before getting reimbursed. Many insurance or government systems work this way: the pharmacy assumes upfront costs for delivering goods or services to patients, then periodically submits 'claims' for reimbursement that can take time to process and result in payment. A typical reason for a 'cash flow crunch' in any business is the length of time it takes others to pay for work already done – and this may be a problem for this pharmacy. On the cash disbursement side, there may also be some red flags. The 'operating expenses and supplies' category is somewhat vague, yet consumes a great deal of cash. Further exploration of what these expenses and supplies are would be warranted to ensure there is no wastage or inefficiency. Payroll expenses represent close to 30% of cash received; in a service intensive business this may be appropriate and necessary but further examination to ensure overstaffing is not an issue might be required. Given other expenses, rent appears somewhat high: perhaps the pharmacy is located in a particularly posh high street location, but this is not reflected in significant additional revenue, and suggests there may be a misalignment between location and revenue that is costing the business money. Furthermore, there is an extraordinary amount being paid on debt servicing through interest on a bank loan. An important way of reducing expenses is to manage debt more efficiently and there may be opportunities to enhance cash flow through more sensible debt payment options.

Financial statements and effective financial management

A core competency for any manager, leader or entrepreneur are the financial management skills necessary to ensure long-term viability and sustainability of the operation. Without solid financial foundations, no business – whether for-profit, government, or non-profit – can survive. While managers, leaders and entrepreneurs will rarely be involved in the actual production of financial statements, they need to be comfortable and confident in interpreting financial statements as a tool for supporting better management. Financial statements contain a treasure trove of information regarding the financial health of an organisation, and should directly influence managerial decisions around purchasing, hiring, inventory control, and other processes. Gaining confidence in interpreting financial statements, and using these statements on a regular basis to guide managerial decisions, is important and will contribute directly to ensuring businesses can survive and thrive.

Further reading

Carroll N. *Financial Management for Pharmacists: a decision making approach*. New York: Lippincott, Williams & Wilkins, 2016.

Gapenski L. *Understanding Healthcare Financial Management*, 5th edn. Chicago: Health Administration Press, 2007.

Handley M. Balance sheets: tools to inform changes in practice. *Perm J* 2005; 9(2): 61–62.

Singh H. *Essentials of Management for Healthcare Professionals*. New York: Productivity Press, 2018.

Wilson A. *Financial Management for Health System Pharmacists*. Maryland: American Society of Health System Pharmacists, 2009.

CHAPTER 7

Budgeting, variance reports and forecasting

Upon completion of this chapter you should be able to:

- understand the role of managers, leaders and entrepreneurs in budgeting, variance reporting and financial forecasting in pharmacy
- explain the four approaches to budgeting for business
- list the four sources of variance in a business
- outline the steps involved in the approach to forecasting.

In both professional and personal life, it is essential to closely monitor and proactively manage finances to ensure small problems do not become big ones, and that sufficient money is available to achieve objectives. While the ability to interpret financial statements is important for managers, leaders and entrepreneurs so they can understand the overall financial health of an organisation or business, they are rarely directly involved in the production or review of these statements. Instead, the main contributions they make to financial planning involves annual budgeting, monthly or quarterly variance reporting, development of annual projections, and production of business plans to support implementation of new programmes and services.

Budgeting

At its simplest, a budget is basically a spending plan for an operation or a business that anticipates needs for spending, investment in new equipment or capital, and costs that will be required to generate revenues. Typically, budgets are done on an annual basis, though some organisations may use longer time frames, and in some cases (for example, in the event of a threat of bankruptcy) shorter time frames may be used. In personal life and for some small businesses, the easiest, but often least accurate, model for budgeting is to simply adjust current spending upwards or downwards for the next year; in this traditional budgeting method, the current year's actual amounts spent on items serves as the starting reference point for the next year's budget. For simple, uncomplicated, and predictable situations, this model of upward/downward adjustments based on last year's actual activity has the advantage of being quick, easy, and intuitively obvious. However, for most businesses this simplistic approach can be problematic as it will unlikely be able to anticipate major changes in the environment, or support any attempts at growth or evolution of the organisation.

There are four commonly used approaches to budgeting for business (both in the public and private sector) which are detailed below.

Incremental budgeting

Similar to the traditional budgeting model described above, incremental budgeting uses the previous year's actual amounts spent as a foundation for projecting next year's budget. Incremental budgeting begins with a careful listing of all expenditures and expenses, including salaries for staff, benefits costs, equipment purchases, supplies consumed, inventory purchased, taxes paid, rent costs, etc. One of the first and important tasks for managers, leaders and entrepreneurs is to carefully and systematically review each and every budget line and category, to ensure it is appropriate, accurate, and sufficiently clear. In incremental budgeting, a line item such as 'purchases' is simply too vague. Instead, it should be broken down in more detail: for example, 'supplies', 'equipment', 'inventory', and 'furnishings'. The more detailed the budget line items, the easier it becomes for the manager to understand and control costs. Of course, there are reasonable limits to the level of detail that is necessary: 'supplies' could be broken down into 'compounding' and 'dispensing' supplies, but there is rarely a need to break it down further into '50 g ointment pots purchased', '100 g ointment pots purchased', '250 g ointment pots purchased', etc. For incremental budgeting, a reasonable and appropriate balance of detailed budget line items allows the budget holder to proceed to the next stage of the process.

For each line item on the budget, the budget holder needs to project and estimate what costs are expected to be for that specific line item next year. Unlike traditional budgeting – where an entire budget is revised upward or downwards based on projections of what will happen next year (for example, based on the rate of inflation) – in incremental budgeting, each individual line item is adjusted upwards or downwards based on factors that influence that specific line item. For example, during the COVID-19 pandemic, supply chain shortages became a significant cost driver due to worldwide production problems; however rental costs in many cases decreased at the same time as property owners feared losing businesses that rented from them due to economic uncertainty. Incremental budgeting would allow a manager to increase the budget line for 'computer purchases' by 15% to account for chip shortages, while decreasing the 'rent paid' line item by 10% due to negotiations with a landowner.

The advantage of incremental budgeting is that it is relatively simple and easy to understand; there are few complex calculations required since current, actual (ideally audited) budget numbers are used and adjusted individually to account for inflation or other changes. It saves time because it is relatively simple but produces more accurate budgets than a traditional across-the-board approach. Incremental budgets may, however, inadvertently perpetuate unnecessary spending as budget line items are repeated year-over-year and rarely removed completely. It can also cause staff members to feel they need to spend everything in that budget line item to prove that it was needed, whether in fact it was necessary or not. Incremental budgeting may not really push to determine the specific value or importance of a budget line item, but instead simply anticipate expected upward/downward price pressures. For example, the 'computer purchases' line item that may have increased by 15% due to chip shortages would not be scrutinised further to determine whether in fact a new computer actually needed to be purchased. Most companies use incremental budgeting because it is straightforward and in businesses that experience little growth or change each year, it may be most appropriate.

Activities-based budgeting

Particularly for service intensive businesses (including pharmacies where clinical/care services are a large or growing part of operations), activities-based budgeting can be a useful alternative approach to forecasting spending for the upcoming year. In particular, where companies do not have a great deal of historical information about spending (for example, a pharmacy where newly permitted clinical services are being introduced), this approach can be a more accurate method than incremental budgeting.

Activities-based budgeting is a top-down approach that begins with a strategic plan aimed at key deliverables and outcomes the business expects to achieve in the next year. For example, if a pharmacy has a strategic objective of generating £250 000 through a new public health screening initiative aimed at hypertension screening, they will first need to identify what human resource, supply, and equipment requirements exist to deliver the service. Services such as this are more person intensive, rather than product intensive. Because there is no historical data on this new service, an activities-based budget uses a top-down approach; the business needs to work backwards from the revenue goal to determine how many screenings will need to be performed, how many staff hours will be required to perform this number of screenings, how much equipment will be needed, and how much marketing/promotion will be necessary to drive this new business. Budget holders need to determine what the costs of all inputs required to generate £250 000 from this new service will be. As this service becomes more mature, stable, and predictable, incremental budgeting could be used in future budgeting cycles.

Activities-based budgeting is most important where little or no historical data exists regarding actual costs. It is forward looking, so provides managers with opportunities to consider operational efficiencies rather than perpetuating previous inefficiencies (a risk with incremental budgeting). It helps businesses stay outcome-focused and determine whether investments made are 'worth it' by the end of the budget year. It is, however, a lengthy, time-consuming process that can become cumbersome and sometimes overwhelming for managers. Experience as a budget holder is usually needed in order to be successful as there are numerous contingencies and 'what-ifs' that need to be considered: for example, if operating a hypertension screening program, how do other existing programs (like new medicine review) scale up or down according to workload? One of the most important issues with activity-based budgeting is the reality that it is not based on historical data but instead on projections which can be unreliable or simply educated guesswork: if not monitored and adjusted closely throughout the year, cash flow issues can quickly emerge.

Zero-based budgeting

Generally more popular in public sector organisations like hospitals and GP practices, zero-based budgeting requires budget holders to create budget categories and justify items and budget projections without reference to last year's numbers. Every item on the budget needs to be scrutinised and justified each year, with no guarantee that simply because it appeared on a previous budget it will perforce end up on this year's budget.

This method is excellent for eliminating unnecessary expenses, and for flagging costs that the organisation could consider operating without; it is usually seen as the best method for finding and reducing unneeded operating costs. It is however, very time-consuming and inherently political, because each year, each budget line must be debated and justified, and this can be stressful and threatening – particularly where budget line items refer to a person's salary. In zero-based budgeting, budget holders are held accountable for costs and waste, and this method can help them to aggressively streamline inflated budgets and help organisations bring costs under control while minimising the actual negative impact on day to day operations. Unfortunately, at its worst, this method also appears to reward short-term thinking rather than long-term strategic planning. For example, in zero-based budgeting, items such as continuing professional development for staff may not be as important or recognised as valuable and consequently might be cut, depriving the organisation of future potential growth opportunities. Further, budget holders may be tempted to use zero-based budgeting as a way of unfairly pressuring staff to do more with fewer resources.

Value-based budgeting

Increasingly viewed as the ideal compromise between incremental, activities-based, and zero-based budgeting, value-based budgeting is an approach that, while time-consuming, helps focus budget holders and workers attention on the fundamental purpose and objectives of the organisation. In this approach, budget holders and staff members work collaboratively to review budgets. For existing budget line items and for newly proposed ones, two questions need to be asked: a) why are we spending this amount of money?; b) what is the value this spending brings to our customers, employees, other stakeholders and (where relevant) shareholders? The underlying philosophy of value-based budgeting is to justify expenses, not simply based on activities performed or money saved, but instead on the value it creates. For example, investing in continuing professional development of staff members by sending them to training programs or providing tuition subsidies to allow them to complete post-graduate diplomas; this would be difficult to justify in zero-based budgeting because the cost/expense occurs in one year, but the benefit/revenue may not be realised until the following year. Value-based budgeting recognises this reality by acknowledging the importance of future value. Other common expenses – for example, social responsibility gestures such as a pharmacy sponsoring a local sports club or community event – can be justified as building goodwill and brand awareness (a strategic value) even though there may not be direct and immediate revenue generation. Where incremental budgeting does not scrutinise each item/category sufficiently, and zero-based budgeting may ruthlessly over-scrutinise each item, value-based budgeting tries to steer a middle path between the two. The collaborative nature of this approach can also be an effective tool for team-building and enhancing staff morale by including them in the process more explicitly.

The main advantage of this approach for budget holders is that it keeps front-of-mind the concept of the organisation's 'value proposition': why does the organisation exist in the first place and what value does it actually bring? It can be particularly useful in a competitive field like pharmacy as it helps individual pharmacies differentiate themselves from one another: for example, one pharmacy may have cost savings for clients as its core value, while another may focus on exemplary customer service, while a third may want to showcase innovative public health initiatives. Having defined a core value for the pharmacy, budget holders can then use the budgeting process more productively to reinforce this value more efficiently and effectively. Of course, 'value' can be subjective and trigger significant debate and disagreement, particularly if the organisation itself does not have a strong and clear strategic plan, vision, and mission for itself. Without these key elements, value-based budgeting can be quite painful and threatening to some individuals.

The method of budgeting used by budget holders needs to align with the business/organisation's strategy and operating philosophy. It is important to be mindful of which budgeting method they are using, rather than simply think managerial budgeting is the same as personal budgeting. The method used will generate significantly different kinds of budget projections and where time permits, it is sometimes a useful activity to create parallel budgets for the same year using different methods/philosophies to realise how important mindful decisions are to the budgeting process itself.

Budgetary management

Simple templates for budgets do exist and can, in some cases, be a useful starting point for budget holders, but care should be taken to never over-rely on such templates as they rarely can capture all financial elements of a specific organisation or operation. When preparing a budget, one can generally consider four broad categories for review: a) Revenues: income from sales, services provided, investments or other sources should all be recorded in a budget. In most cases, gross revenues are reported by category (e.g. income from sales of over-the-counter products or prescription products, or from delivery of clinical services like vaccines). Breaking down projected revenue by source is a useful way for managers to better understand and control where costs are to be allocated. b) Operational expenses: these expenses are the routine costs of running a business, including budget lines such as rent for space, computers/equipment, utility charges, etc. Similar to revenues, operational expenses should be broken down to an appropriate level of detail so managers can better understand and control unnecessary expenses or those costs that do not truly contribute to sustainability and profitability. How and where costs for inventory are allocated to a budget need to be determined – in most cases purchases of prescription and over-the-counter drugs and dispensing supplies would be allocated to operational expenses, even though they 'flow-through' the budget and are directly linked to revenue (income when they are sold). c) Capital expenses: budget holders may often have budgetary responsibilities for investments in the business related to renovation or construction of new space to deliver new services. In many cases, routine maintenance of the physical space within which the business functions will need ongoing attention to prevent small maintenance issues from becoming big operational problems, and sufficient capital expense budget should be allocated each year to ensure ongoing maintenance of space, equipment, furnishings, etc. is possible. d) Personnel expenses: within a care and service intensive business such as pharmacy, employee-related expenses associated with salary, benefits (including health care and pension) as well as investments in continuing professional development and training, are included in annual budget plans.

Learning to budget as a manager, leader or entrepreneur can be a stressful and time-consuming process, and requires significant attention to detail and a willingness to ask questions, dig deeply for answers, and rely upon data (rather than conjecture) in formulating answers. Lazy budgeting practices may save time early on but often end up in poor financial control. Making assumptions based on previous years' performances without truly considering evolving circumstances can also result in costly mistakes. Openness to mid-year budgetary corrections as situations change is essential, as is the need to be constantly monitoring budget projections with respect to actual performance based on variance reporting.

Variance reporting

One of the most important financial management tools available is variance reporting. Variance reports are documents that compare budgeted/planned financial outcomes with actual performance. It is a way of comparing what was expected to happen with what actually happened as a way of analysing differences between budgets (which are best estimates of the future, or projections) and reality. Since budgeting is usually done on a yearly basis, monitoring budgets monthly (or at least quarterly) through variance reporting is essential to actually understanding how the business is performing.

Variance reporting is usually based on the annual budget, so that for each budget category and each specific line item on the budget, a 'budgeted' amount can be compared with an 'actual' amount. This applies to both revenue and expenses. For example, a pharmacy may have budgeted for £250 000 annually in revenue from a new hypertension screening program, translating into £62 500 each quarter (three-month period) since no seasonal variation in hypertension screening was anticipated. A quarterly variance report may note that in the period of April 01 – June 30, the pharmacy earned £30 000 from this service, a variance of £32 500. If that performance were to persist for the remaining three quarters, the total revenue for this budget line item would only be £120 000 for the year, a shortfall of £130 000 from the annual budget projection. Knowing early in the financial year that this service is not as financially successful as first imagined can help the budget holder make important decisions: perhaps more work/time/money needs to be invested in marketing this service to try to 'catch up' and meet the revenue projections by the end of the budget year. Alternatively, perhaps the target was too ambitious and revenue projections need to be scaled back accordingly – meaning associated expenses for staffing and equipment for this new service might also need to be cut back proportionately. While these are not easy decisions for budget holders to make, having data to support difficult decision making is essential. The value of regular variance reporting is that it provides sufficient time to analyse a situation and adjust budget and performance expectations accordingly, before the end of the budget year where significant losses might be a major problem.

Variance reports are usually easiest to use if they are formatted in the same way as the budget itself, so that the same category names and same individual budget line items are compared as 'budgeted' versus 'actual'. In reality, however, this can be difficult, expensive, and time-consuming to produce every three months, so in many cases, budget holders receive variance reports that only compare budget categories (such as 'employee expenses' or 'operational expenses') rather than individual line items within these categories. This introduces a unique challenge for managers, leaders and entrepreneurs to try to interpret what the problem actually is and how best to proceed. For example, if a variance report only compares budgeted to actual 'revenue' without specifying where that revenue came from (e.g. dispensing medications versus vaccination services) it might be difficult to understand what the problem is and how best to address it. Budget holders may find themselves in the difficult situation of trying to forcefully advocate with accounting departments or others to provide more detail on monthly or quarterly variance reports to allow them to have a better insight into financial performance. In other cases, where accounting departments are unable to produce sufficiently detailed variance reports, individual budget holders may find it necessary to actually produce 'shadow logs' or keep their own approximate records of performance in specific areas to help them to understand what is going on. Though common, the use of shadow logs is a controversial practice since managers, leaders and entrepreneurs have neither the time nor expertise of accounting departments to accurately track revenues and expenditures and compare back to budget projections. Still, the real world limitations of accounting processes mean that, in some cases, limited and approximate data is better than no data and such techniques provide at least some useful insight into financial performance.

There are four main forms/sources of variance in a business such as pharmacy:

1. Sales/revenue variance or the difference between planned/expected sales of goods and services and what actually happened. Sales price variance occurs when sales are made at a higher or lower price than expected. For example, the business may have purchased too much inventory of cough and cold products and as the winter season ends, they simply want to get rid of it quickly so discounts are offered to consumers. In contrast, sales volume variances reflect differences between the expected amount of sales (or services delivered) and planned/budgeted amount. For example, the pharmacy may have planned on administering 750 flu vaccines each month but because of concerns over pandemic conditions, ended up administering 1500 in a single month. Sales/revenue variance helps budget holders understand how projected/expected financial performance differs from actual and can guide decisions regarding what needs to be changed to get back on track financially; if twice the number of flu vaccines were administered than were budgeted for, then more staff will need to be brought on board...and the additional revenue from these extra vaccines should pay for and offset the increased costs of more staff.

2. Direct material variance describes the difference between expected costs/quantity of inventory materials compared to actual costs and quantity. Purchase price variance describes the difference between expected and actual costs of supplies and materials (including medications, vials, labels, etc.) used. Material yield variance reflects the difference between the quantity of materials expected to be used for the provision of services and the actual quantity used. For example, the manager may have budgeted a specific amount of personal protective equipment and supplies (e.g. gloves, disposable masks, etc.) to dispense the expected number of vaccines in the pharmacy, but a quarterly variance report indicates less than half of this amount has actually been used despite being on track to meet vaccination targets. This might indicate staff are taking shortcuts (e.g. not changing gloves each time another person is vaccinated), and this could require additional training or monitoring of staff.

3. Labour variances describe differences between budgeted and actual costs for staffing, including wages and benefits. Labour variances reflect the efficiency of the workforce and are an important indicator of workload related issues when compared to sales, revenue, or other output focused measurements. For example, if the number of vaccines administered is twice the budgeted amount, yet there is no labour cost variance, this could indicate staff are over-worked, at risk of burnout, and potentially at risk for errors. Managers should not look at this situation as a source of price ('great – see how efficient my staff can be?') but instead an early warning indicator of potential risk and harm. Matching labour variances with output indicators is important; short-term profitability should not be seen as an advantage if it leads to long-term problems. Another important kind of labour cost variance relates to the seniority of staff – in general, long-standing employees get paid more than junior employees, but may not necessarily produce a greater output despite being paid more. Careful monitoring of labour cost variances can help managers better understand when workforce renewal is important to ensure ongoing sustainability of the business.

4. Overhead variances reflect a large category of fixed, variable, direct, and indirect costs associated with running the business and providing goods and services that are purchased. Overhead variances include costs such as utilities (electricity, heating, telecommunications) as well as other expenses associated with keeping a business operational. In some climates, overhead variances are expected – seasonal costs for heating and air conditioning may make utility charges uneven across the year. Smoothing overhead variances through the use of equalised billing options offered by utility provider companies, can help better manage cash flow over a year long time frame and make it more predictable.

Some organisations require formal explanations of significant variances, using statistical techniques to define thresholds: for example, a budget-to-actual variance of more than 10% might require documentation. In some cases, organisations may allow budget holders some flexibility in reallocating budget lines within a category: for example, under the employee expenses category, it may be possible to shuffle some percentage of budget lines from full-time employees to locum/contract employees provided the total amount of employee expenses does not change, even if the budgeted amount for full-time employees drops and the amount for locum/contract increases by the same amount. It is rarely permissible to reallocate across different budget categories: for example, if operational expenses are lower than expected because rent prices have dropped, this 'saving' should not be reallocated to employee expenses and more people hired. Reallocation across budget categories creates confusion and reduces transparency of the budgeting process and so is rarely useful. Reallocation within budget categories based on variance reporting can be productive as it helps budget holders understand and have options for responding to changing business circumstances.

The objective of variance reporting is not to put managers, leaders or entrepreneurs on the spot to test how prescient and accurate their budget projections were. Instead, variance reporting simply provides data to allow them to examine the actual performance of the business in a way that allows for mid-stream course corrections, to avoid having more costly and potentially catastrophic problems emerge at the end of the budget cycle.

Projections

Budgeting and business planning frequently require budget holders to make 'projections' regarding financial performance and outputs/productivity. This can be a significant challenge and in some cases managers, leaders and entrepreneurs feel they are just pulling numbers out of thin air with no solid foundation to defend them. In budgeting and planning there is an expression called 'GIGO' – garbage in, garbage out – meaning that budgets, forecasts and plans are only as good as the data used to base projections upon.

When asked to 'project' sales revenue and volumes for the next budget year, or to 'predict' employee costs and staffing levels, managers need to have a system or process in place to ensure GIGO does not adversely impact on budget and planning. Financial forecasting refers to the process of developing justifiable and defensible projections regarding future outcomes and financial plans. Forecasting is both an art and a quantitative science and findings ways of blending these effectively will govern its accuracy, usability, and success.

At the core, forecasting requires analysis of past financial and performance patterns, current/actual realities, and integration of reasonably expected contextual and environmental changes on future expectations. A systematic stepwise approach to projections and forecasting should include the following:

- *Define assumptions:* The first and arguably most important step is to define the fundamental issues that will likely impact any projections. This requires an understanding of the overall economic, social, and political environment within which the business operates: for example, it is relatively clear in most jurisdictions that downward financial pressure on dispensing fees will continue, while increasing expectations of revenue generation through clinical services provisions will be the norm. The specifics of these may change during a year, but the general concept that more revenue will be generated from clinical services than dispensing in the years ahead is a useful and reasonable starting assumption. In defining assumptions, several key questions need to be considered including: a) What is the time horizon for the forecast? Typically, a budget cycle runs over a 12 month period, but changes in assumptions may evolve over a multi-year period, and this might need to be reconciled as part of the planning process. b) What is the objective of forecasting? In most cases it will be to provide a financial foundation for maintaining a business over the course of a year, but in some cases, the objective may be related to a major growth initiative (e.g. building a new hospital, or developing a new primary care delivery system). 'Maintenance' versus 'growth' forecasts have different time horizons and assumptions that need to be considered. c) What are the political, legal, and societal issues that will influence the forecast? This is amongst the most difficult, but important questions to answer as these issues are usually completely beyond the control of managers. For example, in February 2020, no one could have projected the world-changing impact of the COVID-19 pandemic and its financial impact on pharmacies large and small. It may be easier to account for anticipated changes related to the scope of practice evolution of pharmacists and regulated technicians, introduction of new medicines or technologies such as home diagnostic tools, as well as greater integration of pharmacy into primary care. Translating this understanding into concrete financial projections with respect to staffing, equipment/supplies, and other budget line items is challenging but central to forecasting. d) Ensure current revenue and expense categories in the budget are appropriate and relevant to future needs. Broad budget categories such as 'employee expenses' and 'revenue from clinical services' are likely to always be part of a pharmacy's budget and planning processes. However, in forecasting, new categories may become more commonplace – for example web presence. As the COVID-19 pandemic has demonstrated, virtual care has become more commonplace, and the infrastructure to support virtual care delivery may be quite different than a bricks-and-mortar pharmacy. Anticipating evolving needs and identifying both broader category changes/evolution that may be required, as well as specific line items (e.g. 'development of pharmacy-specific android and iPhone compatible app') will be necessary as part of forecasting.
- *Gather relevant data:* Forecasting should not be a fantasy sports league game, but a data-driven process that requires research. Use of statistical data (for example, the number of virtual consultations performed annually) can guide decisions regarding the future trajectory of an organisation. Forecasting models are never perfect but are strengthened significantly if there is a foundation of data to support decisions.

- *Define contingencies:* The essence of forecasting is to try to control the uncontrollable – which of course is impossible. One useful approach can be to create multiple scenarios – each with their own budget – to understand the ramifications of different choices/decisions. For example, a pharmacy may want to create a forecast in which 50% of new medicines consultations are delivered virtually, while another scenario involves 0% delivered virtually. Comparing revenues, costs, expenditures, etc. with these different contingencies provides decision makers with a band of financial information, rather than a specific single budget figure, and this can enhance flexibility in responding to changes during the budget cycle.
- *Use statistical methods to project previous actuals into the future, accounting for anticipated contingencies:* In some cases, it may be possible to use extrapolation or regression methods to help support forecasting. These statistical-analytical tools often assume that past performance predicts future outcomes; while this is usually considered an erroneous assumption, it can provide a 'status quo' contingency option, but also the opportunity to apply contingencies to historical data and determine how this might influence outcomes. Budget holders may be hesitant to even think about using daunting methods like 'linear regression' to project future budget needs; importantly, commercially available software (such as Excel) provides fairly robust functionality to apply statistical-analytical tools and generate various different outcome scenarios based on changing assumptions.

Today, most budget holders must generate multiple budgets based on different forecasts and assumptions, resulting in a band or range of outcomes to select from. Ultimately, a budget should only have one single discrete amount of money allocated to each line item; however, using these methods to generate a range of options, then selecting the option that best approximates future projections based on stated assumptions can provide the most accurate pathway forward for forecasting.

In generating forecasts, the credibility of the forecaster is essential. An important way of establishing credibility is to be clear and transparent with respect to justification and reasons for assumptions made, and clarity in terms of how assumptions influenced final calculations. For experienced budget holders, it is also important to monitor and honestly report on previous accuracy with forecasts, and to use this data to self-reflect and self-calibrate for future forecasting needs. While forecasting is an imperfect science at best, it is an essential competency for managers, leaders and entrepreneurs. The fact that it will be imperfect does not reduce the need to undertake forecasting in a systematic way, learning from previous mistakes and inaccurate predictions, and being transparent and clear in communication to staff and other stakeholders.

Summary

Budgeting, variance reporting, and forecasting are daunting but essential business tasks. A systematic approach to each of these helps to build confidence and is more likely to lead to accuracy rather than random guesswork. While all budget holders – as human beings – have some experience in these tasks in their personal lives, it is important to recognise that business planning is different to personal financial planning. While more systematic, data-driven processes may be needed, businesses will usually have resources and support available to access, and these should be used and fully integrated in the work of managers, leaders and entrepreneurs.

Further reading

Carroll NV. *Financial Management for Pharmacists: a decision making approach*. New York: Lippincott Williams & Wilkins, 2016.

Gapenski LC. *Understanding Healthcare Financial Management*, 5th edn. Chicago: Health Administration Press, 2007.

Handley M. Balance sheets: tools to inform changes in practice. *Perm J* 2005; 9(2): 61–62.

Singh H. *Essentials of Management for Healthcare Professionals*. New York: Productivity Press, 2018.

Wilson AL. *Financial Management for Health System Pharmacists*. Maryland: American Society of Health System Pharmacists, 2009.

CHAPTER 8

Justice, equity, diversity and inclusivity

Upon completion of this chapter you should be able to:

- understand what is meant by the term JEDI
- list the JEDI principles
- understand the importance of JEDI in organisations
- explain the role of managers, leaders and entrepreneurs in implementing JEDI principles.

In the 'Star Wars' movie franchise, the Jedi are the main heroes, working alongside both the Old Galactic Republic and later supporting the Rebel Alliance. They are seen as honourable, academic, meritocratic and guardians of order and truth, wielding a supernatural power known as The Force to achieve positive, virtuous outcomes. In this way, the Jedi have considerable and recognised moral power.

In most organisations today, there is considerable discussion about JEDI – justice, equity, diversity and inclusivity – as not simply legal requirements for businesses but as moral obligations to communities, workers, and society as a whole.[1] For many managers, leaders and entrepreneurs, the concept of JEDI may be completely reasonable and something that can be embraced. However, the way in which JEDI principles are actually enacted and 'lived' in an organisation can cause considerable debate and dissent, and can sometimes be a fractious and difficult thing to actually manage.[2]

What are the JEDI principles?

Justice, equity, diversity, and inclusivity are terms that may sound similar but they do connote different important concepts that help shape organisational policies, practices and governance. As such, it is important for managers, leaders and entrepreneurs to understand and be able to effectively communicate what these principles are, how they are similar yet distinct, and why they are important to different stakeholders.

Justice is at the core of why organisations are interested in these principles.[3] Justice speaks to fairness, impartiality, objectivity, and transparency of processes, especially those related to important decisions such as hiring, promotions, and pay increases.

- *Fairness:* One of the most important attributes of a modern society is fairness, both in processes and in results. The term 'fair' can be difficult to precisely define but in most cases individuals can recognise and acknowledge (sometimes grudgingly) when things are fair and when they are not. Attributes of fairness include having a clear and defensible reason for decisions, relying upon evidence rather than emotion, and ensuring arms length processes for making decisions that prevent favouritism or nepotism.

- *Impartiality:* Subjectivity, bias, and pre-judgement are realities of human nature and decision making, and can perpetuate injustice and unfairness. A key element of justice is processes to ensure impartial, objective decision making that is free from unconscious (or conscious) bias. Sources of bias could include conflict of interest, stereotyping, or lack of respect for individual differences. Impartiality is usually advanced through training programs that help individuals surface, identify, and articulate their unconscious biases, group deliberation/decision making processes that include different perspectives and experiences, and clear penalties or sanctions if conflict of interest or bias, influences behaviours.

- *Objectivity:* In JEDI, objectivity is a goal that focuses on the consistency of decision making, regardless of the person actually making the decision – or the person who is the subject of the decision. Reliability and validity of tools used to support decision making can enhance objectivity (for example, the use of standardised interview questions for applicants). Objectivity frequently implies some form of measurement or quantification of data to allow for demonstration that it has been achieved and sustained.

- *Transparency:* One of the most important JEDI principles – and one that is most often under the control of managers, leaders and entrepreneurs – is transparency, or clarity and openness in communication with all stakeholders. From a management perspective, transparency means that all job vacancies are posted and that a formal interviewing and hiring process is undertaken, rather than having some people simply appointed to a new role. Transparency also means ensuring clear and plain language is used in all communication to support full understanding and to not make English language fluency a barrier for some individuals. Transparency also benefits from constant commitment: ongoing, regular, frequent communication is preferred over a single, long, dense message, as a way to ensure individuals are not surprised by a new policy or a recent decision.

These four JEDI principles help us to better understand each of the four components of JEDI itself:[4]

- *Justice:* The overarching aim of programs, initiatives and philosophies of JEDI is to recalibrate and address historical inequalities and restore fairness and balance in organisational life. The notion of 'justice' embraces the concept of moral rightness and appeals to each individual's sense of fair play. It also acknowledges that, even in the recent past, societal bias and unfairness has resulted in the unjust treatment of some individuals through no fault of their own, and in many cases simply because of demographic or other characteristics that are intrinsic.

- *Equity:* The terms 'equity' and 'equality' are sometimes (and mistakenly) used interchangeably, reflecting broader misunderstandings of important issues faced by individuals and groups that have been historically disadvantaged. In some cases, treating everyone equally (the same, or 'equality') actually simply reinforces or maintains inequity or unfairness. This is primarily due to the fact that some individuals have more challenging barriers to overcome when accessing resources or opportunities than those from historically advantaged or privileged groups.

For example, an individual who speaks English as a first language will simply find it easier to communicate in English than someone who has learned English as an adult. Having to constantly and consciously translate words and concepts is cognitively exhausting and gives the appearance of work to others. Non-English speakers may hesitate slightly in responding to questions as they try to find the right word to explain a concept; such hesitation may be misinterpreted as evasiveness or even a lack of intelligence. Equity recognises that the native and non-native English speaker start from different positions of strength but because of a specific intrinsic characteristic, end up in different places. Fairness (or equity) demands that we understand these different starting places and do not subconsciously, unconsciously, or consciously bias against the non-English speaker in our decisions. The non-native English speaker may be just as intelligent, just as motivated, and just as competent as the native English speaker but it simply takes them a little longer to formulate a sentence due to their different starting point. Equity involves specific techniques designed to help equalise individual's chances for success. For example, in a job interview, it is becoming increasingly common for all candidates to be provided the interview questions in advance of the actual interview. This way, non-native English speakers are given a bit more time to reflect and formulate sentences as responses rather than have to translate on-the-spot. Native English speakers are also given the questions in advance so they are not disadvantaged in any way. This form of equity serves to level the playing field so the real thing being tested in the interview is an individual's thinking and answers – not their ability to speak glibly on the spot.

- *Diversity:* In many organisations today, diversity initiatives have focused on external demographic characteristics (such as ethnicity or race). Terms such as BIPOC (in North America, signalling Black, Indigenous, or People of Colour) or BAME (in the United Kingdom, signalling Black, Asian, or Minority Ethnic) have become ways of sorting individuals. The spirit of diversity as a JEDI concept recognises there are important ways that individuals differ from each other, and that organisations and workplaces are strengthened when they are more representative of the populations they serve. A homogenous workforce composed of individuals with substantially similar backgrounds is less likely to be creative, adapt to environmental change, and be responsive to the diverse clients they serve. Terms like BIPOC and BAME may have some use in alerting organisations to examine diversity practices, but should not be considered a complete solution. Diversity is often considered along four different dimensions: internal, external, functional, and philosophical. Internal diversity is described as characteristics over which individuals have little or no choice, including race, ethnicity, or age. In some cases, internal diversity may be readily visible (e.g. race) while in other cases it may be hidden (e.g. sexual orientation or gender identity). External diversity describes characteristics based on more conscious decisions and choices individuals make, for example religious faith/beliefs, or marital status. Perhaps controversially, external diversity is also usually the place where socio-economic factors (including level of education attained) are also included. Functional diversity speaks to individual skills, talents, interests, and emotional intelligences – for example, the ability to sing well or rapidly do mental arithmetic may not be evenly spread through the population but reflect innate individual talents. Finally, philosophical diversity addresses individual's worldviews and personal understanding of the ways in which societies function. This includes political beliefs or social beliefs (e.g. on topics such as abortion or same-sex marriage). The diversity of 'diversities' is an important consideration in JEDI and highlights the ways in which intersections of identities are increasingly important in understanding the unique qualities of each member of a workforce.

- *Inclusivity:* Perhaps paradoxically, many organisations may appear to be diverse but are actually not very inclusive. It is sometimes said that diversity is like an invitation to a party, while inclusion is being asked to dance once you've arrived. Inclusivity speaks to the feeling of being seen, acknowledged, and actually valued rather than simply being a bystander watching everyone else having fun but you. Simply having a diverse workforce in no way assures inclusivity. Instead, inclusivity requires conscious management decisions and policies. For example, this could include building time for prayers and allocating meditation/prayer room spaces in a business, or implementing 'family friendly' parental leave programs to support young parents. It also means contributing to and actively supporting local LGBTQ2S+ activities so 'family' is not defined in an inequitably narrow way. Managerial practices supportive of inclusivity breed employee loyalty and engagement, and have been described as one of the best recruitment and retention strategies an organisation can invest in. Beyond that, employees who feel included will generally be more creative and productive and this can support organisational strategic priorities.

Why is there interest in JEDI?

The roots of JEDI in organisations is connected to evolving societal awareness of the negative impact of bias on individuals, communities, and society.[5] Bias is generally described as an inclination, feeling, or behaviour rooted in stereotype or prejudice that results in unfair comparison between members of one group over another.[6] The corrosive nature of bias is the story of human history: at different times and in different ways, different groups have been 'othered'. Othering is a psychological process by which individuals devalue, diminish, and dehumanise individuals from groups outside their own.[7] The foundation of othering is frequently (but not exclusively) based on demographics or characteristics rather than on individual behaviours. One of the most enduring and widespread forms of othering relates to sex and gender: many societies and cultures (and individuals) hold beliefs that women are 'lesser-than' men and consequently should not be in positions of authority, power, or responsibility. In part, this has been justified because of physical characteristics (i.e. women are generally smaller and may not be as fast or strong as men) which of course denies the reality that other characteristics (intellect, judgement, values) are frequently far more impactful than the ability to merely lift heavy objects. Othering can also involve, for example, the notion that the primary destiny of women should be child-bearing and child-rearing and that women who choose not to have children have somehow failed. These beliefs derive from false and corrosive thinking related to demographics and characteristics but have lead to centuries of oppression, abuse, degradation, and – from a human resource perspective – underutilisation of women around the world. Similar forms of othering are rooted in racial bias/stereotype, attitudes and beliefs regarding sexual orientation/identity, and outrageous views regarding the 'value' of individuals with different forms of psychological or physical handicaps.[8]

Othering is not inconsequential and has produced some of the most horrific outcomes in human history. The othering of Africans produced slavery; the othering of Jewish people produced the

Holocaust, and the othering of gays and lesbians has led to stigma and suicide. While some may justify their othering in religious terms, or as freedom of speech or expression, the reality of course is that othering is a way for a dominant group to keep and consolidate its own power by creating a false enemy. While it is tempting to believe that the 21st century has expunged othering from our thinking and behaviours – of course, it has not.

The overarching premise of human resource initiatives related to JEDI start from the historical understanding of unfairness experienced through othering, and the reality that individuals come to organisations from very different starting places.[9] JEDI is an attempt to establish fairness in organisational processes and decisions that account for the historical experiences of discrimination, abuse, and dehumanisation that many continue to experience today.[10] It recognises that certain individuals have 'privileges' that were unearned and simply due to accidents of birth that endowed them with certain racial, sexual, religious, socio-economic, and ability-based powers.[11]

The backlash against JEDI

The well-reasoned and well-intentioned foundations of JEDI have recently been weaponised by those who reject the fundamental problem of 'othering' and instead claim that 'fairness' means everyone should be treated exactly the same regardless of their historical experiences and background.[12] Dismissing JEDI in pejorative terms such as 'wokeness' or 'political correctness', they claim that JEDI attempts to address historical unfairness against some groups by perpetrating new unfairness against other groups.[13] Lamentations regarding the inability of 'straight white men' to get jobs because they aren't black Jewish lesbians in wheelchairs attempts to caricature JEDI as a system-wide plot to emasculate and control one group at the expense of another.[13] This has given rise to some of the most problematic developments in the world today in terms of social cohesion, belief in governments and institutions, and faith in the legal system and processes. It has produced bitter political polarisation and made government and organisational governance extremely challenging.[14] In some cases, it has led to physical assaults, violence, and mass shootings.

At the core of the backlash against JEDI may be the perception by some that they are being unfairly disadvantaged in the name of redressing historical wrongs that they personally did not commit.[13] For example, some may claim, 'I don't have anything against gay people – some of my best friends and relatives are gay – but why do they always have to be in everyone's face about it, flying flags, talking about pride, kissing in the streets! We need a straight pride parade!'. This disingenuous statement clouds the reality that for millennia (and into the current century) many (if not most) gays and lesbians have been explicitly targeted by their families, their communities, their politicians, their religious institutions – and their workplaces – simply because of who they love and who they are. The choice has been a dire one – supress, deny, hide and reject who you are at your core in order to 'fit in' and not make waves. In the process, self-loathing, depression, helplessness, and in some cases, suicide will follow. Today's move from acceptance and towards embracing and actively affirming sexual diversity amongst most major organisations and businesses in the world, recognises this historical experience. It cannot change the past but it can signal hope for the future where individuals can be free to be who they truly are and truly love. Concerns by some that gays and lesbians are getting 'special treatment' at their expense are unfounded: no one is persecuting and diminishing 'straight pride' by proclaiming 'gay pride'.

For managers, leaders and entrepreneurs, this is an incredibly challenging situation to manage effectively and humanely. JEDI tends to provoke extraordinarily and disproportionately strong emotional responses on both sides. Attempts to mediate or discuss it rationally can frequently lead to amplified polarisation and recriminations. Strong emotional labels such as 'bigot' or 'racist' may be used which further entrench divisions, while questioning JEDI in any way can be seen as a return to othering ways which leads to fear for safety and progress won to date.

The business case for JEDI

For some managers, leaders and entrepreneurs, philosophical discussions around the need for JEDI can be uncomfortable or even irritating. Whatever one's own opinions or feelings may be, the vast majority of organisations today have recognised the economic benefit and value of embracing JEDI in strategic planning.[15,16] The 'business case' for JEDI highlights the ways in which JEDI can be positive in different ways for organisations, including:

- *Attracting the best and broadest talent base:* It is clear that talent, skills, and knowledge relevant to organisational success is broadly distributed across the population.[15] Historically disadvantaged groups – including women, BIPOC/BAME individuals, LGBTQ2S+, and disabled people – have much to contribute to organisations. JEDI practices that support inclusivity of these groups in the workforce mean greater opportunities to bring forth these talented individuals to contribute to a business's bottom line profitability.[16] Large corporations such as Apple, Disney, and HSBC have all recognised that full-throated support of JEDI objectives and embedding these within organisational practices leads to better hiring.
- *Retaining the best talent:* Individuals who feel excluded from their workplace culture will rapidly seek other employment options to manage this discomfort.[15] Inclusivity is an important tool for retaining skilled workers – satisfied employees are less inclined to change jobs or leave organisations. Given the time, expense, and complexity of recruitment and hiring, business tactics that aim to retain a workforce and ensure they are happy, contribute directly to the profitability of an organisation.[16]
- *Productivity growth:* Satisfied employees are generally more creative and productive than unsatisfied employees, and are more willing to go the extra mile and help build on an organisation's strength.[15] Particularly in fields where interpersonal skills, communicative competency, and problem-solving are necessary, inclusivity can be essential to unleashing potential and productivity.[15,16]
- *Positive organisational culture:* Workplaces that are inclusive typically demonstrate more positive cultures focused on teamwork, honesty, and open communication and these can help support organisational success.[16] Lack of diversity in a workforce has been shown to actually reduce creativity in problem-solving and foster group-thinking that can be damaging and counterproductive for success.[15,16] For example, where women are more represented and included in organisational decision making, there is a less likelihood of fraud or criminal behaviour occurring than when only men are charged with decision making.[16]
- *Corporate leadership in society:* As discourse around JEDI has coarsened in society, and

politicians have weaponised inclusivity for political gain, corporations have increasingly taken the lead role in advocating for justice, equity, diversity, and inclusivity within society. Corporate leadership in JEDI is increasingly seen as an essential counterweight to populist rhetoric that is threatening societal civility and order.

JEDI in organisational life

The complexity of this issue is often beyond the capacity of any individual, even a CEO, to manage through persuasion, cajoling, or even punishment. As a result, the approach taken by most organisations, governments, and businesses is to recognise that individuals cannot be relied upon to adhere to uphold JEDI principles simply out of goodwill and altruism, or off the side of a desk while doing other jobs.[17]

In many parts of human life, there is a recognition that the worst instincts and behaviours of human beings need to be contained in order to promote peace, stability, security and fairness – otherwise, the law of the jungle and survival of the fittest will emerge.[17] In many parts of the world, there has been a generations long effort to raise awareness and change minds and hearts regarding othering, privilege and our understanding of fairness. It starts in primary school and carries through social activities, organised sports teams, and religious organisations. It has been a focus of the media and popular culture. The idea that education, media, social pressure, and other persuasion techniques of this sort would change the minds and hearts of the population and raise awareness about the dangers of othering, would ultimately lead to broad acceptance of JEDI principles without question or dissent.

Sadly, today, we know this is not the case, and as a result, a more muscular, directive and legalistic approach has come to dominate JEDI implementation in many organisations: attempts to change minds have had mixed success and so now, we simply legislate appropriate and acceptable behaviour in this area.[17]

For managers, leaders and entrepreneurs, this approach can sometimes be challenging. People of good intention may broadly agree with philosophical aims of JEDI but may feel personally penalised if (for example) they are seen as being 'an insufficiently diverse candidate' to warrant promotion or hiring. Well-intentioned attempts to embrace inclusivity by – for example – having organisations participate in local gay pride parades may be offensive to those with sincerely held religious beliefs – and these people also contribute to the workplace. JEDI principles may make some individuals feel they cannot speak freely or truly share their thoughts on controversial issues for fear of being labelled intolerant or biased, and in turn may start to complain about 'wokeness' or 'political correctness' dominating business decisions.

One of the most difficult challenges can be balancing competing perspectives regarding JEDI while maintaining a civil and productive team or organisational culture.[18] This challenge reflects broader social trends that have evolved in the last decade. On the one hand, with the rise of social media and populist political rhetoric, there is greater societal indifference towards reprehensible racist, sexist, homophobic, transphobic, and Islamophobic speech and behaviour than ever before and this actually threatens the fabric of civil society itself. On the other hand, public acceptance of same-sex marriage, inclusion of disabled people, and ethno-cultural diversity has never been greater: consider the growing number of women and BIPOC/BAME individuals at the most senior levels of government and the growing number of gay and lesbian political and business leaders.

In most cases, managers, leaders and entrepreneurs themselves will only have limited scope for developing, framing, or defining JEDI policies and practices within their organisation, but will have significant responsibilities for actually implementing, defending, and building support for them. This balancing act requires them to be intentional, authentic, and self-reflective. Those who only grudgingly 'follow-the-rules' but don't actually buy into JEDI objectives, risk creating a team or organisational culture that is subversive and polarising. A manager or leader who truly does not agree with or accept the JEDI principles they have been tasked to implement or defend will be unsuccessful. Authenticity is integral to success and inauthentic managers, leaders or entrepreneurs are immediately transparent to those they manage.

If you have responsibilities around JEDI implementation (including defending it to skeptical colleagues), but have personal reservations (for whatever reason) about the task, it is essential to engage in authentic self-reflection and transparent communication with your own managers/supervisors and colleagues. Unsuccessful JEDI implementation is most frequently linked to ambivalent or negative opinions about JEDI among those responsible for putting it into operation and defending it. Techniques to support those who have reservations about JEDI objectives could include appointing inclined team members who are non-managers/leaders as JEDI champions, providing for more gradual/incremental implementation, or transferring responsibilities to supervisors above the manager/leader. In some cases, organisations may be tempted to opt for a 'nuclear solution': remove the disinclined manager/leader from their role entirely as a way of demonstrating commitment to JEDI. Such a draconian solution may be appropriate but it will also come at a significant organisational and cultural cost and should be considered very carefully and strategically. In most cases, transparent communication and dialogue may result in ways of addressing this situation without escalating to these levels.

JEDI in pharmacy

As health service and care providers, pharmacists must be conscious of the impact of systemic bias and discriminatory behaviours on the health and well-being of their patients, their colleagues, and their staff members. Allyship refers to the actions, practices, and behaviours used by managers to demonstrate their support for those who have been historically disadvantaged through systemic bias. While allyship involves beliefs and feelings, it is most focused on actual behaviours: kind words and sympathetic gestures towards hurt feelings can provide some support and reassurance but ultimately those who have the power to change organisations and systems – people like managers – need to consider ways of changing these thoughts into actions. Small but meaningful practices (such as placing a pride-progress flag in a prominent location during Pride month, or posting signs signifying zero-tolerance for abuse or discrimination) are an important first step for pharmacy managers. Modelling positive allyship behaviours with staff to help create a workplace culture that moves beyond grudging tolerance or reluctant acceptance of diversity and towards active affirmation by (for example) recognising and celebrating different religious holidays, is important. Careful monitoring of recruitment, hiring, and promotion practices within the organisation is necessary to ensure unconscious bias is not influencing staffing decisions in ways that misalign employees with the populations they serve.

Managers also have opportunities to provide staff training and development to support more equitable and inclusive patient care practices. For example, consider accessibility issues in many high street community pharmacies and the ways in which narrow doors and aisles, steps, and crowded floorplans make it difficult for those requiring mobility aids to even physically enter the pharmacy. Further, consider the ways in which those with limited sight or hearing may not feel welcomed due to distracting ambient noise or insufficient lighting. In many cases, accessibility issues such as these will require expert assessment and recommendations for change, not simply well-intentioned but amateur interventions from pharmacy managers. Committing time and resources to actually ensure workplaces that serve the public are in fact accessible to all members of the public is a strong demonstration of allyship.

For some pharmacy managers, the overwhelming weight of historical discrimination and the magnitude of changes required in order to begin to address these issues can lead to a form of paralysis and a feeling of helplessness. It is essential for managers to recognise that their allyship is not about changing all historical wrongs overnight, and that small, incremental, steady improvements that align with JEDI principles can have significant impact on individuals, and can help shift the culture within a workplace in meaningful ways. Even the least observant of managers will recognise traditional behaviours and patterns that are built upon unconscious bias and that continue to disadvantage historically disadvantaged individuals: simply starting somewhere, with one problematic issue and consciously working to address it, can have a positive impact for staff and patients, and help to create a culture of allyship within the workplace that will accelerate in the future.

Being a JEDI defender

In most cases, those charged with implementing JEDI will be personally and philosophically supportive of objectives and most interested in successfully putting principles into practical operation. Doing so may require them to overcome indifference, resistance, or even outright hostility within a team or with specific team members. Where religious objections are cited as a reason for rejecting JEDI principles, this can become even more complex from a human rights legislation perspective.

In such cases, fairness, objectivity, transparency and impartiality are useful principles to apply in communicating with team members. As a manager, leader or entrepreneur it will be necessary to be mindful of the natural tendency to make assumptions and stereotype those who are ambivalent or resistant as 'intolerant' or 'biased'. Beginning from a perspective of genuinely wanting to engage with these individuals to understand reasons for resistance implies a listening – rather than a telling – form of communication. The nature of JEDI sometimes means education and logic alone are insufficient to overcome deeply held beliefs or strong emotional responses. While logical argument and education/awareness raising should be tried, it is also realistic to expect they will have limited success. Non-judgmental exploration of alternatives – for example, what accommodations could be made for those with sincerely held religious objections to certain JEDI objectives? – is important. In order to avoid potential litigation, documentation of conversations and this exploration is usually helpful in case disagreements escalate into law suits. Exploring 'what can we all live with' options rather than fully embracing JEDI elements can sometimes yield compromises that are acceptable to all.

It is important, however, for everyone to recognise that 'compromises' of JEDI principles for individuals who are resistant can also send powerfully negative messages to others about the true commitment of the organisation. In attempting to navigate dissent with one team member, this could create ruptures in many other ways as well, with accusations of 'favouritism', 'kowtowing' or 'not really being committed'. This is a politically difficult and sensitive balancing act, that will sometimes mean accommodation and compromise may not actually be possible.

Where compromise and accommodation are not possible, risk mitigation and damage control become the central concern of the manager and the organisation as a whole. Consumer boycotts of large corporations embracing JEDI principles (e.g. Disney and its support of 'gay days' at certain theme parks) can be both reputationally and financially damaging. Similarly, acquiescing to resisters of JEDI can trigger equal and opposing blowback from supporters. In an ideal world, honest and open communication and sincere efforts to understand the multiple diverse perspectives on complex human interactions should yield acceptable compromises...but given the politicised nature of JEDI and the polarised societal fabric of today, this is sadly not always realistic. In such cases, managers, leaders and entrepreneurs need to recognise the limits of their authority, responsibility, and locus of control, and ensure consistent, clear, timely and accurate reporting of developments to senior leaders who will have responsibility for managing these incredibly complex issues.

Summary

Justice, equity, diversity, and inclusivity are not simply noble ideals but necessary business activities that promote organisational success. While managers, leaders and entrepreneurs may not be directly involved in articulating and framing JEDI principles within organisations, they frequently have significant responsibilities for implementation and defending them. This requires honest self-reflection, authentic and inspirational leadership, and excellent communication skills in order to navigate the increasingly polarised and politicised environment within which JEDI is practiced. While this can be frustrating, exhausting, and emotionally draining, the benefits for individuals and organisations – and the satisfaction of simply doing the right thing under difficult circumstances – can be a significant reward.

References

1. Hammond JW *et al* (2021). *Why the term JEDI is problematic for describing programs that promote justice, equity, diversity and inclusion.* New York: Scientific American Online. https://www.scientificamerican.com/article/why-the-term-jedi-is-problematic-for-describing-programs-that-promote-justice-equity-diversity-and-inclusion/#

2. Shields B. Justice, equity, diversity and inclusion curriculum within an introductory bioengineering course. *Biomed Eng Education* 2022; 3: 39–49. https://doi.org/10.1007/s43683-022-00086-z

3. Gambill J, Giovengo K (2020). *Justice, Equity, Diversity and Inclusion (JEDI) Report.* Georgia: Marine Extension and Georgia Sea Grant/University of Georgia. https://repository.library.noaa.gov/view/noaa/38592

4. Simpson D *et al* (2022). *Assessing what matters: a milestone focused on justice, equity, diversity & inclusion.* AAMC Group on Education Affairs Regional Spring Conference April 20-22 2022 Virtual Meeting. https://institutionalrepository.aah.org/faculty/125/

5. Ayala MJ *et al*. Belonging in STEM: an interactive, iterative approach to create and maintain a diverse learning community. *Sci Life* 2021; 36(11): 964–967. https://doi.org/10.1016/j.tree.2021.08.004

6. FitzGerald C, Hurst S. Implicit bias in health care professionals: a systematic review. *BMC Med Ethics* 2017; 18(19). https://doi.org/10.1186/s12910-017-0179-8

7.   Canales MK. Othering: towards an understanding of difference. *Advances in Nursing Science* 2000; 22(4): 16–31. https://doi.org/10.1097/00012272-200006000-00003

8.   Powell JA, Menedian S. The problem of othering: towards inclusiveness and belonging. *Othering and Belonging* 2018; 1: 14–40. https://www.otheringandbelonging.org/the-problem-of-othering/

9.   University of North Carolina School of Medicine and Health Sciences (2022). *Justice, Equity, Diversity, and Inclusion Toolkit*. North Carolina: University of North Carolina School of Medicine and Health Sciences. https://www.med.unc.edu/healthsciences/about-us/diversity/jeditoolkit/

10. Katz JH, Miller FA. No going back – raising the bar on addressing inclusion, diversity, and systemic change. *Organization and Development Review* 2021; 53(3): 8–17.

11. BeLue R *et al.* Uplifting black organizations to uplift the black community. *Organization and Development Review* 2021; 53(3): 18–24.

12. Rath E, Raheja A. Diversity and inclusion during crisis: An archetypal perspective. *Organization and Development Review* 2021; 53(3): 32–40.

13. Walker KA. Understanding and disrupting white supremacy at work: An action and inquiry guide for OD practitioners. *Organization and Development Review* 2021; 53(3): 41–47.

14. Applegate B, Patterson S. Making good trouble, necessary trouble in the field of OD: an invitation to the work of decentering whiteness. *Organization and Development Review* 2021; 53(3): 48–55.

15. Robinson G, Dechant K. Building a business case for diversity. *Academy of Management Executive* 1997; 11(3): 21–31.

16. Morley T. Making the business case for diversity and inclusion. *Strategic HR Review* 2018; 17(1): 56–60. https://doi.org/10.1108/SHR-10-2017-0068

17. Ely RJ, Thomas DA. Getting serious about diversity: enough already with the business case. *Harvard Business Review* [online] 2020. https://hbr.org/2020/11/getting-serious-about-diversity-enough-already-with-the-business-case

18. Arya V *et al.* Systemic racism: pharmacists' role and responsibility. *J American College Clinical Pharmacy* 2020; 3(7): 1265–1268. https://doi.org/10.1002/jac5.1338

CHAPTER 9

Human resource management: Job descriptions, recruiting and hiring

Upon completion of this chapter you should be able to:

- detail the role of managers in successful recruitment and hiring in pharmacy
- understand the value of job descriptions
- explain the elements of a good job description
- demonstrate an understanding of a strong interview process.

One of the most challenging but important parts of professional life as a pharmacist involves interpersonal interactions. Whether formally named or not, most pharmacists need basic competencies in supervision and management of other staff, including pharmacy assistants and regulated technicians.[1] The service orientation of pharmacy means that a key input for any business are the people who are recruited and hired.[1] Thinking of professional and technical staff as business inputs may seem somewhat ruthless, but effective operations management in pharmacy is often built upon a solid foundation of effective and humane human resource management.

Human resource management (HRM) consists of a variety of different specific tasks, but a critical element of successful HRM involves finding and hiring the best possible staff to support attainment of strategic priorities.[1] Three particularly important elements of this task include crafting effective job descriptions, a thoughtful recruitment process that will make an organisation attractive to the best prospective candidates, and an interviewing/hiring process that is both discerning and welcoming.

Crafting job descriptions

One of the first and most important tasks for human resource managers is defining the skill sets and competencies needed for the organisation and formalising this in a job description. A good job description acts as both an internal record to guide performance assessment and express mutually agreed upon objectives for the role, as well as a recruitment tool designed to excite prospective candidates about the workplace.[2] The job description begins with an understanding of where a specific position fits within a broader organisational structure (usually depicted in an organisational chart).[3] The organisational chart describes how specific jobs relate to one another (for example, who reports to who). Smaller organisations such as community pharmacies may have no need for a formally documented organisational chart, while larger organisations like hospitals will have very elaborate models. Based on where a position fits within an organisation, it becomes possible to develop a job description that highlights responsibilities, outcomes, accountabilities and reporting relationships. Even in the smallest of organisations, undocumented or informal job descriptions can be a problem: without formal written documentation there will be uncertainty regarding expectations and this can lead to both practical and legal problems if different individuals have different ideas of what their job is. A formal job description is strongly recommended for every individual in an organisation, no matter how large or small that organisation is. Key components of a job description should include:[4]

- *Job title:* A brief, concise summary highlighting the purpose for the job, formal/legal labels, and an encapsulated summary of the scope of the role. Examples of a clear job title include: 'supervising pharmacist – dispensary' or 'clinical pharmacist – infectious diseases'.
- *Job remit:* A statement of the purpose or remit of the role should provide everyone in the organisation with a common and clear understanding of the role itself, the level and scope of responsibility and what key deliverables are expected. The job remit should answer the question, 'why does this job exist in this organisation?'.
- *Duties/Responsibilities:* Often this is the longest part of a job description; it contains details of the specific activities and functions that are expected to occupy the employees time and attention. Essential duties should be clearly highlighted.
- *Required qualifications:* In the context of a job description, qualifications are not necessarily academic or educational but instead focus on specific credentials. For example, not everyone with a pharmacy degree may be capable of prescribing; if a prescriber is needed, this qualification should be stated along with a description for how the credential or proof of capability can be demonstrated by the candidate.
- *Educational background:* Regulated professions such as pharmacy require certain academic backgrounds and these requirements should be included in the job description. It is important, however, to carefully assess how these are presented; for example, if an individual from another country (like Canada) has a BScPhm or a Pharm D degree, and is still able to meet regulatory standards for registration, does it make sense to include 'MPharm' as an educational background requirement? Instead, 'MPharm or equivalent degree, recognised by regulatory body' may be more appropriate and allow internationally educated pharmacists opportunities to take on new roles.
- *Experience:* Many jobs, particularly those with supervisory responsibilities, may require some kind of real world experience to complement education and qualifications. This is often described in terms of years. While this may be legitimate, it is important to not discriminate against those who may have overseas experiences that are equivalent; it is rarely defensible to require 'local' experience, and candidates should have the chance to explain how their non-local experience provides substantially similar opportunities for demonstration of real world competencies.
- *Working conditions:* Many job descriptions include a section describing working conditions and physical demands of essential job duties and responsibilities. This could include, for example, requirements for evening or weekend shift work, physical issues such as lifting heavy boxes, and expectations regarding travel or on-call requirements.

- *Salary and benefits:* Job descriptions should include information regarding remuneration in a transparent manner. In most cases, salary bands/ranges may be cited; if these are negotiable, this should be stated clearly.

Increasingly, in an effort to expand representativeness of the workforce, job descriptions include explicit acknowledgement of the desire to identify members of traditionally under-represented or disadvantaged groups to expand the workforce.[5]

For smaller organisations in particular, there may be a temptation to overlook or under-invest in the development of a job description – 'we're hiring a pharmacist here, and everyone knows what that means, right?'. It is important to note that job descriptions also play an important legal role within employment relationships; where performance of an employee is not satisfactory, a well crafted job description can provide the basis for coaching and remediation or – at worst – dismissal.[6] Sufficient attention to the details of a job description ensures the organisations interests and objectives are clearly outlined, but it should not be so overburdened with minutiae that professional judgement and creativity are stifled.

Job descriptions should be reviewed on an annual basis and where necessary updated to reflect evolving organisational priorities. The best time to review and update job descriptions is usually as part of an annual performance assessment process, where managers and employees can discuss accomplishments, challenges, and specific elements of the role itself. Employees should be encouraged to regularly review job descriptions to ensure alignment with day to day work, and to help remind them of the criterion upon which their success will be judged.

Recruitment

Employers recognise how complex and important recruitment of the best possible candidates can be: most organisations do not want simply a warm-body-with-a-pulse, but instead a high-performing, energetic and committed individual to help grow the organisation. It is sometimes said that leaving a position vacant is preferable to hiring the wrong person: poor recruitment efforts often will lead to bad hiring decisions, and this can be costly, exhausting, and sometimes fatal to an organisation.[7]

Recruitment is sometimes described as a marketing process and many of the most widely used recruiting techniques for professionals like pharmacists have their roots in traditional marketing efforts.[8] Recognising that the best candidates for a job will often have multiple attractive offers means that managers need to 'sell' and actively promote the benefits of their organisation to attract the best applicants.[9]

Since the COVID-19 pandemic, there has been considerable concern regarding the state of the health care workforce in general, and the nature of the pharmacy workplace in particular. In many parts of the world, a 'great resignation' occurred during the years of the pandemic in which many experienced and dedicated professionals left the workforce in large numbers due to exhaustion and burnout, and those who remained became even more demanding of certain workplace requirements.[10] As a result, recruitment efforts have evolved considerably, in a manner similar to online dating: there is a recognition that recruitment is about trying to find the best possible fit or match between a workplace and a potential employee. Similar to online dating, it is a complex interplay of different techniques that attempt to showcase significant advantages of a workplace in ways that generate interest and excitement, but that are also honest and filled with integrity. Employers who use less-than-transparent recruitment techniques, or who are making promises to potential employees that are not being kept, will quickly generate a bad reputation in the professional community, which will hamper recruitment efforts for years to come. Ultimately, recruitment is a two-way dialogue with prospective applicants scrutinising organisations as closely as organisations are evaluating them for the right chemistry and 'fit'.

Recruitment strategies that are most frequently used today include:[11]

- *Social media:* In most fields, including pharmacy, social media has become the most frequently used way organisations of all sizes find and target potential employees. Commercial sites including LinkedIn and Indeed can be useful, as can pharmacy-specific sites (including Facebook pages and communities). Twitter is increasingly used as a way of advising prospective applicants of an opening.
- *Your website:* Most prospective candidates will do their own diligence regarding the suitability of your workplace, and will look for a web presence of some sort. A professional and engaging customer-facing website is also a powerful recruitment tool. Many strong candidates may actually avoid working for an organisation with a clunky (or non-existent) website since it signals the management is out-of-date and not particularly dynamic.
- *Consider a compensation package rather than just a salary:* All prospective candidates are interested in remuneration and in general, the more talented candidates will expect a higher salary. It is important, however, to recognise that salaries by themselves are not the sole motivator; an interesting and customised compensation package can be a powerful recruiting incentive. Increasingly, strong candidates are looking for a workplace that provides independence, creativity, engagement, fun, and opportunities for work-life balance. Beyond simply salary, compensation can include sabbatical or study-leave provisions, work-from-home flexibility, control over specific new initiatives or other elements that are appealing to a prospective candidate. Up-front signalling, as part of recruitment, of the employers openness to craft a bespoke compensation package (beyond standard salary and benefits) will be intriguing to many candidates.
- *Use technology to support more efficient recruitment:* In most organisations, the recruitment process relies heavily on technological mediation, including email (for communication), Dropbox (for the exchange of documents such as degrees or certificates), Doodle (for scheduling appointments), etc. Many applicants will rely on mobile phones, rather than computers, to connect with prospective employers so ensuring seamless use of these technologies makes it easier for applicants to provide the information you need, and will enhance the organisation's reputation.
- *Don't dawdle:* Where technologically enabled, recruitment processes can and should move quickly. Prior to launching a recruitment process, planning is required to ensure the organisation and its hiring managers can respond and decide expeditiously, so as to minimise wait times for applicants. Minimise time delays between scheduling and holding interviews, or completing interviews and making hiring decisions. Being clear with applicants about expected timelines – and actually achieving them – demonstrates managerial effectiveness.
- *Use internal networks more effectively:* One of the most powerful but often overlooked recruitment strategies involves full engagement of the current workforce. Friends and colleagues of current employees may provide valuable access to talented professionals.

Further, a recommendation from a friend who works within and can vouch for the organisation is likely one of the most powerful recruitment inducements available. Engaging current employees and providing supports or rewards for successful candidate referrals is increasingly useful in recruitment, especially where competition with other employers exists.

- *Treat unsuccessful applicants well:* An overlooked component of recruitment is the exposure it provides to diverse applicants. In most cases, many individuals may apply for a position but only one person is hired. Unsuccessful candidates may become an excellent pool from which to recruit for future positions. Treating all candidates respectfully throughout the process is essential. Clearly explaining why a candidate was unsuccessful, and offering to keep their documentation on file for future positions, is a goodwill gesture than can support successful future recruitment. Where possible, avoid imperious statements such as 'only those candidates selected for interview will be contacted', and try to establish contact with all applicants as a way of building a talent pool for future hiring. Where candidates have been interviewed but were unsuccessful, provide feedback, encouragement, and signal that future opportunities may arise. Treating candidates in this way sends a strong signal regarding managerial competency and positive organisational culture.

- *Engage with professional and industry associations:* Professions like pharmacy rely heavily upon diverse professional organisations and associations like the Royal Pharmaceutical Society or the UK Clinical Pharmacy Association. These types of organisations are invaluable for peer networking but also support recruitment. As an employer, being visible and contributing meaningfully to professional associations, highlights an organisational culture dedicated to professional practice – and also provides opportunities to engage with potential applicants before the recruitment process begins. Most associations offer online 'job boards' and events such as conferences and networking sessions provide direct access to the broadest possible talent pool.

Your organisation's reputation is the most important recruitment tool: pharmacy is a relatively small and well-connected profession. Reputational strength of an organisation is possibly the single most important recruitment tool available: a strong, professional presence coupled with a track record of success, innovation, creativity, flexibility and a commitment to employee development and wellbeing, will mean the best applicants will be interested in working with you in the future.

Increasingly, recruitment agencies are being used particularly where positions are difficult to fill or where there is some sensitivity around a role (for example, with a senior executive position). Where international candidates are specifically sought, recruitment agencies familiar with different countries can be a great asset. Recruitment agencies have networks and strengths that can be leveraged, but they can be expensive, typically charging between 15–25% of the role's annual salary for their services. At their best, recruitment agencies not only help to save time, they provide access to the best possible applicants. In many cases, they can support practical/logistical problem-solving around citizenship and visas, housing and relocation. They can also act in a more discrete way in approaching potential candidates and in undertaking compensation discussions.

At the heart of the recruitment process is the development and communication of a compelling 'employee value proposition' (EVP).[12] EVP is more than simply job descriptions, salaries, and benefits. The EVP requires employers to insightfully articulate why their organisation is indeed an excellent place to work, to learn, and to develop. Finding words to explain the EVP and making the case in a clear, honest, and interesting way is a useful activity for any manager, and can serve as a powerful recruitment tool. For example, the Unilever company describes its EVP as 'Unilever is the place where you can bring purpose to life through the work you do, creating a better business and a better world. You will work with brands that are loved and improve the lives of our consumers and the communities around us...We develop leaders for Unilever, and Unilever leaders go on to be leaders elsewhere in the world.' The power of such an EVP – and the ways in which it can inspire the most talented applicants to consider working for your organisation – should not be underestimated.

Interviewing and hiring

The purpose of recruitment is to gather the best and most diverse pool of prospective applicants; a successful recruitment process can sometimes lead to a difficult interviewing and hiring process. In presenting themselves for employment consideration, applicants will of course put their best face forward; managers must then consider what is the best way to screen and assess individuals during an interview to identify who will be the best person for the job. Recently, there has been considerable interest in this issue, particularly given the reality that something as important – yet subjective – as 'fit' between applicant and organisation is subject to unconscious bias.[13] Every manager needs to consider how the interview process can be used to make defensible and well-informed decisions in ways that are effective, efficient, fair, transparent, and minimise conscious and unconscious bias.[14]

Screening who to interview

A successful recruitment process will yield many more possible applicants than can be actually interviewed. A screening process is needed to determine who will proceed to interview. Preliminary screening should be done in a way that minimises risk for bias. A helpful technique can be to develop a weighted checklist – based on the job description itself – that quantifies the organisation's hiring priorities. The checklist ensures a consistent interpretation of applicants' CVs and alignment with what the organisation actually needs. For example, if training of students is a key feature of the job description, 20 points out of 100 points can be allocated to previous experience (e.g. 1 point per student supervised). Alternatively, if professional networks are important to the job description, 10 points can be allocated for membership in professional associations (e.g. 2.5 points for each association). Reviewing the job description to identify 'must-have' elements versus 'nice-to-have' elements, then assigning a numerical weighting to these must-have elements provides a fair and consistent way of assessing CVs. It also minimises the risk that distraction elements (e.g. an applicant whose hobby is golf, which also happens to be the hobby of the manager) will unfairly influence decisions. When screening CVs it is necessary to be mindful of implicit or unconscious bias, particularly with respect to internationally educated pharmacists. If a pharmacy degree is a requirement for the role, there must be a compelling and defensible rationale for why a particular country's pharmacy degree is favoured over another. Facile reasons that are actually rooted in bias or stereotype should not be used.

A criterion-and-points driven checklist that is used to assess all applicants equally, will allow for an initial ranking of candidates; from there the top five or seven can be selected for the next stage of the process. It is important to recognise not simply the time and work involved in an interview for a manager or hiring committee, but also the hope and energy that is involved for the candidate. Do not meaninglessly interview candidates who have little chance of success or who 'we want to meet just in case'. Careful quantitative screening using job description based criterion should prevent unnecessary interviews and signpost the most promising candidates for interviewing.

Pre-interview activity

Once a short list of 5–7 candidates to proceed is established, it is increasingly common to ask these individuals to do or produce something asynchronously that can then be used to further narrow the list of who will actually be interviewed. Pre-interview activities provide opportunities for applicants to dedicate time and attention to a specific job relevant task. For example, if patient education is an important element of the job description, these candidates could be asked to record a 20 minute patient-oriented presentation which can be reviewed by the hiring manager or committee. This provides a first-glance at the candidate doing a task that is essential for the role. It provides the candidate with time to prepare and to best position themselves for success. Prior to reviewing all the candidate's pre-interview submissions, a scoring rubric or similar checklist should be developed. The hiring committee or manager should identify their priorities for what 'success' in this activity looks like and grade all the applicants accordingly. Based on this score, a refined short list of 2–4 candidates can emerge, and these individuals can be invited for an interview.

If using pre-interview activities as part of the screening process, it is essential that clarity is provided to candidates regarding the task itself and what is expected. It is most reasonable to actually provide the candidates with the grading/scoring checklist itself so they understand how they will be judged. Clear instructions regarding timelines, delivery format, recording requirements, etc. should be given. It is also important to acknowledge the time and effort that the candidate invests in this process. Be prepared to provide unsuccessful candidates with supportive and constructive feedback on their activity – this may be useful if you want to recruit them in the future. In some cases, it may be important to acknowledge intellectual property rights, and explicitly state that the pre-interview activity remains the property of the candidate and will not be used by the hiring organisation for any other purpose.

The interview

Wherever possible, interviews should involve a panel of managers and peer employees rather than simply a single individual. This is important for reducing unconscious bias.[13] The interview panel should be the same for all candidates interviewed. The panel should be provided with all relevant documents and pre-interview activities; however, the panel need not be provided with checklist scores or grades as this may introduce bias into the hiring process. Once selected for an interview, all candidates should be on equal footing during the interview process itself. The lead of the interview panel should collaboratively develop a standard bank of interview questions that all candidates are asked in a consistent way to facilitate comparisons.

Care must be taken in developing interview questions. Only questions that are relevant and essential should be asked; certain questions cannot legally be asked (for example, relating to family planning or marital status).[15] Interview questions should connect clearly and directly with the job description itself, providing applicants with an opportunity to discuss their suitability for the role. A balance of questions that explores a candidate's biographical/employment/educational history, their real world behaviour in experienced situations, and their projected behaviour in hypothetical situations should be used.[14] In most cases, avoid simple 'yes/no' answers and ask open-ended questions that encourage discussion and dialogue. See Table 1 for some example questions commonly used in interviews.

Table 1: *Commonly used interview questions*

Type of interview question	Sample question	Rationale
Biographical	'What do you see as some of your most impactful professional accomplishments?'	Looking for authentic and verifiable accomplishments listed on a candidates CV, and to understand the individual's philosophy of practice in terms of 'impact'
	'Tell us about your last two positions and what led you to change roles?'	Trying to understand employment stability and capacity to work within an organisation
Historical behavioural	'Tell us about a time you made an important decision you later thought was incorrect?'	Assessing self-reflection capacity and the ability to accept – and respond appropriately – to mistakes
	'How have your previous managers described your performance?'	Understanding relationships and interactions with previous supervisors; this can be verified through post-interview reference checking
Hypothetical behavioural	'What do you see yourself doing three years from now?'	Insight into longer term personal, career, and strategic thinking and planning; this can help assess interest in career laddering
	'In this role you will be dealing with a very diverse patient population. How will you manage the cultural and language differences to ensure best possible patient care?'	Workplace-specific issue; can help identify suitability for the organisation, flexibility/adaptability and willingness to learn

Hiring

An effective interview process should identify preferred candidates for hiring. The hiring process itself is frequently governed by organisation-specific policies (for example, reference checks). Importantly, unsuccessful candidates should be afforded the respect of a debriefing conversation (rather than a simple email) to allow them an opportunity to learn from the experience.

Once the preferred candidate is identified, it is customary to undertake a negotiation process regarding role-specific elements. Careful documentation of what is agreed upon is necessary to prevent misunderstanding. Most frequently, this documentation takes the form of a legal contract outlining expectations of both employer and employee. Depending upon the role itself, negotiation and contracting will cover diverse topic areas, but at minimum should include:[1]

- terms of employment (e.g. full time, part time, temporary, probationary period, hours, work-from-home provisions, scheduling, breaks, etc.)

- compensation (salary, pay frequency (e.g. bi-weekly, monthly))
- benefits (e.g. pension, education allowance, sick time, annual leave, etc.)
- non-financial benefits (e.g. creative control over new programming)
- time-away practices (e.g. paid versus unpaid leaves of absence, family leave, statutory holiday policies, etc.)
- non-disclosure, confidentiality, or non-compete agreements (where relevant)
- liability issues (e.g. whether the employer or employee is responsible for insurance coverage, where relevant)
- regulatory requirements (e.g. annual licensing and continuing professional development fees and expectations)
- equipment and supplies (particularly where work-from-home is involved – who is responsible for computers, internet access, etc.)
- termination and severance (in the event the employment relationship breaks down, what rules govern the end of the relationship, and are these aligned with local/national employment legislation and standards?).

In some cases, organisations may have formal human resource departments that manage the contracting process, but in all cases hiring managers must be directly involved to ensure alignment with workplace expectations and organisational needs. Though awkward at times, it is essential that informality and assumptions be avoided at this stage: careful documentation of expectations in the form of a contract is an important safeguard for both the employer and the employee and will reduce burden in the future in case there are issues.

Hiring should also include careful attention to onboarding, the process by which newly hired individuals are integrated into the workplace.[1] Starting a new job is both exciting and stressful, and it is incumbent upon managers to make the integration process as enjoyable and seamless as possible to optimise the likelihood of success. Pre-planning is needed to ensure the workplace is ready on day one to welcome a newly hired person. This includes clear directions in terms of preliminary medical tests and screening that are required (e.g. TB testing, criminal background checks, etc.). It is usually helpful to set up payroll, tax, and benefits prior to day one, to ensure smooth entry into the workplace. Managers should ensure necessary accounts and logins are set up prior to day one to minimise inefficiency and maximise productivity. A newly hired individual's electronic footprint in the organisation should be in place and ready to use as a way of signalling strong managerial competence and positive organisational culture. Ensuring physical items such as computers, keys, fobs, and a functional workspace is available also smooths the transition. It is usually most helpful to actually plan, schedule, and publish a formal onboarding or orientation program, including a tour of the workplace, meetings with key individuals, etc.

Perhaps most importantly, a welcoming tone needs to be established immediately: onboarding of a new employee also means communication with existing staff so they are ready to welcome a new colleague. Facilitate introductions, sponsor a getting-to-know-each-other lunch or coffee break, and schedule one-on-one meetings with important colleagues on the first day. Small gestures such as a welcome bag with company branded materials like t-shirts or caps, or a card signed by the staff, can help to set a positive tone for what is hoped to be a productive future working relationship.

Summary

Amongst the most important things that managers typically do, is to hire the best possible people to help the organisation achieve its strategic objectives. The process of hiring involves many steps but starts with a clear job description aligned with company priorities. Formal processes for recruitment, hiring, and onboarding can ensure successful workplace integration. It is essential that managers are mindful of the ways in which unconscious and implicit bias may interfere with good, defensible decision making and institute policies and practices that are designed to reduce subjectivity that may disadvantage some applicants. Ultimately, with careful planning, this process can help organisations hire the best possible candidates to help support long-term success.

References

1. Austin Z. *Human resource management in pharmacy: managing and motivating staff to excel.* Washington DC: American Pharmacists' Association, 2022.

2. Al-Marwai SA, Subramaniam ID. A review of the need for writing and updating job descriptions for 21st century organizations. *European J Social Sciences* 2009; 12(2): 241–251.

3. Smith T. It's time to rethink job descriptions for the digital era. *Harvard Business Review* [online] 2021. https://hbr.org/2021/12/its-time-to-rethink-job-descriptions-for-the-digital-era

4. Pontika N. Roles and jobs in the open research scholarly communications environment: analysing job descriptions to predict future trends. *LIBER Quarterly: The journal of the association of European Research Libraries* 2019; 29(1): 1–20. https://doi.org/10.18352/lq10282

5. Society of Human Resource Management (SHRM) (2022). *How to develop a job description.* Society of Human Resource Management (SHRM). https://www.shrm.org/resourcesandtools/tools-and-samples/how-to-guides/pages/developajobdescription.aspx

6. Muskovitz MJ. The importance of job descriptions. *National Law Review* [online] 2011; 1(108). https://www.natlawreview.com/article/importance-job-descriptions

7. Breaugh JA. Employee recruitment. *Ann Review Psychology* 2013; 64: 389–416. https://doi.org/10.1146/annurev-psych-113011-143757

8. Cappelli P. Your approach to hiring is all wrong. *Harvard Business Review* [online] 2019. https://hbr.org/2019/05/your-approach-to-hiring-is-all-wrong

9. Wardlaw MK. Effective Human Resources Recruiting and Hiring Practices for Improving Organizational Performance. Minneapolis, Minnesota: Walden University, 2019 (dissertation). https://scholarworks.waldenu.edu/cgi/viewcontent.cgi?article=8847&context=dissertations

10. Cook I. Who is driving the Great Resignation? *Harvard Business Review* [online] 2021. https://hbr.org/2021/09/who-is-driving-the-great-resignation

11. Society of Human Resource Management (SHRM) (2022). *Recruiting and attracting talent: a guide to understanding and managing the recruitment process.* Society of Human Resource Management (SHRM). https://www.shrm.org/hr-today/trends-and-forecasting/special-reports-and-expert-views/documents/recruiting-attracting-talent.pdf

12. Verlinden N (2023). *The employee value proposition: All you need to know.* Rotterdam: Academy to Innovate HR. https://www.aihr.com/blog/employee-value-proposition-evp/

13. Purkis SLS *et al.* Implicit sources of bias in employment interview judgments and decisions. *Organizational Behaviour and Human Decision Process* 2006; 101(2): 152–167. https://doi.org/10.1016/j.obhdp.2006.06.005

14. Trull SG. Strategies of effective interviewing. *Harvard Business Review* [online] 1964. https://hbr.org/1964/01/strategies-of-effective-interviewing

15. Goodale JG. Effective employment interviewing. In: Eder RW, Ferris GR, eds. *The Employment Interview: Theory, Research, and Practice.* Washington DC: Sage Publications Inc, 1989: 307–323.

CHAPTER 10

Performance assessment and management, and feedback

Upon completion of this chapter you should be able to:

- define the terms performance assessment and performance management
- understand the structure of performance assessment
- detail the role of a manager in performance assessment and management
- explain what is meant by SMART goals
- understand the different types of feedback and how and when to deliver them.

One of the most important activities of managers involves monitoring staff and providing supportive, corrective direction as necessary.[1] At times, this can be challenging for managers who may themselves feel unconfident about their feedback skills, or who are concerned that they may irritate or alienate staff.[2] Further, in a profession like pharmacy there is a tradition of self-appraisal and self-monitoring, and performance management may appear or feel like it is diminishing professional autonomy. Regardless of the size of the organisation or the nature of the practice, all individuals require and benefit from periodic opportunities to have their performance reviewed and appraised in an objective manner, and will appreciate coaching, mentoring, and supportive feedback to improve and enhance their practice.[2,3]

What is performance assessment?

Though daunting, the term 'performance assessment' simply refers to a structured and regular review of an individual's performance on the job. Effective performance assessments are systematic, criterion-based, and involve a predictable/standardised approach so as to avoid unpleasant surprises.[3,4] The structure of performance assessments will vary based on organisation specific factors, but in general should include:[1,5]

- *Clear and specific statements of what outcomes are expected:* While the job of 'pharmacist' or 'technician' is generally understood by all, performance assessment requires managers to clearly and specifically define what activities and outcomes are expected of individual employees. These in turn should be based on strategic planning priorities identified by the organisation. For example, a 'pharmacist' may believe that their central job and key outcome is safe and efficient dispensing of medications, and as a result may spend most of their time, energy, and effort focused on technical dispensing activities. The employer may want the pharmacy to move in a more clinically oriented direction, allowing technicians to assume greater dispensing responsibilities, freeing up pharmacists to provide minor ailments consultations, immunisations, public health interventions, and educational sessions for the community. The manager has the responsibility of translating the organisation's strategic priorities into clear and specific statements that can be agreed upon with the pharmacist – particularly if the pharmacist has a different philosophical stance or understanding of what their role should be. Rather than simply saying, 'be a pharmacist', performance management starts with statements such as 'completes 20 medication reviews monthly' or 'delivers 2–4 group education sessions with patients monthly', or 'provides clinical supervision to 7–10 MPharm students annually', etc. Clear and specific statements usually provide a quantitative target (or range) as well as specific task-focused outcomes. Prior to performance assessment, the pharmacist and manager should have reviewed and agreed upon these statements, and attempted to identify and address potential barriers to success.

- *Clear criteria for evaluating the attainment of objectives/outcomes:* As part of the discussion and negotiation of performance goals, the manager should involve the employee in defining what metrics and criteria will be used to evaluate successful attainment. For example, '20 medication reviews monthly' could be completed on healthy, non-smoking young women taking only oral contraceptives or on vulnerable non-English speaking elderly patients with multiple comorbidities and taking 20–30 medication doses daily. The work involved, outcome and value of medication reviews in these two cases will be very different, so managers and employees need to have clarity on the criterion used for evaluating success. Once again, this is a discussion that should occur well before performance assessment is actually undertaken so there is a common and agreed upon understanding of expectations to prevent any unnecessary surprises.

- *Performance assessment should be regular, not simply annual:* In most organisations, performance assessment is viewed as an annual one-off activity, but in high performing workplaces, performance assessments are regularly, if not constantly, being undertaken. Informal check-ins with employees, along with encouragement and motivation will let them know they are on track for success, or whether a course correction might be needed. Regular informal communication with employees will prevent unnecessary surprises during formal performance assessment touchpoints; ideally, an annual performance review session should simply be a restatement of what the employee and the manager already know, rather than be a time where new information is presented.

- *Provide motivational feedback and coaching throughout the year:* A key role of managers is to provide emotional support for employees to be at their best. This means staying positive and connected throughout the year, celebrating successes, acknowledging challenges, and respectfully suggesting alternatives when barriers emerge. Performance assessment is a specific type of manager–employee relationship that needs to be based on consistency, trust, and respect, rather than a fear driven annual process that is simply endured then forgotten.

- *Assess performance, not personality:* Many managers find it difficult to separate performance from the person: for example, a reserved, less-social individual may actually be a star performer based on defined outcomes and targets, but because they don't portray a certain kind of personality, they may be overlooked. Similarly, an internationally qualified pharmacist who may not have English as a first language and may not be completely well versed in typical local cultural norms, may not be given the credit they deserve for performance success. Managers undertaking performance assessment must be conscious of implicit bias, and carefully separate personality from performance where the two are not directly connected. Avoiding the use of personality labels (e.g. 'immature' or 'overly emotional') is also important as these imply judgement and will likely only trigger a defensive response. Instead, focus on the actual results of specific behaviours and how these may be counterproductive to performance targets and expectations.

- *Align incentives with performance assessment:* Most organisations use performance assessment as a tool for allocating bonuses, salary increases, and other employment related incentives. Performance assessment should provide opportunities to directly compare individuals with similar jobs to identify best and promising practices within the organisation. Transparency in how incentives are aligned with performance assessment is essential, so employees trust both the manager and the system to be fair and impartial. Where clear quantitative targets are established for employees, these can be used as the trigger for the allocation of incentives; ultimately, the employee themself should already know what to expect in terms of incentives based on their performance, as this has been transparently communicated in advance.

- *Use annual performance assessment data to drive short-, medium-, and long-term planning:* Data from individual employee's performance assessments can be useful to provide coaching and mentoring for improvement, but aggregating data across an entire organisation can be invaluable to support strategic planning and defining organisational priorities. This data should provide senior managers with information regarding actual performance, activities, impacts, and outcomes to help them determine value to the organisation. Sharing aggregate data with the entire staff also supports peer-benchmarking and helps everyone become more invested in the organisation's future plans.

When performance management is needed

Ideally – but unrealistically – a structured and clear performance assessment system should result in alignment of an employee's efforts with organisational priorities.[6] Of course, in some situations, it is not that easy. Despite clear expectations, regular and supportive communication, and attempts to align incentives with performance, an individual employee may simply not achieve targets or may not be meeting expectations. In such situations, a performance management system may need to be implemented.[7]

Performance management is sometimes described as a continuous form of performance assessment, in which the manager maintains more regular communication, monitoring and redirection of the employee to support attainment of objectives.[8] Performance management usually requires setting goals and objectives that are more specific, more detailed, and more circumscribed than in general performance assessments, with less scope for individual variability.[9] It is usually invoked in circumstances where an individual's performance is deemed to be unsatisfactory or below expectations.[9,10] Performance management requires a sophisticated combination of planning and communication/interpersonal skills;

it is difficult to present performance management as 'positive' or 'supportive' since it is usually triggered by unsatisfactory performance assessment, and so emotions and stress can be high.[10] Effective listening and respectful dialogue are essential, to provide the employee with reassurance that the organisation supports them and is trying to work with them to remediate identified issues.

At the core of performance management is the need to establish clear objectives that are understood and accepted by the employee. These are most often described in terms of SMART goals:[11]

- *Specific:* Goals for an employee should be clearly defined and aligned with the job description itself. Where possible, specific wording from a job description can be useful to include in performance management to reinforce the expectation of the organisation.
- *Measurable:* Goals should have some specific metric or quantitative target to provide the employee with a clear focus of what is expected, and the manager with specific criterion to evaluate success. Measurable goals also permit ongoing monitoring and tracking, allowing both the manager and the employee to know what progress is being made towards achieving targets.
- *Achievable:* One of the most challenging elements of performance management and setting SMART goals is ensuring that stated goals are actually realistic and attainable. This is where open communication, careful conversation, and honest negotiation are required. Realistic and attainable goals are directly connected to the cognitive, emotional, and physical load the employee is experiencing at the time: an individual who has had no performance issues in the past may now be experiencing significant stress or problems at home and as a result, may simply lack the bandwidth to perform to previous levels or current employer expectations. This needs to be honestly acknowledged and openly discussed and negotiated to see what compromises are possible. Do not set employees up for failure by setting unrealistic or unachievable goals based on perfect conditions that no longer exist. Encouraging open dialogue in a non-judgemental manner that allows the manager to understand what is truly realistic – then honestly negotiating with the employee to find common ground – is essential.
- *Relevant:* Performance management goals need to be worthwhile for both the employee and the organisation. Once again, the job description can often provide both ideas and vocabulary for setting a relevant goal, one that is targeted at the specific strengths and capacities of the employee but that are also meaningful to the organisation.
- *Time bound:* In performance management, reasonable and realistic time frames for accomplishment must be established and agreed upon; a definitive end date is needed to provide a foundation for accountability, but this end date needs to be contextualised around the employee's current cognitive, emotional, and physical load related issues.

Examples of SMART goals include:

- Complete two accredited self study therapeutics modules within 30 days, focused on asthma and diabetes management, scoring a minimum of 80% on self-assessment quizzes.
- Observe five medication reviews conducted by other pharmacists in the practice and write a one page reflection outlining processes used to effectively and efficiently gather information from patients, to be completed in 15 days.
- Successfully complete the online diversity, equity, and inclusion course offered by the company,

scoring a minimum of 90% on the final quiz, within 20 days and provide a one page report highlighting five specific strategies that will be implemented to enhance openness in the pharmacy.

While such SMART goals may seem surprisingly 'small', it is precisely the bounded/finite nature of these that increase the specificity, relevance, and clarity, which – it is hoped – will enhance employee performance and confidence. Of course, where SMART goals are used, managers have accountability to closely monitor and follow-up to ensure completion – including clear statements regarding next steps should the goals NOT be achieved. Wherever possible, affirmative and supportive communication should be used to encourage individuals but it is important to recognise that the process of performance management is often stressful and distressing for everyone.

SMART goals are usually integrated into a personal improvement plan (PIP) or a personal development plan (PDP), a written document akin to a contract that outlines expectations for both managers and employees.[1,12] Such plans should be careful to avoid attempts to 'fix' personality issues: they should be focused on knowledge and skills deficits rather than attempts to change traits or beliefs. Within these plans, statements regarding processes should SMART goals not be achieved should be clearly stated, up to and including potential suspensions or terminations as a last resort. In some cases, the PIP/PDP will actually become a legal document necessary to support dismissal; as such, care must be taken to draft it in a legalistic/professional manner that can withstand legal scrutiny should this ultimately be required. The PIP/PDP should demonstrate a genuine good-will effort on behalf of the employer/manager to work collaboratively with the employee to address specific performance deficits in a fair, impartial, and reasonable manner. The plan should not be punitive in its tone, nor should it be unrealistic in terms of what is expected of the employee. Tracking/monitoring methods should be explicitly described in the document to ensure there is no misunderstanding regarding how managers will be following up to ensure compliance. Part of this involves a mechanism for both manager and employee to summarise and document achievements, articulate new learning or incorporation of new skills, etc. Performance management is never intended to be chronic or long-standing: it is a time-limited, targeted intervention focused on specific performance issues that are essentially remediable within a specific time period. Where successful, performance management should allow both the manager and the employee to re-establish a productive and collegial relationship focused on organisational objectives. Where unsuccessful, performance management may lead to more serious sanctions against the employee and as a result, the manager must ensure sufficient robust documentation to withstand legal challenge.[13,14]

Performance assessment and management are integral to managers' roles and necessary for organisational success. Collegial approaches emphasising respectful communication, coupled with clear planning, monitoring, and follow-up are essential elements of these processes. Demonstrating interest in the employee's development and growth is an important foundation for enhancing chances for success.

Delivering effective feedback

Arguably the most important task of any manager is delivering effective, supportive feedback to employees. At its core, feedback is simply the provision of data/information to an individual that is used as a tool to enhance quality and to facilitate improvement. Of course the word 'feedback' can also be used to refer to the screeching or disturbing humming noise that results from an amplifier or microphone being placed too close to a speaker – highlighting how tone is an essential component of effective feedback. Sometimes, feedback that is intended in one way can reverberate in unexpected and negative ways.

There are many different types of feedback, but managers generally rely on three particular styles: a) formative feedback, designed to be informal, conversational, and focused on coaching and future oriented improvement; b) summative feedback, which typically involves the presentation and analysis of data to evaluate or judge performance based on specific criteria; c) constructive feedback, emphasising techniques and strategies to address identified performance shortfalls.

Formative feedback

Formative feedback is the everyday, informal feedback managers provide to employees to help them develop more accurate self-assessment competencies to allow them to accurately appraise the quality and value of their work. It is important that formative feedback be consistent, supportive, and behaviourally oriented (rather than personality focused). Formative feedback works most effectively when it is embedded in a warm and collegial relationship between manager and employee, so reciprocal trust and mutual understanding are present. When delivering formative feedback, it is essential that managers remember to clearly praise and recognise success and positive behaviours as frequently as highlighting areas for improvement; where formative feedback is only delivered in situations of suboptimal performance, it acquires a negative or punitive tone which undermines both the impact of formative feedback and the quality of the relationship between manager and employee. Incessant or over-the-top praise for minor accomplishments is not necessary and can be grating – but balancing positive and negative formative feedback is essential.

Formative feedback should be delivered in a way that encourages dialogue, not simply downloading information or a hit-and-run of factoids. Encouraging the employee to self-reflect and self-appraise provides opportunities to learn more about that employee's perception of workplace success, and can open other avenues for dialogue. In professional fields like pharmacy, it is often helpful to emphasise learning and continuous professional development as a key feature of formative feedback; rather than judging the success or failure of a situation, asking a question like 'what did you learn from this for the next time?' can be both supportive and encourage deeper reflection.

There is no specific formula or one-size-fits-all approach to formative feedback; instead it should be customised to the needs and wants of both the employee and the manager, with an emphasis on keeping it informal, making it conversational, and emphasising collegiality and peer-to-peer interaction rather than top-down managerialism. One approach that some managers find helpful to emphasise education, learning, and conversation, involves the use of three prompting questions rather than simply 'telling' an employee. These three questions usually involve some variation of: a) what did you do well?; b) what could you have done differently?; c) what did you learn from this that will change the way you do things in the future?. This kind of 'questioning' approach allows the employee to actually reflect and talk rather than simply listen to information. The use of three open-ended questions should encourage dialogue and conversation, and the nature of the questions themselves is non-judgmental, emphasising learning and development. Of course, simply repeating these exact three questions each time formative feedback is provided will become stale quite quickly, but the use of open-ended questions oriented toward professional development (rather than 'let me tell you what I think about you') highlights the way in which formative feedback can be implemented.

A crucial element of effective formative feedback involves tone. Tone describes a cluster of verbal and non-verbal communication cues that conveys to one individual the emotional intent and state of the other person involved in the conversation. Tone includes elements such as body language, eye contact, tone of voice, intonation, as well as things such as distractedness. When engaged in formative feedback it is important to actually focus one's attention on the other person; avoid checking a mobile phone, reading another document, or responding to an email. Positive tone means demonstrating clear interest in the other person, and providing them with your undivided attention. Being distracted from a conversation sets a tone and sends a signal of disinterest which means the other person becomes less interested in the content of the conversation itself.

Tone is also conveyed through other non-verbal cues that can sometimes be challenging to consciously manage. For example, in using open-ended reflective questions focused on learning and development, it may happen that the person answering the questions demonstrates erroneous self-assessment or clearly does not understand the point you were hoping to make. In such situations, a 'tell', or subtle non-verbal response (such as a look of surprise or concern on the face, a heavy sigh, or a scowl) can convey a judgement that is the opposite of what formative feedback is supposed to be about. Being particularly attentive to your own non-verbal tells and trying as much as possible to withhold non-verbal judgement is important in delivering truly formative feedback.

Summative feedback

Summative feedback is typically a more formal kind of feedback, focused on the sharing of data or measurements and using this as a foundation for discussing performance. Summative feedback is generally structured with a specific end-point or objective in mind, and is more problem-and-solution focused than formative feedback. Typical sources of data or measurements that are used in summative feedback include dispensing error rates, sick days, frequency of delivery of clinical services such as medication reviews, etc. Such data can be used in a comparative way, to allow the manager to highlight how an individual employee performs vis-à-vis peers, and use this as a springboard for quality improvement discussions.

Summative feedback, by its nature, tends to be less conversational and more formal or managerial in tone. As a result, it can sometimes be more intimidating or frightening for employees. There may be less of a tendency to emphasise self-assessment and self-reflection and instead focus on accurately defining or describing a data-driven, data-identified problem and looking for possible solutions to implement. Care must be taken to not overly formalise summative feedback to the point where it becomes impersonal or even dehumanising. Managers need to recognise the stress that is inherent in summative feedback and continue to use effective listening and other communication tools that reinforce support, care, and concern.

Crucially, it is essential that managers clearly differentiate circumstances where they are providing formative feedback versus times where summative feedback is being delivered. It can be confusing to employees if they are not clear what kind of feedback is being delivered; they may underestimate or overestimate the importance of comments from managers if they are not clear, and this can impair the delivery of successful feedback. Summative feedback is rarely delivered spontaneously or in the spur of the moment: instead, booking a formal time for a conversation, providing data or other information prior to the appointment, and signposting in advance what the conversation is meant to be about, can alert the employee to the more formal nature of summative feedback, as well as give them time to psychologically prepare for the discussion. Further, receptivity to all forms of feedback – and summative feedback in particular – can be diminished if the listener isn't ready to actually hear the message being conveyed. Confirming in advance that the employee actually has the cognitive and emotional capacity to engage in summative feedback is important.

Summative feedback still relies upon the use of open-ended questions and collaboration: it should not be about the manager telling the employee all their deficiencies and then telling them what needs to be changed. Using data as a foundation for defining or describing a problem or situation, then collaborating around potential reasons and solutions is most helpful. Like formative feedback, not all summative feedback should be negative or corrective. Using summative feedback in a positive way, to praise and affirm successes, is important for both morale and the strength of the relationship between manager and employee.

Prior to delivering summative feedback, it is important for managers to carefully plan the direction of conversation, including how data is to be presented in ways that will optimise the likelihood for acceptance and conversation. It is useful for the manager to have an end-game or goal for the conversation in mind, rather than expecting to simply ask the employee 'what are you going to do about this now?' As with formative feedback, attentiveness to tone and non-verbal cues is essential. Wherever possible, summative feedback should be delivered in a private room, away from the earshot of others. Work to minimise distractions and concentrate attention on the individual. Provide time for the individual to hear and process information and ask reflective check-in questions to assess how receptive they are to the data being presented. Be mindful that in cases where data reveals performance gaps, the employee may be experiencing embarrassment or stress – being sensitive to this is important.

Summative feedback can be provided through multiple consecutive meetings rather than all at once. It may be helpful to schedule a first meeting to share data and discuss the 'problem', then give the individual some time to digest and reflect on the conversation before scheduling subsequent meetings to discuss reasons and possible solutions. Trying to do all of this in a single conversation may trigger defensiveness or resistance, and does not give the individual sufficient time to process the data and information being presented. Summative feedback needs to stay focused on data, and not drift into multiple different areas or devolve into personality or trait discussions. Remaining focused should be the responsibility of the manager initiating the discussion, not the employee, and using gentle redirection techniques to ensure everyone stays on task is important.

Annual performance reviews represent one type of summative feedback, but summative feedback should not be a once-a-year event. Instead, establishing a pattern of delivering positive (and where needed, less than positive) summative feedback throughout the year helps employees know you are interested in their work and are actually using data – not simply inference – to help them meet their objectives.

Constructive feedback

Constructive feedback represents a blend of formative and summative feedback mechanisms and is often described as a process of providing employees with observation based comments derived from multiple qualitative and quantitative data sources. It is designed to foster self-reflection, encourage dialogue and stimulate what-if alternative hypothesising using verbal and non-verbal communication techniques that clearly signal support rather than criticism.[1]

Occupational studies across many different fields of work – and from educational programs – indicates that most people feel they do not receive enough feedback about their work to know if they are performing well or not.[13,14] Most of the feedback they receive appears to be summative and negative, thereby making it difficult to positively reinforce the things they are doing well. Worse, this creates a culture where 'feedback' of all sorts is perceived as punitive and corrective. Constructive feedback aims to address this issue by adopting a coaching perspective, using data to highlight issues but emphasising professional and personal development in a non-judgmental, employee-focused way.

Critical to success in constructive feedback is effective and appropriate word choice. In order to maximise opportunities for employees to actually accept, internalise, and ultimately change their behaviour, carefully chosen words are necessary. For example, if a pharmacist is sabotaging team dynamics and relationships by consistently talking over others at meetings or interrupting them, it is important to frame the message positively for constructive feedback. Rather than stating 'you're always interrupting people and they think you're a know-it-all', it would be better to say, 'it's great you are so passionate about your work, but many of us, when we're excited about something, will sometimes forget to leave space for others to share their thoughts too – have you noticed this?' Alternatively, rather than belittle an employee who has a higher-than-average dispensing error rate by saying 'you work too fast and make too many mistakes', it may be more constructive and palatable to say 'I've always been impressed by your big picture thinking. Sometimes when we're so focused on the big picture, it's easy to overlook some of the smaller details – any thoughts on that?' Constructive feedback requires careful word choices that support face-saving in difficult situations. One important word to avoid overusing in constructive feedback is 'you', particularly when that word is connected to accusatory or judgemental elements.[1]

Constructive feedback can sometimes be used to address less concrete performance related elements that are not behavioural but instead rooted in personality or attitude. Great care must be exercised in framing these issues respectfully and supportively, not in ways that are demeaning or dehumanising. Emphasising the notion of being more successful and more capable of achieving and exceeding expectations helps an individual think about these difficult topics in a less threatening manner.

Ultimately, constructive feedback should emphasise the concept of autonomy and provide people with options and choices in terms of changes they want to make. Telling someone to change their behaviour is less likely to succeed than helping that person understand how their behaviour is interfering with success, then developing a menu of options designed to increase the likelihood of success. In constructive feedback, avoid the temptation to come across as an expert who has the right answer, but instead, work collaboratively to strategise around alternatives and options. This often requires considerable pre-planning and deliberation, even rehearsal, in order to minimise the risk that conversations will go in unintended and hurtful directions.

When well delivered, constructive feedback can be one of the greatest gifts a manager can offer an employee, and one of the most impactful interventions managers can make. Planning and attentiveness to verbal and non-verbal communication are essential for successful constructive feedback, and for building stronger relationships. Clearly distinguishing and differentiating between summative, formative, and constructive feedback, and ensuring the employee is clear as to what kind of feedback is being delivered at a specific time, is crucial.[14]

Delivering effective feedback is both an art and a science, and it can take years to practice and develop this important skill. The principles described above are a useful starting point, but all managers spend much of their careers honing and improving. Like their employees, they too will benefit from receiving formative, summative and constructive feedback in order to continuously improve.

Summary

Performance assessment, management, and feedback are crucial parts of a manager's responsibility, but these are not skills that are necessarily easy or natural for many. In most cases, structure, organisation, and planning are required to prevent unanticipated or unwanted consequences of well-meaning but ham-fisted feedback. Careful word choice and attentiveness to verbal and non-verbal communication cues are essential for all forms of performance assessment and feedback. Listening and asking the right kinds of questions can generate productive conversations that allow employees to grow and develop, while simultaneously strengthening relationships with managers.

References

1. Austin Z. *Human Resource Management in Pharmacy: Managing and Motivating Staff to Excel.* Washington DC: American Pharmacists' Association, 2022.

2. Gesme DH, Wiseman M. Performance appraisal: a tool for practice improvement. *J Oncol Pract* 2011; 7(2): 131–134. https://doi.org/10.1200/JOP.2010.000214

3. van Woerkom M, Kroon B. The effects of strengths-based performance appraisal on perceived supervisor support and the motivation to improve performance. *Front Psychol* 2020; 11: 1–12. https://doi.org/10.3389/fpsyg.2020.01883

4. Cappelli P, Conyon MJ. What do performance appraisals do? *ILR Review* 2018; 71(1): 88–116. https://doi.org/10.1177/0019793917698649

5. Balu L. Best practices in performance appraisal. In: SDM Institute for Management Development. *6th International Conference on Managing Human Resources in the Workplace.* Mysore, 2017.

6. Sanchez CR *et al.* Does effectiveness in performance appraisal improve with rater training? *PLoS ONE* [online] 2019; 14(9): e0222694. https://doi.org/10.1371/journal.pone.0222694

7. Brown TC *et al.* Performance management: a scoping review of the literature and an agenda for future research. *Human Resource Development Review* 2019; 18(1): 47–82. https://doi.org/10.1177/1534484318798533

8. Talbot C. Performance Management. In: Ferlie E *et al.* eds. *The Oxford Handbook of Public Management.* Oxford: Oxford University Press, 2007: 491–518. https://doi.org/10.1093/oxfordhb/9780199226443.003.0022

9. Awan S *et al.* Effectiveness of performance management systems for employee performance through engagement. *SAGE Open* 2020; 10(4). https://doi.org/10.1177/2158244020969383

10. Osmani F, Maliqi G. Performance management, its assessment and importance. *Procedia – Social and Behavioural Sciences* 2012; 41: 434–441. https://doi.org/10.1016/j.sbspro.2012.04.052

11. Aghera A *et al.* A randomized trial of SMART goal enhanced debriefing after simulation to promote educational actions. *West J Emerg Med* 2018; 19(1): 112–120. https://doi.org/10.5811/westjem.2017.11.36524

12. Society for Human Resource Management (SHRM) (2022). *Performance Improvement Plans (PIP).* Society for Human Resource Management (SHRM). https://www.shrm.org/resourcesandtools/tools-and-samples/exreq/pages/details.aspx?erid=586

13. Gnepp J *et al.* The future of feedback: motivating performance through future-focused feedback. *PLoS ONE* [online] 2020; 15(6): e0234444. https://doi.org/10.1371/journal.pone.0234444

14. Auh S *et al.* Frontline employee feedback-seeking behaviour: how is it formed and when does it matter? *J Service Research* 2018; 22(1): 44–59. https://doi.org/10.1177/1094670518779462

CHAPTER 11

Creating and managing high performance teams

Upon completion of this chapter you should be able to:

- define what is a high performance team
- understand the role of a manager in creating high performance teams
- detail how managers aid the formation of a high performance team
- list the characteristics of team dysfunction that a manager should monitor for
- explain the influence of managerial mindsets in supporting high performance teams.

In almost all organisations today, individuals work in groups (or teams) to meet objectives, share workloads, and contribute complementary skills and talents.[1] A crucial task for managers involves creating and managing teams that work effectively, efficiently, and harmoniously in order to achieve strategic objectives and organisational targets.[2] Within a professional workforce involving pharmacists and regulated pharmacy technicians, 'creating' teams does not mean simply throwing random individuals together based on credentials and expecting it to all work out, and 'managing' teams does not work if it is based on top-down authoritarian decision making.[3] A central management principle of a professional workforce is the role of the manager in creating conditions that allow for the fullest expression of each team member's talents, strengths and interests.[4] Motivation and engagement are essential to professional work – and creating and managing teams means finding ways of determining, channelling and supporting each individual's talents and aspirations in ways that align with organisational priorities and objectives.

What is a 'high performance team'?

A team is generally defined as a group of people working together to accomplish objectives beyond individual self-interest or gain; from this perspective it is clear that not all groups are actually teams.[1,5] Further, placing different individuals together and simply expecting them to 'figure it out' and work as a team is both unrealistic and unhelpful. Learning to transcend individual self-interest and work effectively towards common goals and objectives – rather than simply following orders from above – is difficult but essential for organisational success.

'High performance' teams demonstrate several key attributes, including:[3]

- members possess an internalised sense of purpose aligned with organisational goals
- each member has a bond with and commitment to other team members – and a desire to see them succeed
- members recognise that their personal success is contingent upon the success of others in the team – when one team member succeeds, the entire team succeeds
- a clear understanding of each others' responsibilities and roles
- a personalised sense of accountability to other team members to perform to the best of each individual's capabilities
- a diverse range of skills, education, background, life-experiences, and interests that complement one another
- a shared sense of interdependence
- trust in one another
- predictability, stability, and an ability to cohere as a team over time.

As can be seen, many of the attributes of a high performance team are strongly emotional in nature: a sense of accountability, trust, and interdependence all speak to intangible but essential human factors that govern how effectively individuals can work together. These intangible but essential qualities can make creation, formation, management and motivation of high performance teams challenging as the inherently qualitative nature of human inter-relationships makes quantitative measurement and approaches difficult.[3]

Despite these difficulties, the reality in all types of organisations today is that teamwork is central to modern life – including workplaces and health care. High performance teams have significant advantages over the work of individuals because each team member can contribute unique ideas, talents, skills, and viewpoints.[6]

Creating high performance teams

One of the most important tasks of management involves hiring and assembling workplace teams. In virtually all organisations, each new person who is hired becomes a member of an existing team. The hiring process frequently involves careful scrutiny of 'fit' – the extent to which a prospective new employee has values, behaviours, and attitudes that align with existing cultural norms and expectations in the workplace. In many cases, managers focus on 'fit' more than they may on qualifications or technical skills: in some cases, this can lead to bias in hiring or blatant discrimination (for example, when internationally educated health care professionals with superior qualifications, are denied jobs because they did not graduate or qualify from 'here').[6]

Organisational psychologists have identified the central, pivotal role of creating a shared vision and articulating common goals, as key to the creation of high performance teams.[7] Through the hiring and team creation processes, managers need to emphasise these rather than focus on processes and procedures. Within a pharmacy context, this means clearly and boldly articulating a vision or an ideal of why the organisation exists and what it is setting out to do for its communities. Unfortunately, many managers may have difficulty in this area, and instead overemphasise procedural issues or day to day logistical challenges in the hiring decision. A key finding of research in teamwork highlights the problems that arise when managers focus on details and dictate or micromanage processes: it leads individuals to simply lose interest in broader organisational goals and priorities, and assume a more passive 'tell me what hoop you want me to jump through, and I'll jump' role in the organisation.[8,9]

Micromanagement is toxic to high performance teams because it removes opportunities for individuals to actually share their talents, skills, and experiences and drive innovation.[9] Micro-management is incapable of actually focusing on vision and shared goals as it is too preoccupied with immediate details and problems. In contrast, managers who create high performance teams start with the belief that individual team members working together can unleash their own talents more effectively to solve logistical issues and problems, and in the process, this creates a psychological energy within the team that heightens interpersonal connectivity, interdependence, and trust.[3]

Creating high performance teams relies heavily on managers modelling the interdependence and trust they expect of their team members. Managers recognise that their success in an organisation is directly connected to the productivity and outputs of the teams they manage: in some cases, this leads managers to fret and micromanage as a way of controlling outcomes. In contrast, managers who trust their teams to deliver outcomes recognise their personal interdependence with these team members, and create psychological conditions for each team member to trust in return.

For managers who can overcome the tendency to micromanage, this means clear and transparent communication, respectful and affirming feedback, and intentional emphasis on motivating and engaging team members rather than simply 'telling' them what to do. Especially in the context of a professional workforce as in health care and pharmacy, telling or ordering educated and skilled individuals will simply lead to disengagement, demotivation, and suboptimal outcomes in return. For managers, this means intentional and mindful self-reflection and constant vigilance to ensure micromanagement tendencies are held in check, and that big picture, vision and goals thinking and conversations, guide the creation of teams.

The formation of high performance teams

Effective managers recognise the importance of their own mindset in creating high performance teams, but also acknowledge that the process of team formation is not random or unstructured. While micromanagement can be problematic, simply leaving team members to their own devices to 'figure it all out' can result in issues. Tuckman has described the process of team formation using five different stages, each of which provides managers with unique and important opportunities to support and – where appropriate – intervene to create better outcomes.[10]

1. *Forming:* The forming stage of team development involves the initial 'getting-to-know-you' process where individuals, who are strangers to one another, are sussing each other out, learning about each others values, interests, and strengths, and trying to develop a team culture. Forming can be difficult because each individual may have their own preconceptions about what the team is supposed to do, how they are supposed to interact with each other, and what the culture and rules governing interactions should be. During the forming stage, there is generally a need for managers to be directly involved and present, as a way of transmitting and reinforcing broader organisational cultural norms and objectives to the team. It may also be necessary during forming for managers to ensure that the more naturally extroverted, talkative or Converger type

of team member, does not dominate at the expense of others. Managers can support forming by modelling inclusivity and effective listening, by clearly articulating organisational values and cultural norms (and enforcing these), and checking in with all team members regularly to ensure they feel heard, cared for, and cared about. This may require more time and attention early in the team formation process as individual team members test boundaries of acceptable behaviour with one another and simply start to learn about, and from, their team colleagues.

2. *Storming:* The second stage of team development is often characterised by the testing of boundaries, conflict and disagreement, and management challenges. As forming proceeds, individual team members start to define for themselves where boundaries exist and what cultural rules or norms are dominant. In many cases, there will be a desire to test these boundaries, and this can lead to discord. During the storming phase, managers need to be vigilant and ready to intervene in ways that do not demonstrate favouritism but instead are clearly and consistently linked to organisational values, mission, and vision. Failure to intervene in a timely manner can send the wrong message and can demotivate individuals and lead to further storming. Finding a balanced and consistent way to support proportionate and reasonable testing of team and organisational boundaries as a prelude to innovation, without permitting a free-for-all undisciplined team culture, can be difficult but is helpful in building a high performance team.

3. *Norming:* The third stage of team development involves the acceptance and firming of a unique team culture that should be aligned (but somewhat distinct from) broader organisational norms. Where team culture is too tightly aligned with the rest of the organisation, it may be a symptom of micromanagement. This can lead to the squelching of innovation as individuals are simply aping what they see around them, rather than positively contributing to the emergence of a new team dynamic. In contrast, where the norming phase involves the emergence of a team culture that is significantly misaligned with organisational values and norms, this may be a sign that greater manager involvement and direction is needed and that 'storming' has been unsuccessful. Finding the right balance to encourage innovation can be tricky, but is usually clear during the norming stage. In this stage, managers may find that they are less involved and spend less time directly with their teams, but they need to be ready to quickly intervene in a clear and principled manner as boundaries are pushed and tested. During norming, interpersonal relationships amongst team members will solidify and mature, and this can help support further evolution of the team and productivity in the future.

4. *Performing:* During the first three stages of team development, managers are usually required to be more present and involved, closely monitoring and carefully navigating different situations in a balanced and proportionate way. Knowing when to be directive and when to allow the team to sort itself out is a managerial art that takes patience, reliance on observation, and continued commitment to a positive mindset. During the performing stage of team development, the dividend of this work and insight should become apparent. In performing, teams have developed a positive group culture that is sufficiently aligned with organisational values and norms, but still leaves scope for individual expression and innovation. With performing teams, managers often find it is possible to have minimal day to day oversight or contact and trust teams to simply get on with their tasks. In this stage, it is still essential that mangers find effective ways of recognising, rewarding, motivating, and engaging team members. A significant risk during performing is that team members start to feel stagnant or bored and may look for other

opportunities or jobs, thereby dismantling the team. Managers working with teams at this stage need to develop techniques for refreshing enthusiasm, and recognising the value and impact of both individual team members and the collective output of the group.

5. *Adjourning:* The final stage of team development represents moments where teams experience transitions, usually due to people leaving jobs, changing roles, retiring, or in other ways changing the structure of the team. Adjourning refers to the process by which the collective self-identity of the team must constantly evolve, as the context and environment around the team changes and as its internal members move on. It is important for managers to be present and fully engaged during adjourning: team members who are accustomed to performing may experience doubt, fear, and anxiety during these transitions. One person leaving a team can quickly become a mass exodus if other team members feel their best days are behind them and new opportunities await. Skilful management of these emotional responses of remaining team members is essential, along with ongoing commitments to motivation, engagement, reward, and inspiration. Managers need to provide reassurance that even though a team may be changing, their high performance can continue albeit with a different team configuration.

The team evolution process is continual, but managers have different roles to play during the process. Skilful, balanced, and proportionate interventions at different stages of team evolution can help accelerate progress towards high performance; of course, micromanagement, ham-fisted, or impersonal/formulaic responses can alienate and demotivate individual team members and result in underperformance. Adjusting management roles and interventions based on the stage of team formation is crucial, along with ongoing commitments to a trusting/interdependent mindset, and alignment to broader organisational values, mission, vision, and goals.

What can go wrong with teams – and what managers can do

At any point in the team formation process – but more likely prior to performing – teams may encounter difficult situations that threaten common vision and may undermine a collective culture.[11] There are several characteristics that may be early warning indicators of team dysfunction that can undermine performance; managers need to be attuned to these characteristics and utilise effective redirection strategies to help teams re-establish positive forward momentum.[12,13,14]

- *Non-participation:* When team dynamics and processes evolve in a way where individual team members are disengaging and not actually contributing to discussions, activities, or decision making, it is often an indication of disgruntlement. While interpersonal differences (e.g. introverts versus extroverts) may influence, to some degree, the pattern and extent of contributions to a team, all team members – regardless of emotional intelligence – should have pathways available within the team to freely express, dissent, and fully participate. Where non-participation is observed by a manager, it should not be discounted, or ignored, but actively pursued. Speaking to the non-participating team members is essential, to understand their perspectives and experiences and to identify options for addressing this issue. It is equally important to speak with more dominant members of the team to understand their perspectives. Ultimately, the manager should try to find solutions based on the common understanding that all team members should and are expected to participate fully in the team. Rather than finding blame or fault with individuals, exploring reasons and barriers to full participation should be the objective. As a manager, a non-negotiable 'bottom-line' expectation of full and free participation can provide motivation for all team members to address the barriers collectively rather than focusing on personality differences.

- *Ineffective intra-team communication:* In virtually all teams, communication is the lifeblood that sustains relationships and drives productivity. Managers may observe a variety of different 'pathologies' in team dynamics and communications that can be early warning indicators of team dysfunction; frequently, communication problems are the starting point for broader interpersonal problems that can extend the storming period and prevent norming and performing. Examples of ineffective communication in teams include: a) hogging, or the tendency for one or a few individuals to constantly dominate conversations and meetings; b) fogging, or the use of vague terms and commitments as a way of hiding true opinions and beliefs; c) frogging, or the tendency to jump from one topic to another in a disorganised or illogical way, as a technique to avoid conflict or making decisions; d) flogging, or a team's need to constantly second guess its decisions and behaviours and unhelpfully revisit previous actions without productive outcomes; e) bogging, or the inability of a team to find consensus on difficult issues, or to 'get over' previous disagreements by continuing to hold grudges with one another and attempt to get even; and f) 'dead buffalo sitting in the middle of a table', or the tendency of teams to ignore obvious interpersonal and communication problems within the group, hoping they will magically disappear. Team managers should pay close attention to both the quality and quantity of communication between and amongst team members as it can provide a useful insight into the health of a team's dynamic. When communication problems such as these are noted, it is imperative that they not be overlooked or laughed off – small communication problems often presage bigger team dysfunctions. Equally, it is essential that managers do not over-react and instead be proportionate and balanced in how they address these issues: attempting to micromanage communication problems will alienate the entire team and produce subversive responses. In most cases, individual conversations with team members to allow confidential and safe exploration of issues, followed by full team meetings to report and discuss ways of addressing problems, can be useful, but only if individual team members are confident that their honest discussions with the manager will remain confidential. Rather than the manager 'solving' the team's problems, there should be a focus on presenting data to the team, then facilitating a discussion that allows them to determine options for solving their own problems.
- *Lack of inclusivity:* Modern workplaces are characterised by the diversity of the workforce. High performing teams recognise that team diversity is a characteristic of success and should be valued. Where interpersonal tension arises in ways that exclude, marginalise or diminish others because of who they are, there is a need for managers to act in a principled manner. Lamentably, there may still be individuals (even with professional designations) who hold unacceptable personal biases and treat individuals from historically disadvantaged communities in unprofessional ways. In some cases, these individuals may be savvy enough to not be obvious or overt, but still clearly demonstrate disdain through application of microaggressions. Lack of inclusivity and acceptance of microaggressions within a team

dynamic, are signals that the team is dysfunctional. In most organisations, human rights legislations and corporate policies will be relevant and may override the manager's capacity to manage these issues informally. Where discrimination (overt or subtle) exists, zero tolerance for this behaviour is essential. Where team behaviours do not rise to this level – but inclusivity is still lacking – managers have professional and moral responsibilities to intervene in constructive ways. Most often, this means engaging in dialogue, modelling inclusivity, and using performance management techniques to ensure appropriate behaviour prevails. In some cases, there may be a need for stronger managerial action, including discipline or, where needed, termination. Inclusivity in workplace teams is a strong signal of not only the health of teams but also the quality of organisational culture, and should be monitored and defended accordingly.

- *Inability to manage conflicts effectively:* Dissent and disagreement are part of human life and part of any team's work. Through the process of addressing dissent, better outcomes frequently emerge because different perspectives are valued and considered. Managers need to be vigilant and carefully monitor – without actually getting directly involved in – the ways their teams manage their own disagreements. Key indicators include the way dissent is communicated (verbally versus non-verbally), how team members take turns expressing their views, and what processes are used to address disagreement (e.g. majority-wins versus trying to find compromise solutions). Equally important will be teams where conflict and disagreement never occurs – the absence of conflict is often a worrying sign of team dysfunction. In some cases, this might mean people are disengaged and simply don't care enough to disagree with one another, or that domineering individuals on the team have complete control so dissent is not allowed. Dissent, disagreement, and conflict are all natural and expected parts of all human interactions, including workplace teams. Managers should neither expect nor want to eliminate conflict; instead, the objective should be productive management of conflict in ways that do not impact group cohesion or engagement. Where issues with conflict exist within teams, it is important that managers find ways of understanding individual team member's perspectives and experiences in a safe and confidential manner, then find ways of engaging the entire team in group directed problem-solving, focused on transparency and effective communication when disagreements occur.

- *Problems in decision making:* In most organisations, teams are trusted (and expected) to not simply discuss and debate issues but actually make decisions and act on them. It is important for managers to understand team-based decision making processes to ensure they are appropriate, proportionate and aligned with organisational values and objectives. Sometimes, teams may make decisions too quickly without adequate deliberation, often resulting in a 'risky shift' (the tendency of teams to make decisions that are actually more risky than any single individual might make, because of the perception that no individual is actually responsible). In other situations, teams may become paralysed and unable to make decisions at all, constantly referring back to the manager to decide on their behalf. In both cases, this represents a team dysfunction that needs to be addressed by the manager. In cases where teams demonstrate problematic decision making, it is essential that managers do not resort to micromanagement or take on the role of making decisions instead of the team – doing so renders the team somewhat useless. Instead, an approach that allows the manager to reflect back to the team what processes they are using for decision making – and how these may or may not be most appropriate – can help the team openly discuss how to improve to allow for more independent, effective, and efficient decision making in the future. It is important to recognise that there is no one-size-fits-all decision making model that works for a team in all cases: sometimes a consensual approach involving compromise may be appropriate, while in other cases, a majority-wins approach may also be appropriate. In general, it is important that – regardless of the decision or the outcome – all team members felt they had an opportunity to contribute to conversation and present their views freely as a way of signalling inclusivity and being valued by other team members.

Managerial mindset for high performance teams

As has been described in this chapter, one of the most important lessons for managers with respect to the creation, formation, and management of high performance teams, involves their own self-perception of what it means to 'manage' or 'lead' a group of professionals. Managers have an enormous influence on the development of a nascent team culture and team dynamics.

A managerial mindset to support high performing teams is difficult and complex. Team managers are rarely presented in a heroic or positive way; where books, movies, plays or television shows portray team mangers, it is often in a comedic, disparaging, or disdainful way. Managers are often seen to be enabling others' bad behaviours or covering up nefarious schemes. There is an entire franchise of movies titled 'Horrible Bosses' and in both the UK and the USA, the television programme 'The Office' depicts team management in less than flattering ways. While it may be tempting to believe all managers are narcissistic and horrible, the reality is that teams do need leaders. A 2021 study described an experiment in which teams took part in an 'escape room' challenge, in which the team had to solve clues to find a secret exit under time pressured conditions.[15] Some groups were asked to nominate team managers in advance of the task, while other groups were manager-less. Over 63% of those teams with a manager completed the task, while only 44% of those without managers were successful. From this study we can see that while management may be a thankless task at times, it is necessary and managers do not have an easy job. In the context of managing high performance teams, this can mean having to meet unreasonable expectations of those below and those above, whilst always maintaining a positive attitude and a smile.

As noted in this chapter, a managerial mindset for high performance teams involves a carefully calibrated balancing act. It means shifting away from attitudes and behaviours associated with micromanagement and task-dictation, and towards granting team members greater freedom to meet outcome objectives without having processes dictated in advance. A managerial mindset means demonstrating you care for and are concerned about each team member as an individual, but still be willing to draw lines in the sand and potentially dismiss individuals who demonstrate behaviours at odds with organisational values. A consistent practice for those with a managerial mindset is willingness to listen and suspend judgement until multiple data sources confirm a belief. Perhaps most central to this mindset, is the recognition that managers of high performing teams cannot – and should not – solve the team's problems for them, but instead should support the team in collectively determining the best pathways forward. This can be challenging because, in many cases, team members may simply assume that 'good' managers solve all their problems. Resisting the temptation to intervene and micromanage, and instead working to empower and motivate team members to determine their own problems and find their own solutions, is one of the most important ways that managers can help create, nurture, and manage their teams to perform to the best of their potential.

Summary

High performance teams are the cornerstone of organisational success in most workplaces today, and managers of teams have complex and sometimes contradictory roles and responsibilities in creating, supporting and nurturing them. A managerial mindset focused on empowerment rather than ordering, and focused on motivation rather than punishment, can help unleash the potential of individuals and the collective power of a team. There are times and circumstances where proportionate and appropriate redirection techniques will be necessary to help teams evolve in a productive manner; recognising and responding appropriately in these circumstances is essential, and requires managers to find the right balance between team control and team autonomy.

References

1. Cohen P, Levesque H. Teamwork. *Nous* 1991; 25(4): 487–512. https://doi.org/10.2307/2216075

2. Tarricone P, Luca J. Successful teamwork: a case study. In: *Quality Conversations, Proceedings of the 25th HERDSA Conference*. Perth: Higher Education Research and Development Society of Australasia, Inc, 2002: 640–646.

3. Austin Z. *Human resources management in pharmacy: managing and motivating staff to excel.* Washington DC: American Pharmacists' Association, 2022.

4. Rosen MA *et al*. Teamwork in healthcare: key discoveries enabling safer, high-quality care. *American Psychologist* 2018; 73(4): 433–450. https://doi.org/10.1037/amp0000298

5. Schmutz J *et al*. How effective is teamwork really? The relationship between teamwork and performance in healthcare teams: a systematic review and meta analysis. *BMJ Open* 2019; 9(9): e028280. https://10.1136/bmjopen-2018-028280

6. Williams J, Mihaylo S. How the best bosses interrupt bias on their teams. *Harvard Business Review* [online] 2019. https://hbr.org/2019/11/how-the-best-bosses-interrupt-bias-on-their-teams

7. Somboonpakorn A, Kantabutra S. Shared leadership and shared vision as predictors for team learning process, synergy and effectiveness in the healthcare industry. *Int J Innovation and Learning* 2014; 16(4): 384–416. https://doi.org/10.1504/IJIL.2014.065545

8. Collins SK, Collins KS. Micromanagement – a costly management style. *Radiol Manage* 2002; 24(6): 32–35.

9. Delgado O *et al*. Micromanagement: when to avoid it and how to use it effectively. *Am J Health Syst Pharmacy* 2015; 72(10): 772–776. https://doi.org/10.2146/ajhp140125

10. Tuckman B, Jensen M. Stages of small-group development revisited. *Group and Organization Studies* 1977; 2(4): 419–427. https://doi.org/10.1177/105960117700200404

11. Lencioni P. *The Five Dysfunctions of a Team: A leadership fable*. New York: Jossey-Bass, 2002.

12. Clutterbuck D. Towards a pragmatic model of team function and dysfunction. In: Clutterbuck D *et al*. eds. *The Practitioner's Handbook of Team Coaching*, 1st edn. London: Routledge Press, 2019.

13. Greer L *et al*. The dysfunctions of power in teams: A review and emergent conflict perspective. *Research in Organizational Behaviour* 2017; 37: 103–124. https://doi.org/10.1016/j.riob.2017.10.005

14. Coutu D. Why teams don't work. *Harvard Business Review Magazine* [online] 2009. https://hbr.org/2009/05/why-teams-dont-work

15. London School of Economics and Political Science (2023). *Do escape rooms help understand workplace behaviours?* London: London School of Economics and Political Science. https://www.lse.ac.uk/PBS/News/Press-release/Do-escape-rooms-help-understand-workplace-behaviour

CHAPTER 12

Challenges in human resource management

Upon completion of this chapter you should be able to:

- understand why managers can find human resource challenges difficult
- list the principles for the management of difficult situations
- explain the role of managers in handling workplace incivility
- detail the principles involved in investigating workplace bullying
- discuss the role of managers in the implementation of reasonable accommodation requests
- understand how to manage mental health issues in the workplace.

For many pharmacists, one of the major barriers to considering a managerial role are the responsibilities associated with difficult human resource situations.[1] Anyone who has ever worked in an organisation before, recognises the complex nature of workplace relationships and the difficulties that can occur when strong personalities collide, mental health issues affect colleagues, or toxic workplace situations, such as bullying, escalate.[2] Some pharmacists will specifically avoid all managerial responsibilities simply due to a lack of confidence in their own abilities to deal with these difficult, interpersonal situations.[3]

It is important to recognise that difficult situations are to be expected and are somewhat routine for managers in all fields. It is equally important to not catastrophise, over-emphasise, or amplify/distort the 'unsolvability' of these difficult problems.

Why do managers find human resource challenges so difficult, and what can they do about it?

Management, by its very nature, involves problem-solving and compromise.[4] Certain management problems may be more technical in their orientation (for example, budget allocations or technology purchase decisions) and as a result may be very important, but may not have the same emotional weight as human resource challenges. Most managers find human resource challenges the most difficult to deal with, precisely because other people are so directly involved.[5] The social and interpersonal nature of human resource challenges means that strong emotional responses – in both managers and staff members involved – are inevitable. It is this emotional entanglement that can make lucid decision making difficult and can influence people negatively away from management careers altogether.[5,6]

The ways in which emotions govern our perceptions of a situation, our prioritising of issues, and our analysis of alternatives, can be significant. For example, as noted in Chapter 2, the emotional intelligence of many pharmacists inclines them towards perfectionism and a strong need to be liked by others. Solutions to most human resource challenges will never be perfect and will often result in some individual or groups being angry or disliking the manager. Failure to recognise how one's own emotional state, biases, and assumptions influence or impact on decision making can result in poor judgment – for example, thinking that the best answer is to simply avoid conflict entirely and ignore a situation, hoping that it will magically disappear.

Successful management of human resource challenges requires managers to be self-aware and constantly engaged in self-monitoring of their own emotional state and responses to difficult conversations and situations. Responding emotionally to a negative comment, or overly-personalising disrespectful, non-verbal communication can escalate problematic situations, leaving both the manager and the staff members feeling even more angry, helpless, and demoralised.

Self-monitoring of emotional state and response is a skill and competency that can be learned, rehearsed and improved. It generally begins with a form of reflection that emphasises clear diagnosis or assessment of one's mood and state of mind. One of the challenges all human beings (including managers) face in dealing with strong emotions, is that they rarely come with a guidebook. Inaccurate labelling of an emotional state can lead to the wrong thing being said or unhelpful behaviour being demonstrated. For example, if a manager needs to decide who must work on Christmas Day, an unpopular decision will, in all likelihood, have to be made. If a staff member who is assigned to work Christmas Day sneers or expresses unhappiness at that decision, it may be easy for the manager to mis-diagnose this response as 'you don't like me' as opposed to 'you don't like the decision I had to make'. The emotional experience of 'you don't like me' can be devastating: it can bring back memories of alienation in childhood, or surface negative self-esteem issues. If the manager frames the response in such personal terms, they are likely to become defensive, depressed, anxious or angry. In contrast, if the same response from the staff member is framed as 'you don't like the decision I had to make', this implies 'a difficult decision had to be made, there was no alternative, I'm sorry it had to be you, but we need to move on'. It is neither the manager's fault nor the manager's personality defect that produced the outcome – it simply was a hard decision someone needed to make (and that someone happened to be the manager).

The way managers frame responses, interactions, and interpersonal communication is integral to successful management of the manager's own emotional response. This response, in turn, will greatly influence whether difficult situations escalate further and provoke even stronger emotional responses. Learning to accurately assess and appropriately frame one's own emotional response when dealing with difficult situations is central to helping better control and manage emotion laden interpersonal communication. Using self-reflection as a way of guiding one's thinking, and running through alternative rationales to explain what is being observed, can help emotionally de-escalate complex situations and allow managers to focus on problems, not personalities, and find acceptable solutions, not perfect answers.[7,8]

One particular challenge – especially for young managers – is the tendency to ruminate about difficult situations. Rumination describes a psychological state in which individuals shift beyond productive reflection and self-assessment, and instead end up fixated or overly focused on details in an unhelpful manner.[9] Rumination involves replaying – over and over again – specific conversations or actions in a vain attempt to find perfect solutions for imperfect situations. Rumination is cognitively and emotionally exhausting, and over time can lead to mental health challenges for the manager.[10] Breaking the cycle of rumination can be difficult but most frequently requires external support or help – for example, a sympathetic friend, a supportive peer, or a supervisor that can be trusted. Most pharmacists have high personal quality standards and can have difficulty accepting imperfect compromises. If at risk of rumination, these individuals may sometimes need 'permission' from a trusted person to simply let go of failures and accept that in most cases, 'good enough is good enough'. Recognising for oneself the trap, risk, and experience of unhelpful rumination is also important: classic symptoms of rumination include difficulty sleeping, concentrating, or eating, turning to substances (alcohol, illicit drugs), or disproportionate emotional outbursts at innocent bystanders (e.g. family members, friends, or other staff who are not involved in the problematic situation). When such behaviours start to occur, finding techniques to stop the rumination cycle will be essential to avoid exacerbating problems further.

Principles for the management of difficult situations

There are some general principles for managing human resource challenges that are usually applicable to most situations. These principles include transparency, objectivity, impartiality, and fairness.

- *Transparency:* Rules, policies, and procedures that guide workplace decision making need to be clear to everyone so that individual preferences or biases do not influence decision making. Transparency requires that policies and procedures for dealing with difficult situations (e.g. workplace bullying) are written in plain language so they are easily understood, exist as a policy and not just in someone's head as an idea, and are easily accessible to everyone. It also requires that where staff members have concerns or problems, there is a clear and established pathway for raising them in a respectful way with managers and others. For example, if a pharmacist is concerned that a staff member may be arriving at work drunk – but has no specific data or evidence to prove this – what are the pathways for raising the concern without being accused of bullying, harassment or over-reacting? Being transparent both in processes and as processes are being applied/implemented, is essential.
- *Objectivity:* Consistency of decision making across different situations is crucial and a hallmark of objectivity. Individuals need to believe that they will be treated in substantially similar ways to others, and not targeted/singled out because of who they are. Depersonalising problems means focusing on behaviours, not personalities. For example, different individuals may have different personalities – some may be quieter while others are gregarious, and some may be more direct/forceful in communication while others are more indirect/circumspect. Direct communicators can sometimes come across as intimidating or bullying even though they do not intend this. Rather than framing this situation as 'you are too intense and need to dial it back!', it is more objective to state 'overly direct communication can interfere with the listener's ability to hear and internalise the message being conveyed'. The first way emphasises a personality defect while the second focuses on a behaviour and its impact. Objectivity in communication means avoiding focus on personality traits and instead emphasising how specific behaviours influence outcomes.

- *Impartiality:* Decisions made by managers need to be free of bias, and this requires managers to carefully reflect and honestly acknowledge implicit or explicit biases that may be tainting interpretations of a difficult situation. Sources of bias could include previous personal ties/relationships to staff members involved in a disagreement, inappropriate stereotyping based on sex, gender identity, sexual orientation, or ethnicity/race, or beliefs about the connection between intelligence/competency and level of education. Strategies for better managing impartiality often include specific training of individuals, or the use of committees to make decisions rather than individuals. Development of clear and transparent policies and procedures using checklists are also a useful tool for enhancing impartiality, as this can reduce the likelihood of subjectivity or personal preference inappropriately distorting decision making.
- *Fairness:* It is often difficult to precisely define fairness, but most people recognise when managers are being unfair. Fairness speaks to issues of policies, processes and procedures being proportionate and equitably applied. It also speaks to recognising that not everyone starts from the same position of privilege, incorporating principles of justice, diversity, equity, and inclusivity in decision making (described in Chapter 8). Fairness also means managers must be efficient in gathering information and making decisions, and must focus only on the issues at hand rather than broaden inquiries in an uncomfortable manner.

Adherence to these four principles can improve confidence and skills in managing difficult situations, and improve outcomes for everyone.

Microaggressions and workplace incivility

Like all human relationships, workplace colleagues must find ways of interacting with one another productively. The social lubricant of interpersonal relationships is civility, a form of politeness and courtesy in behaviour and speech. Importantly, civility need not necessarily cover thinking and beliefs: for example, individuals who have negative opinions about certain groups can still behave in a respectful, polite and civil way towards these individuals.

Microaggression describes recurrent or occasional verbal, behavioural, or environmental actions (whether deliberate or unintentional) that communicate derogatory, demeaning, or unfairly aggressive attitudes rooted in stigma of historically marginalised groups.[11] Microaggressions can, at times, have a veneer of positivity despite the inherent derogatory nature of the action: for example, saying to a colleague, 'my goodness you speak English so well considering where you came from' is exclusionary and insulting. Other examples may include statements like, 'wow, those Asians are so great at math!'. Importantly, microaggressions may not be deliberate on the part of the speaker but still have the effect of dehumanising the recipient of the comment. It can be a challenge to address microaggressions due to the high level of emotions and feelings for both the speaker and the recipient of the comment.[12]

Workplace incivility is usually described as a pattern of relatively low but increasingly frequent negative or anti-social behaviours towards individuals or groups with ambiguous intention to harm, dehumanise, or demoralise. Uncivil behaviours are usually rude and discourteous but may not rise to the level of downright offensive or illegal. They are management challenges because they trigger strong emotional responses, can escalate quickly, but are infrequent, subtle, and ambiguous enough that they often fall through the cracks of existing policies related to harassment. Examples of workplace incivility could include verbal or non-verbal communication that indicates lack of respect for individuals who require dedicated prayer times and space, or demeaning comments regarding reasonable accommodation for a disability, or refusal to address a colleague by a preferred pronoun. The problem of workplace incivility has grown dramatically in the last few years, with over 70% of American workers indicating they had personally witnessed or been the victim of incivility. Incivility has negative impacts on workplace culture, productivity, employee outcome and can lead to burnout, resignation, increased errors, and organisational dysfunction.[13]

The challenge in managing workplace incivility is its ambiguous nature and that in many cases individual uncivil actions – viewed in isolation – may not rise to the threshold required in policy and procedure for disciplinary action. A person using a homophobic slur to describe a colleague would definitely be disciplined – but what about a person who refuses to acknowledge a colleague's same-sex spouse but doesn't actually say or do anything more than ignore them?

Managers may be tempted to overlook or shrug shoulders at individual incidents of incivility or microaggression, but this is a mistake, as it risks escalating or giving a 'free pass' to further incivility. A key strategy in managing workplace incivility is to respect and accept the victim's account of the situation and then to be systematic, transparent, impartial, and fair in gathering data and analysing a situation. Clear documentation of incidents over time can help build a paper trail to demonstrate that incivility is not a single occurrence but a disturbing pattern. Triangulating experiences by gathering corroborating evidence from others can help enhance impartiality and objectivity of analysis. Ensuring all parties involved in the incivility accusation (the accuser and the accused) are aware of the situation and are aware that data is being gathered, can also help to prevent minor incivility from escalating further.

The key to effective management of workplace incivility is to not wilfully ignore or overlook small or microaggressions, hoping they will go away. Equally, it is important to not laugh-off problems and provide advice to 'toughen up' to the victim. These avoidance techniques send strong messages of acceptance of incivility throughout the organisation and will result in escalation. Using triangulated data of specific occurrences that focus on behaviour (not just beliefs) conforming to principles of objectivity, transparency, impartiality, and fairness to both parties, is essential. Equally important is the need to be aware that clear violations of human rights or workplace regulations must be swiftly and clearly dealt with in unambiguous terms.

Bullying

When poorly managed, workplace incivility can produce conditions that lead to workplace bullying, defined as a persistent pattern of mistreatment in the workplace causing physical and emotional harm. In most cases, bullying relies upon a variety of verbal, non-verbal, and psychological abuse techniques aimed at diminishing or dehumanising others.[14] Workplace bullies can often accomplish their aims covertly, making it difficult for managers to actually observe specific instances in real time. Researchers suggest historically disadvantaged groups – for example, women, LGBTQ2S+, new immigrants, BIPOC/ BAME members, or disabled individuals – are at highest risk of workplace bullying but equally may be the least likely to ask for help or defend themselves.[15] Studies in both Europe and North America suggest that 10–15% of the workforce has experienced bullying to varying degrees.[16]

Unlike incivility or microaggression, bullying is usually (but not always) more overt, consistent, and threatening. Examples of bullying workplace behaviour can include spreading untrue and malicious innuendo/gossip about a colleague, excluding or isolating an individual socially or professionally, the use of physical means to intimidate, undermining an individual's reputation or authority, establishing impossible deadlines or outcomes that set individuals up to fail, or using profanity or discriminatory language. In group meetings, bullying will often involve interrupting or preventing individuals from getting a point across, the use of dismissive or dehumanising language in expressing disagreement (e.g. 'that's a dumb idea, only an idiot would say that!'), or taking credit for someone else's work or ideas. While many jurisdictions have workplace or human rights legislations that protects individuals from 'harassment' based on personal/demographic characteristics, there are far fewer legislative protections against bullying – as a result, organisations and managers must be far more vigilant and proactive in managing these issues.

Most organisations today have zero-tolerance policies for bullying – where corroborated, the bully is usually punished swiftly and severely through all manner of sanctions available including demotion, suspension or even termination. While such policies send strong signals about organisational culture, the way they are actually implemented by managers can sometimes diminish effectiveness.

Principles of objectivity, transparency, impartiality, and fairness must be used in investigations of suspected/reported bullying and in examination/analysis of data. The 'reasonable person' test is often used in such situations: would a reasonable person, completely unconnected from the individuals involved, interpret the behaviours in question as bullying? Careful documentation of collected evidence and rationale for decisions must be undertaken by the manager as there are legal implications of decisions related to the assessment of workplace bullying complaints. Importantly, simply separating bullies and victims into different work groups and hoping that stops the problem is rarely successful: in some ways, this actually implies a reward for the bully since the underlying behaviour has not been addressed. Further, the victim can continue to be victimised since the individual remains proximately employed. Bullying is most prevalent in highly competitive workplaces (for example, sales and marketing) where employees must constantly jockey for contested and rare rewards. This kind of structure – designed to motivate employees to excel – may inadvertently create a culture favourable to bullying, implying that the organisation has some responsibility for the behaviour as well.

Complaints or observations related to bullying must be dealt with swiftly, fairly, and clearly managed to avoid workplace toxicity and potential legal issues. Where organisations have no formal policies/procedures for how to investigate and adjudicate bullying allegations, these should be developed and enacted in order to enhance transparency and impartiality of processes. A 'friendly word', an 'invitation for a cup of tea', or other informal mechanisms for resolution should be avoided as they may demonstrate favouritism. Similarly, responses about 'toughening up' will be unhelpful.

Workplace bullying is far more common than most managers realise, and while it is tempting to want to overlook or informally manage it, this must be avoided.[14] It takes time, patience, and tenacity to impartially investigate and adjudicate complaints and observations of bullying, but organisations need to be willing to dedicate the appropriate resources to manage it effectively. The costs and consequences of ineffective management of bullying behaviour (in terms of legal escalation, demoralisation of staff, and knock-on effects to organisational culture) can be severe.

Reasonable accommodation

Most jurisdictions have legal requirements related to 'reasonable accommodation' requests. Historically, the duty to accommodate has been viewed as an issue related to physical disability or physical/mental illness. Accommodation is usually described as a way of adapting work and workflow within an organisation that respects the dignity of the individual in ways that do not cause undue or unfair hardship for that individual or other workers.[17] Increasingly, accommodation has also been expanded to include other issues, such as religious or spiritual needs and age.[18] Examples of workplace accommodations that are generally considered reasonable include provision of reserved parking spots, removal of physical access barriers (e.g. steps or curbs), or allowing a more flexible work schedule (for example, allowing individuals to leave work prior to sunset on Fridays to accommodate Sabbath).

In some cases, managers and colleagues may erroneously view 'reasonable' accommodation as 'favouritism', particularly if it is implemented in ways that suggest others have fewer privileges as a result. While legislation regarding reasonable accommodation can be helpful in guiding manager's decisions, it is also essential that it does not turn into a purely legalistic exercise, as this can create a more toxic organisational culture.[19]

The term 'reasonable' is, of course, somewhat open-ended and subjective, but it is rooted in legal and historical understanding related to the burden to others that is involved in respecting the dignity of an individual. It is in this context that managers have a crucial role to play in modelling acceptance and respect of accommodation and working to educate all staff on its value and importance. Where managers are seen to be reluctant or negative in implementing reasonable accommodation, this transmits a strong message to other members of staff that it can be 'open season' to complain and be dismissive. Transparent and honest communication with the rest of the team is essential to make reasonable accommodation work: simply 'telling' other team members that one of their colleagues can never work on Friday nights due to religious accommodation requirements, risks creating backlash. Hiding behind legal fog and shruggingly saying, 'hey, it's not my idea that's just the law', further heightens antagonism towards the individual seeking accommodation. Nuanced language rooted in respect, teamwork, and collaboration is required to create a positive and accepting culture of understanding. This will likely involve multiple group and individual discussions in ways that do not single-out or spotlight the individual seeking accommodation, but instead emphasise the organisation's commitment to everyone to create the best, most functional workplace.

Where reasonable accommodation creates division and problems is often where managers fail to engage and speak with other team members and help them to understand the value and importance of collegiality.[19] It is incumbent on managers to not simply grudgingly accept the legal necessity of reasonable accommodation, but to actually be able to articulate and promote a believable rationale for how accommodation is in everyone's best interest as a way of embracing diversity, equity, and inclusivity.[19] Central to success is the ability to frame accommodation in these terms as a way of helping to create a team culture that is positive rather than resentful.

Mental health

As the COVID-19 pandemic has evolved, the mental health needs of the workforce have emerged as a significant managerial and operational issue. Of course, mental health issues in the workplace existed long before the pandemic, but the prevalence, depth and impact of these issues appear to have accelerated significantly.[20]

There are, of course, a wide variety of different mental health issues and concerns that individuals may bring to the workplace. In many cases, these will impact interpersonal relationships, communication, productivity and the ability to concentrate or focus. Speculation and innuendo regarding a colleague's mental health is not only unhelpful, it could also be interpreted as uncivil or bullying.

Managers need to be vigilant about the health and well-being of their workforce, and need to recognise the many ways in which the workplace itself may contribute to or exacerbate mental health issues through occupational stress and burnout. As with other management challenges described in this chapter, principles of objectivity, transparency, impartiality, and fairness need to be applied.

It is imperative that managers recognise that their role as manager does not extend to being psychologists or therapists. Well-intentioned attempts to help team members using some form of psychotherapeutic counselling are usually inappropriate and may be counterproductive.[21] Especially where managers are themselves health care professionals like pharmacists, it is essential to NOT assume a patient-professional relationship with a staff member.[21]

Many organisations provide external supports for counselling referral, known as 'Employee Assistance Programs' (EAPs). EAPs are third party organisations staffed by professional therapists; they are confidential and free services provided by employers to help employees manage difficult challenges. A key role of managers is to familiarise themselves with how staff members can access EAP services and to promote the availability of EAPs within the organisation. Within professions like pharmacy, associations and regulatory bodies also provide free, confidential access to EAP like services for their registrants/members.

Where managers suspect mental health issues are interfering with workplace productivity and success, it is essential to not engage in armchair diagnosis or issue directives such as 'you should really go see a psychiatrist'. This can be both offensive and, in some cases, illegal. Instead, focusing on performance and behaviour and informing individuals of the employer- or profession-based EAP supports available, can be helpful. Managers cannot require staff to access these supports, nor can they follow-up to confirm they have been accessed. Instead, they may be able to work with individual staff members to identify appropriate, reasonable accommodations that can be implemented in the short-term to provide an opportunity to help individuals manage difficult circumstances.

Documentation of these issues should be impartial, avoid diagnoses or labels, and instead focus on observed behaviours and their outcomes on productivity and success. Of course, confidentiality must be respected in any communication with other colleagues in the workplace, especially if reasonable accommodations are implemented. In some organisations, short-term paid or unpaid leave may be possible to allow individuals opportunities to focus on their mental health without day to day pressures of work.

Managers have an obvious interest in ensuring their teams are functioning to the best of their abilities in order to achieve organisational objectives.[22] Mental health issues are a significant barrier to personal and organisational success and must be managed effectively and humanely. Most organisations and professions have an array of different supports (EAPs, short-term leave policies, reasonable accommodation techniques, etc.) that can be leveraged to help individuals find their equilibrium. Familiarising oneself with these supports/resources and developing conversations that allow individuals to understand and select from this menu – without blame, diagnostic label, or shame – is a helpful approach to managing a challenging situation.

Principled disagreement/dissent

Social and societal complexity has increased markedly and this has become a management and workplace issue. As rules and norms governing social interactions have coarsened considerably, behaviours and language that was once considered unthinkable is now lamentably commonplace on the streets, in pubs, in families and in organisations. As politicians have weaponised principles of diversity and inclusivity, it is increasingly organisations and workplaces that are left to be the last bastions of civility and decency in society. Lamenting 'wokeness' or 'political correctness' as impediments to free speech or 'my rights', has created an increasingly polarised and fractious world in which organisations operate.

In some cases, this has led to very difficult and uncomfortable situations where workers claim their fundamental human rights are being impinged upon in the workplace. For example, an individual who has strong pro-life views may cite religious objection (and hence invoke religious accommodation) as a reason to not be involved, in any way, in the provision of certain medications. They may go so far as to claim that even handing-off these cases to other colleagues is tantamount to participating in a religiously objectionable activity, and that their rights to free speech are compromised when they are not allowed to try to convince patients to consider alternatives. Use of religious accommodation and the language of diversity and inclusivity as a defence in these situations can further amplify discomfort for managers and other staff. Similarly, the use of pronouns to refer to colleagues (or even patients) can trigger strong principled disagreement or dissent. Increasingly, claims of 'stifling' free speech by forcing the use of pronouns such as 'they' or neologisms such as 'zhe' have created significant problems in some workplaces.

Principled disagreement that uses the same language and thinking of diversity and inclusivity is an extraordinary and relatively new challenge for managers given the either-or, binary nature of many of these types of issues. Unlike bullying or incivility, traditional approaches and policies/procedures may not be effective in managing these issues. In many cases, reasonable accommodation may not be possible as this introduces unfairness or bias into decision making.

Where principled disagreement begins to create workplace issues – either in terms of workflow or team culture – managers need to address these issues swiftly to prevent further toxicity from spreading. The risks, of course, are enormous. Many organisations (large and small) have been targeted for consumer boycotts or media scrutiny based on how they adjudicate these issues. Where managers are faced with principled disagreements of these sorts, it is important to not improvise solutions or rely upon informal dispute resolution mechanisms. In such cases, corporate leaders and policies will likely be necessary given the organisational risk associated with decision making in such circumstances.

Whilst it is tempting to believe that compromise and goodwill may win the day, and that conversation and education can lead to resolution, the reality, in some cases, is that these situations are fundamentally unresolvable to everyone's satisfaction, since they are premised on strongly and emotionally held foundational views. Increasingly, organisations are recognising it is necessary for them to select and declare a 'side' rather than pretending to remain impartial or disinterested. Recent high-profile conflicts between politicians and corporations illustrate this point: for example, when the state of Florida in the US passed the 'Don't Say Gay' legislation, reducing teachers' ability to provide sex education in schools, the Disney corporation was forced to take a stand against the government despite being one of the largest employers (through Disney World) in the state.[23] Other large employers have withdrawn from states or reduced investment in jurisdictions where abortion access and rights have been curtailed.[24]

In these situations, it will rarely be up to managers to decide how to proceed and how to manage; instead, corporate leadership and guidance is necessary, so managers need to recognise circumstances where their job is simply to alert their own supervisors/leaders to the evolving situation within their team. This is not a case of 'passing the buck' or avoiding a decision; instead, it is a recognition of the complexity of situations such as this, and the risk mitigation/management organisations need to consider in formulating a response to principled dissent within their workforce. The legal, reputational, and operational issues of managing principled dissent are significant and need to be carefully considered. Importantly, however, managers also need to articulate their ideas in ways which are aligned with organisational objectives and inclusivity/diversity/equity goals.

Summary

Management challenges are often a reason why individuals avoid management roles. Fear or lack of confidence in being able to effectively deal with difficult situations and conversations can lead some individuals to simply avoid it all together. Learning to deal with management challenges is a skill that can be practiced and honed over time. A principles-based approach that emphasises objectivity, impartiality, transparency, and fairness can help guide behaviour and decision making in difficult situations. Willingness to invest time and energy in meaningful conversation to explore differences in opinion and perspectives is important. Adherence to legislation, regulation, and policies and procedures is also required, as is alignment with broader organisational objectives and vision.

References

1. Shikaze D et al. Community pharmacists' attitudes, opinions, and beliefs about leadership in the profession: an exploratory study. Can Pharm J 2018; 151(5): 315–321. https://doi.org/10.1177/1715163518790984

2. Priesemuth M. Time's up for toxic workplaces. Harvard Business Review [online] 2020. https://hbr.org/2020/06/times-up-for-toxic-workplaces

3. Schmeltzer B et al. Addressing the pharmacy leadership crisis in Canada: a call to action for a unified approach. Can Pharm J 2022; 155(3): 140–142. https://doi.org/10.1177/17151635221089293

4. Longest B. Management certainly matters and there are multiple ways to conceptualize the process; Comment on 'Management matters: A leverage point for health systems strengthening in global health'. Int J Health Policy Manag 2015; 4(11): 777–780. https://doi.org/10.15171/ijhpm.2015.138

5. Overton A, Lowry A. Conflict management: difficult conversations with difficult people. Clin Colon Rectal Surg 2013; 26(4): 259–264. https://doi.org/10.1055/s-0033-1356728

6. Gregory P, Austin Z. Conflict in community pharmacy practice: the experience of pharmacists, technicians and assistants. Can Pharm J 2016; 150(1): 32–41. https://doi.org/10.1177/1715163516679426

7. Moss M. Less is more: the new management mindset. Nursing Management 1994; 25(7): 88–89.

8. Park H, Faerman S. Becoming a manager: learning the importance of emotional and social competence in managerial transitions. Am Rev of Public Administration 2018; 49(1): 98–115. https://doi.org/10.1177/0275074018785448

9. Smith J, Alloy L. A roadmap to rumination: a review of the definition, assessment, and conceptualization of this multifaceted construct. Clin Psychol Rev 2009; 29(2): 116–128. https://doi.org/10.1016/j.cpr.2008.10.003

10. Joubert A et al. Understanding the experience of rumination and worry: a descriptive qualitative survey study. British J Clinical Psychol 2022; 61(4): 929–946. https://doi.org/10.1111/bjc.12367

11. Williams M. Microaggressions: clarification, evidence and impact. *Perspectives on Psychol Sci* 2019; 15(1): 3–26. https://doi.org/10.1177/1745691619827499

12. Harrison C, Tanner K. Language matters: considering microaggressions in science. *CBE Life Sci Educ* 2018; 17(1): fe4, 1–8. https://doi.org/10.1187/cbe.18-01-0011

13. Velazquez A *et al*. Microaggressions, bias and equity in the workplace. *American Society of Clinical Oncology Educational Book* 2022; 42: 852–863. https://doi.org/10.1200/edbk_350691

14. Bartlett J, Bartlett M. Workplace bullying: an integrative literature review. *Adv Developing Human Resources* 2011; 13(1): 69–84. https://doi.org/10.1177/1523422311410651

15. Rayner C, Cooper C. Workplace Bullying. In: Kelloway E *et al*. eds. *Handbook of workplace violence*. Sage Publications Inc: California, 2006: 121–145. https://doi.org/10.4135/9781412976947.n7

16. Saunders P *et al*. Defining workplace bullying behaviour: professional lay definitions of workplace bullying. *Int J Law and Psychiatry* 2007; 30(4-5): 340–354. https://doi.org/10.1016/j.ijlp.2007.06.007

17. Blanck P. Disability inclusive employment and the accommodation principle: emerging issues in research, policy, and law. *J Occupational Rehabilitation* 2020; 30: 505–510. https://doi.org/10.1007/s10926-020-09940-9

18. Anand P, Sevak P. The role of workplace accommodations in the employment of people with disabilities. *IZA J Labour Policy* 2017; 6(12). https://doi.org/10.1186/s40173-017-0090-4

19. Ferri D. Reasonable accommodation as a gateway to the equal enjoyment of human rights: From New York to Strasbourg. *Disability Equality* 2018; 6(1). https://doi.org/10.17645/si.v6i1.1204

20. Pearman A *et al*. Mental health challenges of United States healthcare professionals during COVID-19. *Front Psychol* 2020; 11: 2065. https://doi.org/10.3389/fpsyg.2020.02065

21. Cleary M *et al*. Mental health and well being in the workplace. *Issues in Mental Health Nursing* 2020; 41(2): 172–175. https://doi.org/10.1080/01612840.2019.1701937

22. LaMontagne A *et al*. Workplace mental health: developing an integrated intervention approach. *BMC Psychiatry* 2014; 14(131). https://doi.org/10.1186/1471-244X-14-131

23. Pendharkar E (2022). *Here's what Florida's "Don't Say Gay" and anti-Woke bills actually say*. Bethesda: Education Week. https://www.edweek.org/leadership/heres-what-floridas-dont-say-gay-and-anti-woke-bills-actually-say/2022/03

24. Hodges L (2022). *Corporate America reckons with its role in reproductive rights*. NPR. https://www.npr.org/2022/07/25/1112599476/abortion-roe-companies-pay-travel-law-ban

CHAPTER 13

Motivating and engaging staff to succeed

Upon completion of this chapter you should be able to:

- explain the three layers of satisfaction and their limitations
- detail the importance of workplace commitment
- list the components of creating professional motivation
- detail an understanding of workplace engagement and its importance
- recognise managerial responsibilities to create a workplace which encourages commitment, motivation and engagement.

The educational psychologist Donald Schön described the unique nature of professional work: to him, professionals are able to deal with 'messy problems' in the real world that defy routine solutions or easy answers.[1] What makes professionals distinct and important in society is their capacity to manage ambiguity, deal with situations where information is unavailable, and still make decisions – knowing they will adjust and adapt as needed.[2] Professionals – like pharmacists – must have some comfort in working under conditions where there are sometimes no 'right answers', only 'least worst alternatives' from which to select.[3]

Managing professionals is complicated by the nature of professional work itself. Not only must professionals meet employer/manager expectations, they are also governed by regulatory/licensing body requirements, legislative frameworks, and codes of ethics. While it is tempting to believe that business, regulatory, legal, and ethical objectives will always align in professional work, the reality, of course, is messier.[4] For example, in many jurisdictions, pharmacists are able to conduct comprehensive medication reviews with at-risk patients to ensure best possible pharmacotherapy and use of medicines. In most jurisdictions where this service is provided, governments or insurance companies reimburse or compensate pharmacists for this professional work. Employers of pharmacists have come to rely on this revenue stream as part of business planning, and as a result, may push pharmacists to complete a minimum number of medication reviews monthly in order to receive compensation that will enhance profitability. This mixed incentive has produced a variety of unintended outcomes: studies from several jurisdictions where pharmacist-led paid medication review services exist, point to the uncomfortable reality that the patients that pharmacists invite to participate in reviews are actually those least in need of this service.[5] Because pharmacists may feel managerial pressure to complete a minimum number of reviews each month, they must juggle complex workloads; the easiest path forward to satisfy management demands is to select the least complicated (and thus least needful) patients for medication review.

This example highlights a central tension and complexity in managing a professional workforce. While quotas and minimum workload requirements may be effective in a factory setting, the use of similar techniques by managers of professionals can produce problematic outcomes.[6] As Schön noted, professional work is characterised by 'messiness' and requires professionals to exert creativity, wisdom, compassion, and judgement in dealing with ambiguous problems. Blunt managerial approaches involving quotas inhibits expression of these important characteristics and reduces professional work to a simple occupation instead.

Professional success

Most managers recognise that workplace commitment, psychological motivation, and professional engagement are all pre-requisites for success in the 21st century workplace.[7] Simply going through the motions and completing tasks in a tick-box fashion will not produce optimal outcomes.[8] Professionals need to be psychologically invested in their work in order to be maximally productive, creative, and resilient in the face of routine daily obstacles and problems.[9] It is unrealistic to assume that simply because someone is a regulated health care professional, they will magically find the commitment, motivation, and engagement necessary to succeed. As a result, there are unique responsibilities and opportunities for managers to support professional success using techniques and strategies designed to unleash each individual's professional potential.

Many organisations take this responsibility seriously and invest considerable resources in monitoring the psychological state of the workforce. One of the most common measurements used is 'satisfaction'. The term itself is somewhat vague and has been used to describe a variety of different psychological states ranging from general contentment with work, to grudging resignation that no other alternatives are possible. Managers routinely use tools such as anonymous job satisfaction surveys or performance appraisals that focus on satisfaction as a desirable objective without actually defining it clearly for themselves or their staff.

Psychologists describe 'satisfaction' in terms of cognitive, emotional, and behavioural elements.[10] The cognitive elements of satisfaction do not address issues of joy or pleasure but instead simply focus on the extent to which the actual day to day tasks and responsibilities of the role align with one's preconceptions and expectations. Cognitive satisfaction exists when the job being done is actually the job a person thought they would be doing. In contrast, emotional satisfaction focuses on the quality of working life, including workplace stress, level of control/autonomy in work, and subjective experiences associated with going to and being at work. Finally, behavioural satisfaction focuses on how cognitive and emotional satisfaction translate into productivity and outcomes: where individuals are both cognitively and emotionally satisfied, this will manifest in better interpersonal relationships, enhanced communication, and a willingness to 'go the extra mile' in order to be more productive at work.[11]

These three layers of satisfaction are often present in routine questionnaires administered by managers to assess the satisfaction of individual workers and the workforce in general, but there are significant limitations to only focusing on satisfaction. The problem of 'presenteeism' occurs when individuals are 'satisfied' but not truly 'happy'.[12] For example, a professional may believe they are fairly paid, they have a reasonable work–life balance, the job is what they expected, and workplace conditions are appropriate. In this case, all three layers of satisfaction would be rated as positive...but this particular individual – while satisfied – may not have any real motivation or incentive to 'fire on all pistons' and bring their best possible self and skills to their work on a regular basis. They are 'present' and appear content and functional, but are not working to the best of their ability. This, of course, means less than optimal outcomes for the organisation.

Understanding commitment

Managers interested in unleashing the full potential of their workforce need to implement techniques designed to elicit commitment in addition to satisfaction. Like satisfaction, commitment is a psychological state of mind demonstrated within a workplace that incorporates three distinct layers: a) affective commitment, in which individuals have an emotional connection to their profession or workplace; b) moral commitment, in which individuals have an internalised sense of duty to serve; and c) practical commitment, in which individuals have invested significant time and energy into building workplace success and connections so the cost of leaving is simply too high.[6,13] Historically, managers of professionals have overemphasised practical commitment as a driver for workplace productivity or success by, for example, using threats like non-compete clauses in contracts to highlight the real world costs of leaving a workplace. More recent research has suggested that one of the most important drivers for professional commitment is affective commitment; in particular, the interpersonal relationships professionals form with each other within a workplace or practice.[14] Emotional attachment to colleagues and a subjective sense of having 'friends' at work is a powerful driver of behaviour, productivity, and innovation, and is the root of recent managerial strategies focused on 'team building' activities.[14] Corporate retreats, workplace perks, conferences, and other socially oriented activities that build camaraderie and personal connection amongst individuals who work together, appear to have a positive psychological benefit in terms of affective commitment which in turn produces positive productivity and business outcome gains.[15] More recently, however, some skepticism has emerged regarding the limits of these team building activities, particularly in an environment where every manager and every organisation utilises them; early success with affective commitment techniques may have reflected their novelty rather than intrinsic value.[14] High profile, costly marquee events like corporate retreats and 'fun away days' may now actually have the opposite and unintended effect on some people, triggering eye-rolling cynicism rather than building affective commitment. Instead, many managers now look to the actual substance of the work itself as a tool for building commitment and use team management strategies (described further in Chapter 11) to organically and authentically create interpersonal chemistry amongst co-workers as they autonomously and jointly solve professionally interesting, challenging, and meaningful problems.

Understanding motivation

Satisfaction and commitment are necessary but insufficient to truly unleash the potential of individual workers and a professional workforce. It is important to recognise that individuals may be satisfied and committed, but still under-motivated to perform to the best of their potential. Like satisfaction and commitment, professional motivation consists of three different layers: dedication, tenacity, and perseverance.[16] Dedication describes observable, measurable elements of motivation connected to workplace performance, including punctuality, attendance record, and success at achieving pre-negotiated outcomes or performance targets. Tenacity describes the psychological motivation necessary to overcome practical obstacles in order to complete tasks and projects as environmental circumstances change. Tenacity is a type of motivation that fosters creativity in practical problem-solving. Finally, perseverance focuses on the motivation to overcome some of the more nuanced, psychological or interpersonal barriers (for example, workplace negativity or toxic culture) that can sap energy for productive work. All three layers of motivation speak to an individual's capacity to 'overcome' or effectively self-manage problems in ways that are productive, energy-building (rather than energy-depleting), and sustainable.

Organisational psychologists have differentiated between 'intrinsic' and 'extrinsic' motivation at all three layers.[17] Intrinsic motivation is usually described as factors leading to dedication, tenacity and perseverance that are related to the work, or the job itself. For example, many pharmacists and health care professionals find their motivation in helping patients manage complex health related issues. They are able to overcome and effectively self-manage obstacles and problems because the greater goal of helping others provides them with the psychological energy necessary to be creative and persistent, and not lose hope or belief in the work itself. Such intrinsic motivation is powerful and usually stems from subjective, emotional, positive responses from patients as pharmacists do their jobs to the best of their ability. In contrast, extrinsic motivation emphasises factors that have little to do with the work or the profession itself – for example, salary, title, or social prestige. Extrinsic motivation is based on a ruthless quantification of how much money (or status) can 'buy' certain kinds of behaviours. In the recent past, managers have erred in believing that money or status were sufficient to motivate professional workers. While, of course, professionals (like all people) expect to and need to make a decent salary for their work, there are limits to the effectiveness of extrinsic motivators typically used by managers. For example, as the COVID-19 pandemic evolved, motivation of the health care workforce changed considerably. In the early days of the pandemic in 2020, neighbourhoods would gather in socially distant ways to bang pots and pans to 'celebrate' the sacrifices of health care workers and National Health Service (NHS) staff. Later in the pandemic as weariness and cynicism grew – and as misinformation about vaccines spread – health care workers themselves were targeted by anti-vax proponents and harassed or abused. After several years of sacrifice, danger, and exhaustion, health care personnel also went from being 'heroes' to 'villains' for some. This lead to incredible de-motivation amongst health care professionals (including pharmacists). A common response from managers during this time was to overemphasise salary increases as a way of re-building motivation. Of course additional money is appreciated, but money alone could not replace intrinsic motivation lost over the course of the pandemic. Focusing primarily or solely on extrinsic motivation can actually be even more demotivating. Instead, management techniques that focused on actual workplace conditions to try to re-energise intrinsic motivation were more successful. Finding ways of allowing professionals to spend more time with patients, hiring additional staff to reduce workload so quality of care could be increased, or reducing bureaucratic workplace requirements to allow professionals to focus on patient care, are all more likely to enhance motivation in a sustainable way, at all layers, rather than simply focusing on extrinsic elements such as salary.

Understanding engagement

Most of the management research focused on satisfaction, commitment, and motivation arose as a result of concerns about worker retention, and an attempt to influence decisions related to staying in or leaving a position. This is understandable, given the cost and time associated with recruiting and filling positions when individuals leave jobs. More recently, researchers have noted the connection between retention and engagement, and the role of optimal/peak performance in enhancing productivity, outcomes, and quality.

Kahn was amongst the first to coin the term 'engagement' to describe a new construct emphasising qualitative aspects of workplace performance.[18] Engagement was used to describe a constellation of psychological, cognitive, and emotional factors that fostered a deep connection to one's work, one's professional role, one's colleagues, and one's workplace. From this perspective, previous constructs such as satisfaction, commitment, and motivation were merely scaffolding or supporting infrastructural elements necessary to enable authentic engagement. Without satisfaction, commitment, and motivation, engagement may not be possible...but those three elements in themselves are no guarantee that engagement will emerge. What is unique about engagement – and what makes it particularly relevant for managers of professional staff – is its emphasis on the unique, creative insights professionals need in order to be at their best. Recall that Schön described professional work as 'messy' because the problems professionals solve are ambiguous, situational, and require not only knowledge and skill, but also wisdom, compassion, and judgement. In many cases, disengaged professionals can appear perfectly competent and effective, but simply not care about the work they are doing. They go through the motions, show up for a paycheque, make no major errors, then just go home. Few of us would ever want a professional we relied on to be this kind of person. Most recipients of professional service recognise the central importance of the professional actually caring about their work and caring about us as their clients/patients. From this care comes a willingness to go the extra mile, 'fire on all pistons', and bring the best of oneself (both professionally and personally) to solving problems in creative, moral, and compassionate ways.

Schaufeli and Bakker described engagement as an active, positive psychological state occurring in the midst of day to day professional practice that was characterised by: a) vigour, or a sustained and sustainable burst of psychological attention that fostered deeper concentration, attentiveness, and physical stamina, all of which lead to the ability to simply work harder; b) invested dedication, a psychological state of interconnectedness between the individual and the work being done in which professional outcomes are perceived as personal success; c) absorption, a psychological state producing heightened sensory capabilities linked to maximal attention and focus in which individuals literally see and hear more, better, and clearer, as a foundation for optimal problem-solving in an intrinsically pleasurable way.[19]

Csikszentmihalyi popularised these concepts and coined the term 'flow' to describe the optimal state of peak performance in human interactions.[20] Sometimes described as 'being in the now', or 'immersive joy', flow describes a psychological state '...in which people are so involved with an activity that nothing else seems to matter; the experience itself is so enjoyable, people will continue to do it... for the sheer pleasure of just doing it'.[20] Researchers interested in professional work noted that a key component of flow was the unleashing of creativity in problem-solving; this lead to interest in what management techniques and strategies could be used to create workplace conditions aligned with this.

The fundamental premise of both flow and engagement is this notion of psychological fuel necessary to sustain creative, professional work.

Within pharmacy as a profession, there has been recent interest in trying to better understand what flow looks like, and what determinants of engagement exist within the scope of practice of pharmacists and the boundaries of the profession itself. One recent study focused on the experiences of award winning pharmacists in Canada.[21] Participants in this study had recently been acknowledged by peers, colleagues, and patients, as being exemplars in their field, winning (for example) prestigious 'Pharmacist of the Year' awards or 'Commitment to Care' awards. A foundational assumption of this study is that these exemplary, recognised pharmacists would be the closest to flow within the profession, and this (it was expected) could provide useful insights for non-award winning pharmacists regarding engagement.

Four key findings emerged from this work. First, these award winning pharmacists described high levels of ambivalence about their profession and professional identity, somewhat variable workplace satisfaction, and inconsistent commitment to pharmacy as a profession. Many of them spoke candidly about struggles they experienced in actually believing being a pharmacist was the right profession for them, and some spoke freely about on-again, off-again lack of motivation that sometimes plagued them. Despite being recognised as 'award winning', they did not necessarily always love their jobs or love their profession; at best these strong emotional feelings were episodic and transient. Second, participants in this study noted the importance of extrinsic motivators and extrinsic reinforcements (including the prestigious rewards they had received) in helping them overcome internalised ambivalence. Significantly, they also noted that while important, extrinsic rewards and motivators only had a short, time-limited, positive impact, and that before too long, another extrinsic reward/ motivator was needed to sustain positivity. Third, participants noted how situationally sensitive and specific their engagement actually was: seemingly small environmental issues (such as an angry customer, a quarrelsome colleague, or a supply shortage) was enough to derail engagement, suggesting motivational characteristics such as perseverance and tenacity were not very strong.

The fourth finding of this study related to the description of determinants of engagement amongst these award winning pharmacists. Six key determinants were identified. Importantly, these determinants provide useful insights for managers to help them create workplace conditions that could help support the emergence of flow in the workforce.

1. *Autonomy:* All participants in this study described how important professional independence and the ability to control and select work was to supporting peak performance and engagement. The ability to self-direct and prioritise, and freedom from micromanagement by supervisors contributed significantly to engagement. Participants described how overly prescriptive standardised operating procedures, or overly involved managers, created cognitive and emotional loads that interfered with engagement: rather than focusing on patients, care, or service, these managerial practices actually ended up triggering a response of 'what hoop do you want me to jump through for you now?'.

2. *Altruism:* Participants in this study highlighted personal and moral beliefs related to kindness and caring, and noted that when, as pharmacists, they could be kind and caring to patients, this actually helped enhance engagement. Being kind and caring to others produced positive emotional benefits that generated its own psychological fuel to support engagement and

overcome environmental obstacles. The need to be kind and to care for others was a powerful motivator and the response from patients to kindness and caring produced its own positive reinforcement.

3. *Admiration:* Perhaps surprisingly, most participants in this study placed a high degree of value on external recognition as a driver for engagement, but not necessarily recognition in the form of the award they had received. Instead, the greatest drivers for engagement were admiration from patients and peers. Being respected and admired for competency, knowledge, skills, and judgement as a pharmacist, by those being served and by colleagues, had an important influence on professional identity and allegiance in ways that supported engagement.

4. *Agreement:* An important determinant of engagement identified in this study was the perceptions of other health care professionals, notably physicians. Being seen as a trusted advisor and colleague of other prescribers appeared to fulfil a strong psychological need for recognition from respected others that supports and sustains engagement.

5. *Alignment:* High performing pharmacists in this study highlighted the importance of feeling like they were part of a broader health care team rather than simply working as a pharmacist in isolation or as part of a pharmacy. Aligning one's efforts with the work of other professional colleagues outside pharmacy was described as an important tool for building intrinsic motivation and commitment, but also of heightening a sense of importance that led to engagement.

6. *Aspiration:* The psychological characteristic of general optimism or positivity was consistently observed amongst participants in this study, beyond the profession-specific determinants described above. Positivity enabled a virtuous upward cycle of success, opportunities – and ultimately awards. Hopeful attitudes and a belief in things simply getting better (not just for the individual, but for the profession and for society as a whole), helped reduce the emotional and cognitive load associated with negative thinking but also supported better interpersonal relationships and communication, which in turn supported greater professional success.

As a manager, there are several important implications to consider from these 6As of engagement. First, they do not provide a comprehensive or detailed playbook for motivating and engaging staff for greater success, but they do provide psychological insights that align with emotional intelligence and can help managers better understand the staff they supervise. The 6As point to the relatively low value of traditional extrinsic motivators in driving engagement, and highlight instead the importance of interpersonal connectivity – with peers, patients, physicians and others – as a valuable tool for supporting engagement. As a manager, finding ways of expanding and enhancing this interpersonal connectivity can be important, for example, by fostering social events bringing local physicians and pharmacists together, or finding ways to individualise pharmacists so patients ask for them by name rather than simply wanting to 'talk to a pharmacist'. A second important insight from this research points to the reality that even these award winning pharmacists had ups and downs with respect to engagement: to be successful as a manager, the objective is not to have full engagement at all times but to recognise that it will wax and wane. Superficial management techniques that oversimplify the power of positive thinking or paint an unrealistically optimistic view of how tremendously important pharmacists are, will be transparently and painfully unbelievable. Minimising enthusiastic cheerleading and simply allowing for ups-and-downs in terms of engagement will be both less exhausting for managers and more impactful for pharmacists. Third, given the important ways in which admiration from patients shapes engagement, removal of bureaucratic and managerial barriers to have greater connection with patients may be helpful. Restructuring workflow in ways that allow pharmacists to have greater autonomy (for example, through independent prescribing) and more opportunities for altruism, without creating burdensome paperwork or bureaucratic requirements, can heighten success and engagement. Finally, small but impactful changes in management strategies and a manager's style of supervision – for example, avoid micromanagement – are essential in creating an environment to foster engagement.

Most of the research undertaken in this chapter focuses on pharmacists rather than pharmacy technicians, assistants or other staff that managers supervise. While there is limited evidence for these different groups, there is no reason to believe that the general principles discussed here would not also apply to these individuals and groups. Regardless of educational background or professional designation, the 6As of engagement will likely be broadly applicable for these staff groups and with similar techniques (e.g. avoiding micromanagement, reducing bureaucratic barriers to altruistic behaviour with patients, etc.) should be similarly successful.

Developing a managerial style to foster engagement

The evolution of understanding workplace psychology has highlighted the necessity but insufficiency of only considering satisfaction, commitment, and motivation, particularly in the context of creative professional work in a field like pharmacy. Importantly, managers have responsibilities to ensure the infrastructure necessary for engagement to flourish is in place, and this will almost always be built on a foundation of a satisfied, committed, and motivated workforce. Managers need to recognise, however, that this is not enough, and that unleashing the full potential of the workforce requires commitment to engaging them in their work, their patients, their place of practice, their colleagues, and their profession.

While managers cannot be responsible for each worker's personal or professional happiness, they can review existing structures, workflow, policies, and procedures to determine how 'the way we always do things around here' may be interfering with the expression of engagement. Honest and open dialogue with staff and the willingness to listen and try suggestions is important; the complex psychological nature of engagement means that most of the best solutions will come from individuals themselves, rather than managers. This requires a managerial style focused on listening, clarifying, and trying, rather than a style that focuses on telling, enforcing and selecting. Demonstrating authentic interest in the satisfaction, commitment, motivation, and engagement of staff – and using conversation and dialogue as a tool to monitor and better understand – sends a strong signal of managerial and organisational support for the creation of a high-functioning, engaged workplace. Avoid the temptation to assume that all or most pharmacists or staff will respond to the same interventions in the same way – customising approaches for the unique needs, interests, strengths, and personalities of each individual is necessary. Be prepared for many conversations with many different individuals, rather than a one-size-fits-all group meeting.

While this may sound daunting and exhausting, there can be significant dividends from this managerial approach. Highly individualised, conversational techniques demonstrate sincere interest in helping individuals achieve engagement and are much more likely to succeed than blanket policy changes that may or may not resonate with each individual based on their specific circumstances.

An engaged workforce is built one person at a time, and this may require changes to traditional management styles that have emphasised efficiency and treating everyone exactly the same.

Summary

A central responsibility for managers is to find ways of eliciting the best possible performance out of the workforce. There has been considerable evolution in understanding how this can be accomplished. Where initially the emphasis was on recruitment and preventing unnecessary staff turnover, work in this area focused on the concept of satisfaction and commitment. More recently, as the unique nature of professional work itself was incorporated into managers' understanding of their role, there has been a shift towards thinking about motivation and engagement. For a professional workforce, there is a general understanding that engagement provides the psychological fuel necessary to unleash peak performance, and that engagement itself is supported by satisfaction, commitment, and motivation.

Managers seeking to foster conditions conducive to an engaged workforce must consider many factors and use individualised means and methods to reach individual professionals. Inauthentic or one-size-fits-all solutions for engagement will likely be unsuccessful. Instead, focusing on workplace conditions and intrinsic motivating factors associated with the profession itself may be more helpful. The 6As of engagement (autonomy, altruism, admiration, agreement, alignment and aspiration) may be a useful conceptual framework to guide managerial decisions and style to support the flourishing of a motivated and engaged workforce.

References

1. Schon D. *The Reflective Practitioner: How Professionals Think in Action*. New York: Basic Books, 1984.
2. Koshy K *et al*. Reflective practice in health care and how to reflect effectively. *Int J Surg Oncol* 2017; 2(6): e20. https://doi.org/10.1097/IJ9.0000000000000020
3. Mantzourani E *et al*. The role of reflective practice in health care professions: next steps for pharmacy education and practice. *Res Social Admin Pharm* 2019; 15(12): 1476–1479. https://doi.org/10.1016/j.sapharm.2019.03.011
4. Quilty T, Murphy L. Time to review reflective practice? *Int J Quality Health Care* 2022; 34(2): 1–2. https://doi.org/10.1093/intqhc/mzac052
5. Dolovich L *et al*. Initial pharmacist experience with Ontario-based MedsCheck program. *Can Pharm J* 2008; 141(6): 339–345. https://doi.org/10.3821/1913-701X-141.6.339
6. Austin Z. *Human Resource Management in Pharmacy: Managing and Motivating Staff to Excel*. Washington DC: American Pharmacists' Association, 2022.
7. Fornes S *et al*. Workplace commitment: a conceptual model developed from integrative review of the research. *Human Resource Development Review* 2008; 7(3): 339–357. https://doi.org/10.1177/1534484308318760
8. McElroy J. Managing workplace commitment by putting people first. *Human Resource Management Review* 2001; 11(3): 327–335. https://doi.org/10.1016/S1053-4822(00)00054-1
9. Rossenberg Y *et al*. The future of workplace commitment: key questions and directions. *European J Work and Organizational Psychol* 2018; 27(2): 153–167. https://doi.org/10.1080/1359432X.2018.1443914
10. Raziq A, Maulabakhsh R. Impact of working environment on job satisfaction. *Proedia Economics and Finance* 2015; 23: 717–725. https://doi.org/10.1016/S2212-5671(15)00524-9

11. Flowers S, Hughes C. Why employees stay. *Harvard Business Review* [online] 1973. https://hbr.org/1973/07/why-employees-stay

12. Widera E *et al.* Presenteeism: a public health hazard. *J Gen Intern Med* 2010; 25(11): 1244–1247. https://doi.org/10.1007/s11606-010-1422-x

13. Herrera J, Heras-Rosas C. The organizational commitment in the company and its relationship with the psychological contract. *Front Psychol* 2021; 11: 609211. https://doi.org/10.3389/fpsyg.2020.609211

14. Aziz H *et al.* Employee commitment: the relationship between employee commitment and job satisfaction. *Int J Humanities and Education Development* 2021; 3(3): 54–66. https://doi.org/10.22161/jhed.3.3.6

15. Rossenberg Y *et al.* An HRM perspective on workplace commitment: reconnecting in concept, measurement, and methodology. *Human Resource Management Review* 2022; 32(4): 100891. https://doi.org/10.1016/j.hrmr.2021.100891

16. White S, Generali J. Motivating pharmacy employees. *Am J Hosp Pharm* 1984; 41(7): 1361–1366. https://doi.org/10.1093/ajhp/41.7.1361

17. Di Domenico S, Ryan R. The emerging neuroscience of intrinsic motivation: A new frontier in self-determination research. *Front Hum Neurosci* 2017; 11: 145. https://doi.org/10.3389/fnhum.2017.00145

18. Kahn W, Fellows S. Employee engagement and meaningful work. In: Dik B *et al.* eds. *Purpose and Meaning in the Workplace*. Washington DC: American Psychological Association, 2013: 105–126. https://doi.org/10.1037/14183-006

19. Bakker A *et al.* Workplace engagement: an emerging concept in occupational health psychology. *Work and Stress* 2008; 22(3): 187–200. https://doi.org/10.1080/02678370802393649

20. Csikszentmihalyi M. *Flow: the Psychology of Optimal Experience*. New York: Harper & Row, 1990.

21. Austin Z, Gregory P. Understanding psychological engagement and flow in community pharmacy practice. *Res Social Adm Pharm* 2020; 16(4): 488–496. https://doi.org/10.1016/j.sapharm.2019.06.013

CHAPTER 14

Workplace design

Upon completion of this chapter you should be able to:

- explain what workplace design is
- detail the relationship between design and cognitive and emotional load
- understand the evolution of workplace design in pharmacy
- list the current key considerations in pharmacy workplace design.

Anyone who has spent time in a pharmacy will know what a busy and chaotic place it can be. Whether located within a community, hospital, or other setting, pharmacies provide a physical space for the provision of a wide variety of professional services and care. The design of workplaces and workspace is often something managers will simply take for granted, as though they have no particular influence over decisions that have been made in the past. Even when new pharmacy spaces are created, pharmacy managers may feel they have little to contribute to the discussion of workplace design as this is the remit of industrial engineers or other specialists.

Those working within pharmacies/dispensaries understand the strong connection between workplace design and productivity, motivation, engagement, safety, and quality. Those managing these environments have unique insights into opportunities to enhance traditional designs to support evolving models of professional practice. Understanding principles of workplace design in pharmacy and using this to improve efficiency, effectiveness, safety, and quality in practice, are all important managerial responsibilities.

What is workplace design?

Workplace design usually refers to the process of organising a physical work environment to optimise the performance of workers and to enhance safe, effective, and efficient delivery of products and services (in the case of pharmacies, this will also include delivery of health care).[1] While high risk environments such as construction sites or chemical laboratories have often been the focus of workplace design initiatives, more recently there has been interest in health care delivery settings and professional workplaces like hospital dispensaries and community pharmacies.[2] Workplace design also includes issues such as air quality and circulation (particularly important as a result of the COVID-19 pandemic), lighting, ergonomics, and placement of equipment. In professional settings, aesthetics are important to consider as these can be used to reduce worker stress, improve workers' moods and temperaments, and make spaces simply feel less crowded.[3] Where intentional and mindful workplace design decisions are not made, deferred, or ignored, random unplanned evolution will likely occur that will result in greater chaos, clutter, and potential inefficiency.[4] Importantly, workplace design is not simply a superficial decorating exercise in making spaces look good – it is grounded in psychology and focused on enhancing engagement and optimising productivity while safeguarding the physical and mental well-being of workers in the space.

Three key elements of workplace design include:[5]

1. *Space planning:* Design goes well beyond how spaces are decorated and begins with understanding functionality and examining efficiency. Functionality requires a clear understanding of current and projected tasks and activities that are to be performed within a space. For example, within a typical community pharmacy setting there are multiple conflicting activities that must co-exist within the same space, including dispensing, compounding, storage of secure physical materials, storage of confidential data, telecommunications (phones, computers) interactive consultations with clients, and direct health care delivery (for example, administration of injections and immunisations or swab testing). A clear understanding of current space needs and reasonable forecasting of the future evolution of needs is essential for effective space planning. One crucial element of space planning involves clarity around public-facing versus private/confidential activities and areas. While there has been a general shift towards 'open concept' and increasingly transparent workplaces where the public observes workers (including professionals) doing their jobs, privacy and confidentiality constraints limits how far this can be applied in pharmacy. Further, the emotional intelligence of most pharmacists may be challenged by too much open concept space and public scrutiny of day to day work, and this can impact motivation, engagement, and can contribute negatively to occupational stress and burnout. Understanding and projecting how work will actually occur in the space and the way workflow will influence the utilisation of different areas within the space is crucial, and an area where managers and staff should have strong input and perspectives.

2. *Aesthetics:* Historically the purview of decorators, the physical 'look' of a workplace is increasingly seen as central to productivity and success, and as a result, industrial psychologists have become interested in how features such as wall colours, flooring textures, lighting features, and equipment fixtures contribute to well-being and productivity in the workplace. While it may be tempting to believe aesthetics are merely a question of subjective taste, it is important to recognise the influence these aesthetic features have on the day to day working life of people in the space itself.

3. *Integration of tools and technology:* Historically, the equipment used within workplaces have been simple add-ons to pre-designed spaces. For example, when computer terminals became ubiquitous in health care, they were simply placed atop counters that were perhaps used for different activities (such as dispensing) because that space was available. Robotic dispensing devices often occupied prime footprint within a dispensary environment, forcing live workers to take additional steps around machines each time, contributing significantly to physical fatigue and causing traffic congestion in tight dispensary settings. Similarly, as virtual conferencing, using systems like Zoom or Skype, became more commonplace during the pandemic, additional monitors were often positioned as television screens rather than as telecommunication tools. Increasingly, workplace design recognises that the tools and technologies that are part of day to day work and workflow need to be more fully, seamlessly, and thoughtfully integrated into design

itself to optimise use and to ensure issues of privacy/confidentiality, ergonomic safety, and even usability (e.g. not placing a monitor close to a window with direct sunlight) are considered.

Workplace design and cognitive and emotional load

The concepts of cognitive and emotional load are of significant importance when considering workplace design, and design can be very effective at reducing these loads.[6] Cognitive load refers to the mental processing required in order to undertake activities and tasks: where cognitive load is high, greater attentiveness to detail and concentration may be required, and interruptions or multi-tasking may significantly compromise quality outcomes or be safety risks.[6] For example, the cognitive load required to calculate a dose of chemotherapy for a severely immunocompromised patient with renal failure, is significantly higher than the cognitive load required to calculate the number of capsules to dispense for a prescription written 'twice daily x 1 week'. Yet, in many typical pharmacy workplaces, both calculations may be completed in exactly the same workspace and place, and this may increase the risk of error when the calculation is more complex. In contrast, emotional load refers to subjective and affective responses to the environment. Crowded, cluttered, dirty, chaotic environments will significantly increase stress and make workers simply 'feel' less confident, competent, secure, and safe. Increased emotional load has deleterious effects on the ability to concentrate, co-operate, collaborate, and communicate. Poor workplace design contributes directly and significantly to both cognitive and emotional load, while more thoughtful design choices can help mitigate against occupational stress that is inherent or intrinsic to the work itself.[7]

Understanding the evolution of workplace design in pharmacy

The story of workplace design in pharmacy is fascinating and connects closely to the evolution of the profession itself. The dispensary has traditionally been the focal point of any pharmacy and was originally intended to be a place for secure storage of restricted materials (medications). As a result, the traditional dispensary was focused on security and storage rather than on providing patient care services, or confidential discussions. The linear design of most dispensaries focused on internal processes rather than on engagement with patients or other health care professionals outside the pharmacy. Technology was extraordinarily limited. As the profession's focus has evolved from a product to a patient orientation, changes to workplace design have been accretive, meaning changing requirements were simply stapled on to existing physical infrastructure rather than fundamentally rethinking or redesigning work spaces. As a result, private consultation rooms were carved out of storage closets and to this day, continue to be awkward and cramped. Computer terminals were simply placed on existing counters in awkward locations, interfering with traffic patterns within the dispensary. As more and more drug products came onto the market, shelving spaces grew taller and more imposing, creating further hazards.

Today, in both hospital and community pharmacy, the design of pharmacy workplaces continues to highlight the vestiges of a compounding-and-dispensing history, with patient care services simply being added on as an afterthought. Further, despite significant advances in technology (including robotics, decision support software and teleconferencing), few pharmacies are set up to actually leverage this potential because their workplaces cannot support the integration of technology into the workflow. While some 'model' pharmacy dispensaries have been pioneered and showcased, these continue to be novel curiosities rather than exemplars for how good workplace design can support better patient care practice. For managers, it is essential to remember that design defines function and activities[8]: the physical infrastructure and layout of a pharmacy will have an enormous influence on the quality, efficiency and effectiveness of all services and care provided by staff members. Further, the physical layout will also directly influence staff morale, attitudes, and organisational culture.[9] Attentiveness to details of physical layout is a managerial responsibility – and an opportunity to positively influence organisational outcomes.

Key considerations in pharmacy workplace design

Whether a pharmacy is being constructed and equipped as a new-build project, or whether it is being renovated after having existed for many years in a specific format, managers need to have a clear understanding of important characteristics for successful workplace design. These include the areas discussed below.

Purpose

What does the organisation want the dispensary and the pharmacy to be? A clear organisational mission and vision are needed in order to define specific goals and objectives. For example, a pharmacy that has a mission focused on compounding of bespoke extemporaneous compounds will have a different purpose than one that is focused on compounding of home intravenous infusions. Similarly, a pharmacy that aims to provide comprehensive travel vaccination programs for its clients will have a different purpose than a pharmacy that provides blister packs/compliance aid packaging for care homes. Historically, pharmacy managers have resisted thinking of organisational purpose, instead they want to have it all – and the possibility of rapidly changing to offer any new service that comes along that may be profitable. Rather than focusing on purpose, they wanted ultimate flexibility in workspace. As a result, highly generic and undifferentiated workspaces have been constructed for generations that are neither fit-for-purpose nor (in reality) actually provide the kind of flexibility that was hoped for. In thinking about 'purpose', managers need to recognise that dispensaries are not built for eternity: instead they are built for a defined period of time (5–10 years) and will likely need to be renovated and retrofitted several times over a person's career, as the profession and its needs evolve. Articulating a clear purpose for the dispensary – one that is aligned with organisational missions, goals and values – can help managers understand the activities that will fulfill the purpose which will drive workplace design.

Outcomes

Having established a purpose for the workspace, it is often tempting to immediately jump to the idea of tasks required to fulfil this purpose. Premature definition of tasks can be problematic, as it may inhibit creative thinking about workspace, workflow, and day to day processes. Instead, it is useful to focus on deliberation about outcomes: how will the manager know the purpose for the dispensary has been actually achieved? Are there specific measurements, metrics, or quantitative indicators of success (for example, number of prescriptions filled daily, number of medication histories completed, number of travel vaccinations administered, or frequency of Zoom based consultations with other health care providers?). Defining the outcomes that are envisioned for the workspace first can help shape the design that is required to achieve these outcomes. It is essential, however, that these outcomes be closely aligned with the purpose, which in turn was derived from organisational mission and vision. There is always a temptation in pharmacy to create a workspace that has the potential to do everything and be all things to all people. The price of this type of design flexibility is frequently inefficiency, ineffectiveness, reduction in quality, and a much more cranky staff who complain about how poorly designed the space actually is.

Activities

Having defined purpose and outcomes, the manager is now in a position to start to define activities that will be undertaken within the dispensary that will help achieve these purposes and outcomes. Particularly where renovation of workspace is being done, consultation with front line staff in this process is critical: a fine-grained understanding of how work is actually completed within the space itself can help to define how the space should be designed. Where renovation of existing space is being undertaken, observation of current activities is very helpful, and in particular, understanding the number of steps required for people to do everyday, frequently occurring tasks. For example, in a compounding-intensive pharmacy, supplies are often kept in a location that is quite remote from the location of the actual compounding. This is an historical holdover from a time where the security of compounding supplies was more important than the efficiency of processes. As a result, each time compounding is required, someone needs to walk 15–20 steps to the other side of the pharmacy to get a supply. Further, a sink may be centrally located in the dispensary so everyone can use it...but in reality, the main users will be those involved in compounding, and this means another 15–20 steps each time. Similarly, a pharmacy that has defined its purpose as including vaccination administration may need to deal with refrigeration issues. In many cases, the pharmacy will have a single large fridge for all such items, including vaccines, insulin, and anything else requiring cold storage. The room where vaccinations actually occur may be on the other side of the dispensary. Rather than purchasing a small, relatively inexpensive second fridge for vaccine storage, pharmacists now must walk 15–20 steps each time to the central fridge. Further, they may need to go to a separate compounding area to pick up needles and sharps containers, necessitating an additional 15–20 steps each time. Over a day, week, or month, these steps add up and create fatigue and frustration for staff – and increase the risk of error. Careful observation and clear understanding of activities required to fulfil organisational purpose is invaluable in helping to reduce unnecessary steps and optimise efficiency.

Technology

The events of the COVID-19 pandemic rapidly accelerated the embrace of technology across health care, and in particular the role of digital consultations. The ubiquity of Zoom and other similar platforms – and the comfort patients of all ages have developed in engaging virtually – means that the clinical consultation activities of pharmacists needs to evolve rapidly. This evolution has been inhibited by the slow pace at which telecommunications technology has been integrated into workspaces. Almost every other industry (including general practitioners) have now shifted to virtual consultation for many situations; at best, in most pharmacies, this is translated as a hurried telephone call in a noisy and interruption driven dispensary with minimal acoustic privacy. Virtual consultations are not the future of pharmacy, but its recent past means that there is significant need to catch up now and provide the right technology (and training) to allow for seamless virtual consultation. Similarly, the advance of robotics (including automated dispensing, IV admixture, and compounding robotics) have resulted in significant decreases in costs. Many of these machines are now affordable by even small and mid-sized pharmacies, but they need to be built-in to workplace planning, not simply thrown on an existing counter to interfere with everyone else's work. Additional technologies – for example, the use of cameras and digital systems to allow pharmacists to verify dispensed prescriptions from a computer screen rather than having to walk 15–20 steps every few minutes to where a technician is working – are increasingly being integrated into workspaces. Managers need to remember that technology is not simply a shiny new toy but an intentionally deployed tool to support purpose, outcomes, and the activities that are required. Technology selection can seem scary and daunting given its expense – but managers need to educate themselves on options, alternatives, costs, and benefits in order to make the best possible technology decision for their workspace needs. Unfortunately, in many cases, fear of making a poor technology decision often means managers choose to make no decision at all, and the potential of technology to enhance practice remains largely unfulfilled.

Personnel

Pharmacy is ultimately a human-focused profession, and this means that people are the most important part of workplace design. While engineers often refer to them as 'users' of workspace, this diminishes their centrality in the workspace design process. Understanding the needs and wants of the people who will inhabit the space (and ultimately, spend more time in this workspace than they do in their own home) helps to integrate thinking about effective design choices. Key design principles when considering personnel include (but are not limited to):

- *Minimise standing and steps:* As described previously above, pharmacy is a strangely physical profession that requires a lot of standing and a lot of walking about in small bursts. This is physically draining and contributes negatively to morale and employment longevity. Careful analysis of activities and technology can help managers design workspaces that more closely resemble other white-collar jobs with lower physical demands, thereby conserving staff members' energy to focus on patients instead.
- *Adequate ventilation:* The COVID-19 pandemic has reminded us of the crucial importance of air quality in workspaces. Adequate circulation and ventilation is important for air quality and must be regularly monitored, especially in pharmacies where volatile solvents are used for compounding. Poor air quality diminishes cognitive capacity and causes drowsiness, and of course can also facilitate the transmission of infectious disease (especially important since ill people will visit pharmacies).
- *Appropriate task lighting:* Eye strain is a significant problem in pharmacy given the amount of reading and the variability in typical font size. While general fluorescent lighting may be fine for some day to day tasks, reading small prescription vial instructions or product monograph

inserts may require specific task lighting to minimise eye strain. Good quality task lighting makes a surprisingly impactful difference on the comprehension of written material and can contribute meaningfully to quality and patient safety.

- *Ergonomics:* This refers to workplace efficiency but is more commonly used to describe design and placement of furnishings (like chairs and tables) to minimise musculoskeletal strain. For example, consider the ubiquitous dispensary counter, found in virtually every pharmacy. It is frequently of a fixed, unchangeable height, higher than a table but lower than a shelf. This height was actually established based on the needs of middle-aged male pharmacists – and today is likely too high for an increasingly feminised profession. As a result, the people using these standard height counters experience micro-straining over time which can lead to occupational injury at worst, and fatigue and frustration at best. Providing counters that can be adjusted by each individual end-user to their height preference is rarely seen in pharmacies, yet the technology is widely available. Similarly, the proliferation of pre-manufactured pharmaceutical products means shelving units in pharmacies have grown taller. Repeated reaching, or climbing up and down step stools to get products, increases the risk of accidents or muscle strain, and again is unergonomic in design. Some pharmacies have responded to this reality by introducing 'fast mover' shelving, in which commonly dispensed products are placed on shelves at a more convenient height. As a short-term fix this is reasonable – but investments in movable shelving units that can easily be shifted to accommodate for an individual's needs, is preferable from a workplace design perspective. Pharmacists engaged in clinical consultations with patients (e.g. administering vaccinations or screening tests, or providing education/undertaking medical histories) need appropriate office space with easy access to computers for documentation rather than awkward closet spaces with a stool placed in it for the patient to sit while the pharmacist stands. Comfortable chairs, tables, good lighting and ventilation, and enough space to maintain appropriate and safe physical distance, are all important ergonomic considerations.

- *Acoustic considerations:* Dispensaries can be busy, chaotic – and loud – spaces. Aural distraction and overload increase cognitive and emotional overload, and may interfere with patient confidentiality and respectful dialogue. Workplace design needs to also consider how sound travels, who can hear what in a typical conversation, and ways to minimise acoustic interference with purpose, outcomes, and activities. Use of sound baffling materials in workplaces can minimise distractions, as can careful placement of more confidential spaces (e.g. consultation rooms) away from busy traffic areas. Understanding how spaces will be used is an essential first step in understanding how to minimise acoustic interference using design and materials.

- *Flooring:* Historically, high foot-traffic environments have utilised flooring materials that are impervious but hard, and this can lead to back strain with repeated standing. Further, materials that make floors easy to clean can also increase the risk of slips and falls in the event of spills. Newer flooring materials that are durable, slip resistant and easier to walk upon have been developed but may be expensive. Use of location-specific mats designed to be stood upon for long periods of time can help reduce back strain. Further, placement of footstools or small footrests to allow one foot to be higher than the other can also reduce back strain. Where possible, reconceptualising space to allow for seated work or a more ergonomic design of counters and tables can also be considered in addition to appropriate flooring choices.

Security and social distancing

The COVID-19 pandemic has highlighted the need to carefully consider how workplace design can be used to ensure staff members feel safe – both physically and from the risk of infectious disease. Early in the pandemic, desperate measures included the erection of plastic/acrylic/plexiglass barriers between patients and staff members which may have inhibited (but not eliminated) the risk of transmission of airborne disease, but also alienated pharmacy staff from their patients. Some measure of physical barrier is likely a semi-permanent change to all customer-facing work environments, but most research suggests adequate ventilation is more impactful than physical barriers of this sort. Workplace design can also be used to this advantage – for example, deeper counters or tables force greater physical separation rather than a narrow counter with a plexiglass divider. Another lamentably important reality has been the need to consider physical security and the safety of pharmacy staff, from theft, physical or verbal assault, or threats. This is a particularly challenging design issue as traditional security interventions usually involve isolative techniques that run contrary to the ethos of the pharmacist-patient relationship. Use of closed-circuit monitors, discrete 'panic buttons', or walled-off areas may send negative messages with respect to care and confidentiality, but may be necessary in some cases. From a workplace design perspective, these are amongst the most challenging issues to manage effectively, particularly since pharmacies are involved in dispensing narcotics, methadone, and other products that may be high risk for theft. Finding ways of balancing patient care philosophy and client engagement with the reality of threats and theft is essential, as is engagement with front line staff to better understand their needs and concerns in space design.

Ambience

Most of the key design features described above have a strongly pragmatic orientation and most workspace design should be rooted in practical realities and business objectives. However, it is also important to consider ambience and décor, given the strong influence these will have on perception, emotion, morale and staff well-being. It is sometimes tempting to dismiss ambience as superficial or merely a distraction, but most of us have had the experience of working in spaces that were overly utilitarian and devoid of spirt or charm, thereby depleting us of energy and enthusiasm. Historically, ambience has been challenging to operationalise in pharmacy workplace design: abstract concepts of 'trustworthiness', 'cleanliness', and 'orderliness' have resulted in somewhat sterile décor focused on the functional rather than the pleasurable. Arguably, pharmacies have been mistrustful of 'decorating' as it may imply a lack of seriousness or scientific rigour. In some cases, corporate guidance will dictate colour schemes and décor choices as a way of reinforcing branding objectives. When considering ambience and décor, it is useful to focus on:

- *Line:* Horizontal, vertical, and variable lines guide an individual's eye and helps to shape a room. The right line selection can make small spaces 'look' larger and cavernous spaces feel cozy. Horizontal lines are usually created by counters, tables, and other surfaces, and convey a sense of stability and efficiency. If there is a need to make a space simply feel wider or longer than it really is, horizontal lines can be useful, though if overdone, it can make a space feel boring and flat. Vertical lines are usually created by structural features of the space including windows and doors. Shelving units in pharmacies can also help emphasise the vertical. When staged well, vertical lines create the sense of volume or height in a room. Diagonal or zig-zag lines can help create a feeling of movement or direction (for example, towards a counselling room); used in small quantities this adds visual interest and breaks up monotony, but can also be distracting or overwhelming if over-used.

- *Form:* This refers to the physical shape of the space, and objects within it. Form is usually described as geometric or organic; geometric spaces have square edges and conventional proportions of length, width and height. Objects within spaces should align with the form of the space, so geometric spaces should have geometric objects placed in geometric orientations. Adding too many organic flourishes into a geometric space often looks 'messy' or disorganised rather than whimsical or creative.

- *Lighting:* The importance of task lighting has been discussed previously, but other forms of lighting include accent lighting (emphasising specific objects) and mood lighting (to help support emotional needs). Accent lighting can be used to showcase specific objects or documents of interest. Mood lighting is essential to consider in workplace design: traditional fluorescent lighting found in many workplaces can be quite difficult for those with illness to manage, given its intensity, frequency and how it may illuminate things that a patient wishes to keep less visible. It is also difficult to manage on a daily basis by staff given its lack of variability and brightness. As a result, it can create a form of cognitive and emotional overload that is difficult to manage. Different lighting sources projecting different kinds and shades/tones of light can be more soothing and create a more positive emotional state.

- *Colour:* One of the most challenging decisions in décor involves colour, and as a result 'beiges' tend to dominate since these are thought to be the least offensive to everyone. The psychology of colour is complex and should not be underestimated in terms of its impact on individuals. Traditionally, greens and blues are thought to enhance calmness while reds expand energy. When considering colour choice, it is important to think about what the space will be used for and activities undertaken – 'decorating' is not an abstract activity but it needs to be connected to function and purpose. It is also essential to think about how light sources will influence the way a colour looks: natural light, fluorescent light, and incandescent light will all bring out different tones and shades depending on the time of day. Traditionally, lighter or brighter colours have been thought to give the illusion of more space, but newer colour palettes and paints available have challenged this assumption.

- *Textures:* Dispensaries do not need to incorporate throw pillows and quilts to enhance the textural appeal of space. Counter surfaces, chair fabrics, and shelving materials all add visual interest to otherwise sterile spaces. Texture is arguably the hardest décor element to incorporate in a professional environment but it can be an important consideration to enhance the appeal and functionality of the space.

- *Patterns:* Paired with colour, the judicious use of patterns can have a similar function to texture in increasing the visual allure of a space. Patterns typically consist of a repeated design (like stripes or pictures). When subtle and balanced, patterns can be visually interesting without being overwhelming. Introducing patterns into small rooms should be carefully considered as this could have the effect of making the space feel even smaller. Complex patterns involving contrasting colours can energise space and make larger spaces feel more homely. As a rule of thumb, no more than 2–3 different patterns should be used in any single contiguous space in order to ensure it does not become overwhelming.

Summary

Workplace design, though often overlooked, is an essential management function that will have enormous implications for organisational success and staff morale. It may be tempting for managers to simply allow corporate designers with limited pharmacy experience to make decisions; historically, this has been the case and the result is a somewhat bland, dysfunctional, and unpleasant dispensary set-up that most individuals experience today. Workplace design is a science and an art, and while pharmacy managers may not be specialists in this area, they have much to contribute in terms of planning – and of course will bear responsibility for outcomes even if they choose not to plan at all. Design is not simply décor, even though décor is an important element of success. Systematic thinking and planning involving all stakeholders but especially front line staff using the space itself, is essential. Managerial ownership and control of the process itself is necessary to ensure the needs and wants of pharmacy staff are embedded in decisions that are made, which will influence day to day working life for years to come. With good design, safe, effective and high quality professional practice are better enabled and this will result in increased morale, productivity, and business success.

References

1. Vischer J, Wifi M. The effect of workplace design on quality of life at work. In: Fleury-Bahi G *et al*. eds. *Handbook of Environmental Psychology and Quality of Life Research*. London: Springer Press, 2017: 387–400. https://doi.org/10.1007/978-3-319-31416-7_21

2. Marmaras N, Nathanael D. Workplace Design. In: Salvendy G, ed. *Handbook of Human Factors and Ergonomics*, 3rd edn. New York: John Wiley & Sons, 2006: 573–589. https://doi.org/10.1002/0470048204.ch22

3. Bangwal D *et al*. Workplace design features, job satisfaction, and organization commitment. *SAGE Open* 2017; 7(3). https://doi.org/10.1177/2158244017716708

4. Salameh L *et al*. Facilitating integration of regulated pharmacy technicians into community pharmacy practice in Ontario: results of an exploratory study. *Can Pharm J* 2018; 151(3): 189–196. https://doi.org/10.1177/1715163518765892

5. Forooraghi M *et al*. How does office design support employees' health? A case study on the relationship among employees' perceptions of the office environment, their sense of coherence and office design. *Int J Environ Res Public Health* 2021; 18(23): 12779. https://doi.org/10.3390/ijerph182312779

6. Hui F, Aye L. Occupational stress and workplace design. *Buildings* 2018; 8(10): 133. https://doi.org/10.3390/buildings8100133

7. Veitch J. Workplace design contributions to mental health and well-being. *Healthcare Papers* 2011; (11): 38–46. https://doi.org/10.12927/hcpap.2011.22409

8. Gutnick L. A workplace design that reduces employee stress and increases employee productivity using environmentally responsible materials. Ypsilanti, Michigan: Eastern Michigan University, 2007 (dissertation).

9. Reiling J *et al*. The impact of facility design on patient safety. In: Hughes R, ed. *Patient Safety and Quality: An evidence based handbook for nurses*. Rockville: Agency for Healthcare Research and Quality, 2008: 167–192.

CHAPTER 15

Workflow management

Upon completion of this chapter you should be able to:

- explain the general workflow design principles that managers should recognise
- list the key principles in pharmacy workflow design
- recognise the areas where managerial decisions will impact workflow
- understand the importance of successful management of workflow design.

One of the most important and practical jobs of a manager involves designing, monitoring, and improving workflow within an organisation. Workflow can be described as the processes undertaken by individuals within organisations to accomplish specific tasks in support of strategic objectives.[1] Within pharmacy, workflow has traditionally described the prescription filling process, but as the profession increasingly pivots towards more of a service and care orientation, workflow principles are applied to a variety of different, non-dispensing activities including the provision of medication reconciliation and new medicines services, delivery of vaccinations, and public health screening.[2] Managers make decisions and supervise the implementation of workflow policies, procedures and practices that fundamentally shape an organisation's culture and directly influence its outcomes.[3] As a result, understanding workflow management principles is integral to success as a manager.

General workflow design principles

Within any business or organisation, workflow design is usually a guideline or ideal rather than a hard-and-fast rule. Workflow design must balance many competing priorities in an organisation, being pragmatic is required. General workflow design principles are often rooted in manufacturing industries where efficiency and cost-effectiveness are central to success. Various best-practices in workflow design exist (for example Lean Six Sigma) that may have some applicability to professional care and services fields such as pharmacy.[4,5,6] For managers, several crucial principles should be recognised and used as a starting point in decision making regarding workflow, including:

- *Workplace design matters:* There is a complex chicken-and-egg co-dependency between workplace design and workflow. Physical layout/infrastructure is directly linked to workflow, and often times workflow ideas can be frustrated by poor workplace design. Limitations in terms of space, lighting, awkward traffic patterns, or inappropriate placement of key equipment will all impinge on workflow. Some of this can be readily changed: for example, a poorly placed computer terminal that blocks communication between colleagues can simply be shifted or replaced by a more streamlined laptop computer. In some cases, workplace design is an insurmountable barrier: for example, it may simply not be feasible to create additional square footage within a space constrained pharmacy to accommodate additional personnel or activities. Ideally, managers are directly involved in both workplace and workflow design so they can be iteratively connected in constructive ways. It is also important to be pragmatic and understand what, in reality, is changeable and what must simply be lived with and worked around.

- *Minimise hand-offs:* Most processes in workplaces involve multiple individuals working in sequence to accomplish a task. For example, in dispensing a prescription, a technician may receive and initially input a prescription into a computer, a pharmacist may then review for clinical appropriateness, prior to handing off to an assistant for filling, who then directs it to a pharmacist for checking, who subsequently passes it to a clerk for filing until a patient appears to collect it. In most pharmacies, the traditional pattern for dispensing prescriptions is both inefficient and potentially compromises patient safety because it involves too many unnecessary hand-offs between individuals. When work has to be undertaken by a group of individuals, workflow should be designed to minimise the frequency of hand-offs and reduce the number of individuals involved in hand-offs as much as possible. Each hand-off increases the risk of error, reduces efficiency, and potentially creates bottlenecks.

- *Minimise waiting time:* Coupled with hand-offs, the issue of bottlenecks and waiting time are a significant concern. Where work moves from one person to another, it may mean that at times there is an asymmetric or unequal workload so that one person moves more quickly than another. Eventually that person will end up waiting for the other team member to catch up in terms of work and this produces inefficient and costly waiting time. Finding ways to minimise waiting time and eliminate bottlenecks in workflow contributes meaningfully to enhanced productivity and profitability.

- *Minimise the number of systems involved in a process:* The prescription dispensing process highlights the problem associated with multiple systems. Prescription processing may require one program for data input and prescription label generation, another system for verification of therapeutic appropriateness, a third system for billing and remuneration, and a fourth system for clinical documentation. While there have been some improvements in pharmacy software in the last few years, in many cases, pharmacy staff will need to work with overlapping systems to complete all aspects of the dispensing process, rather than simply work within one system shell. Similarly, the provision of vaccinations or public health services often requires access to multiple governmental, health service, clinical documentation, and clinical guidance websites or systems. Good workflow design tries to minimise the number of systems workers need to access in order to accomplish routine tasks. Multiple system access is inefficient, unproductive, increases the risk of error, and can produce frustration for workers.

- *Minimise the number of people required to 'touch' an item:* In health care work, issues of security, sterility, and stability are central to questions of safety. The more hands that 'touch' an item (figuratively and literally), the higher the risk exists for contamination, waste, pilferage, or other problems. Workflow should be designed to have the fewest necessary number of people physically come into contact with items (medications, equipment, needles, ampoules, etc.) throughout the process to both enhance efficiency and safety.

- *Minimise need for manual computation:* Manual or mental computation is more likely to produce mathematical errors than automated calculations. Within pharmacy, a relatively simple calculation (e.g. how many capsules should be dispensed for a prescription taken three times daily for ten days?) can easily become complicated if the dose requires two capsules to be taken each time, or if a tapering dosage schedule is introduced. Minimising the need for mental arithmetic – particularly in highly sensitive areas such as chemotherapy dosing calculations – is important for both efficiency and patient safety. In most cases, automation of calculations is readily available and should be embedded in all processes.

- *Minimise need for 'look up' steps:* In virtually every field, there are many details that defy memorisation and will require confirmation through some alternative process. Historically, 'looking up' referred to the process by which individuals would consult an external/authoritative print reference (e.g. a textbook) to confirm a detail that was unmemorised or that was recalled without great confidence. While looking up should be encouraged and is much preferred over simple guesswork, workflow design should minimise the need for individuals to actually stop what they are doing in order to locate a reference and look something up. In many cases, software design can be used to help make this easier, for example, through the use of drop-down menus. In other cases, workflow design that allows individuals an opportunity to gain expertise and confidence through routinisation of work can also minimise the need for look ups.

- *Minimise need for judgement calls:* All professionals encounter ambiguous situations which will require the exercise of professional judgement rather than application of a pre-established rule. Workplace design can be used to minimise the frequency of judgement calls being made, which results in more predictability, efficiency, and safety. For example, where chronic drug shortages exist due to supply chain issues, a policy can be developed that guides pharmacy staff in terms of specific alternatives to follow, rather than relying on situational, subjective judgements. Decision support tools (including software) should be used to provide evidence-based options or answers, rather than off-the-cuff and situationally variable responses.

As can be seen from these principles, a general theme of good workflow design involves 'minimisation' of many things. Fewer hands, fewer subjective judgements, fewer steps, and fewer hand-offs all contribute to more efficient, effective, and safer workflow in both technical and service/care activities.

Key considerations in pharmacy workflow design

Non-pharmacists, who spend any amount of time in a community or hospital pharmacy setting, may be startled by the level of busy-ness, the number of interruptions, the volume of workload, the lack of clear processes and organisation, and the seemingly chaotic traffic patterns of people working in the space. Pharmacy workflow has evolved in a somewhat haphazard manner, in response to the changing scope of practice, roles and responsibilities of staff members, environmental demands, and logistics/ space constraints. This evolution has typically been reactive and organic, defying systematic planning or methodical attempts to predict future needs. In some cases, managers may have the opportunity to 'invent' entirely new workflow designs for new-build pharmacy spaces, but even in these cases, the cultural legacy and memory of pharmacy workflow in other settings has a pernicious effect on planning and design.

The unique design challenge for pharmacy workflow is that it is a service-and-care intensive profession that is superimposed and must co-exist with a highly technical, manufacturing intensive and production oriented dispensing operation.[7] The same individuals who provide service-and-care also generally work in the compounding/dispensing space and toggle between these very different responsibilities frequently and rapidly. While it is tempting to propose bold solutions such as complete separation of cognitive and technical elements of the profession, in reality these are difficult or impossible to actually implement in real world practices. Radical redesign of pharmacy workflow has been attempted but is rarely successful in the longer term, and even more rarely has resulted in the adoption of these practices by other workplaces. In most cases, managers must then consider incremental but maximally impactful changes to workflow design that can focus on a few key principles including:

- *Safety:* Safe and accurate technical and clinical work is the cornerstone of professional practice. Workflow design in a pharmacy must always prioritise safety and include sufficient checks and balances to provide the public with reassurance that the services, care, and products are secure. The safety principle also extends to the safety of the workforce itself: pharmacy staff must work with potentially dangerous products (e.g. chemotherapy or toxic solvents) and so safety of the workforce is an equal priority in workflow considerations. This includes physical security and ergonomic safety in all aspects of work.
- *Quality:* Patients have the right to expect the best possible quality in services, care, and products they receive from pharmacies. Workflow design must be undertaken in ways that optimise or maximise opportunities for high-quality work to be consistently and reliably undertaken. Cutting corners and compromising on quality can quickly lead to safety problems, but it can also lead to suboptimal health outcomes for patients.
- *Effectiveness:* Workflow design needs to prioritise effectiveness – the capacity of the pharmacy and its staff to actually produce/deliver successful outcomes and results. Simply getting through large volumes of work is NOT a measure of effectiveness – productivity without effectiveness is actually demoralising for staff and difficult to justify. Considering how workflow design enhances the actual effectiveness of the work is important and will have ramifications in terms of profitability and economic viability of a practice.
- *Efficiency:* Many outsiders to pharmacy comment on how inefficient workflow appears to the layperson – for example, when patients say, 'it takes 20 minutes for you to dispense my prescription, when you're only slapping a label on a box?'. Efficiency refers to the amount of time/energy/work invested in a task compared to its output. Efficiency optimisation will often require the minimisation of hand-offs, subjective judgements, and minimisation of steps and hands involved in a process, as described in the previous section of this chapter.
- *Sustainability:* In most cases, pharmacies are not transient, fly-by-night operations but institutions and businesses that are integral to communities and organisations and are expected to be in place for many, many years. Workflow design needs to consider the long-term, including long-term motivation and health of the workforce within that workflow. An increasingly imperative element of sustainability includes environmental and planetary considerations related to carbon footprint, heat generation and other activities impacting climate. These will be discussed in Chapter 25.

With these pharmacy-specific workflow considerations in mind, there are key areas where managerial decisions will have significant impact on workflow, including scheduling, multi-tasking, workload, technology, and processes.

Scheduling

A pivotal role for managers involves scheduling staff to work within a pharmacy. This is often one of the most controversial and challenging aspects of management, as it involves balancing fairness with personal considerations. For example, where a pharmacy remains open on Christmas Day – who should work this shift? There are three common scheduling problems managers will face:

1. *Unpopular shifts:* Pharmacies must remain open to serve their communities meaning some pharmacy staff need to work evenings, weekends, and holidays. Scheduling for unpopular shifts has traditionally been built around an informal principle of seniority - the 'older' or more long-standing an employee is, the more likely they are to get priority in scheduling decisions. As a manager, it is important to develop a clear, coherent, defensible, and consistent philosophy of scheduling so that everyone in a workplace can predict and at least grudgingly accept outcomes. Caution should be exercised in simply relying on seniority to guide scheduling decisions as this can 'bake-in' unfairness that will lead to resentment. Alternatives to a seniority-driven scheduling system can include random/lottery selections, annual rotations, or the use of incentives to try to encourage workers to volunteer for unpopular shifts.

2. *Length of a shift:* Some staff members express strong preferences for 12 hour (rather than more typical) shifts, believing that it is 'easier' to work 3 x 12 hour weeks rather than 5 x 7.5 hour weeks, from a child-minding or personal free-time perspective. They may erroneously believe they are just as safe, effective, efficient, and provide quality care after 12 hours of work as after 8 hours of work. Industrial psychologists have noted the deleterious effects of overly-long shifts on human performance and the increased risks of errors, as well as the impact on mental and physical well-being. While personal preference of workers may lead them to want to work fewer, longer shifts to reduce commuting burden or time away from home, this personal preference must be balanced around principles of safety, quality, efficiency, and effectiveness and may (in many cases) need to be avoided.

3. *Scheduling teams, not individuals:* The pharmacy workforce is diverse and consists of many different people with different qualifications and individual quirks. Traditionally, scheduling has focused on individuals, but since most pharmacies work in a team-based environment, there is significant advantage to consider the idea of team (or line) based scheduling. It takes time for individual team members to learn how to work with one another; where the composition of team members changes on a daily basis, the time and cognitive stress required to re-learn how to work with this particular team can be considerable. It is usually more efficient, and generally enhances effectiveness, quality, and safety to have greater consistency in scheduling so team members work with the same other team members on a regular basis. Importantly, this structure also builds social bonds and cohesion, so that team members can watch out for mental health or burnout issues that may be evolving within their teams, in ways that groups of strangers working with one another may not necessarily notice.

Scheduling is as much an art as it is a science, and involves delicate negotiations cajoling, and understanding of how to apply incentives. Incentivisation rather than punishment is a more productive managerial strategy: where emergency shift coverage due to illness is required, simply saying 'you have to work, no one else is available' can breed resentment and reduce loyalty. Instead, managers should anticipate the need to have a contingency fund of perks or money that they can use to create more positive conditions for people to accept schedule deviations. Perks could include additional time off, recognition gift cards, or even merchandise as a way of acknowledging personal time sacrifices made to accommodate last minute scheduling requests. Proactively securing and managing a contingency fund/resources for scheduling is an important tactic to smooth difficult scheduling problems so as not to unduly or unfairly rely upon altruism or professionalism.

Multi-tasking

One of the most distressing hallmarks of pharmacy practice for most pharmacists is the multi-tasking that appears to be inherent in the role. Between answering phone calls, managing technical staff, responding to drug information requests, speaking to patients, etc. the interruption-driven nature of hospital and community practice is both exhausting and overwhelming, and a significant threat to safety, quality, effectiveness, efficiency and sustainability. Many managers simply shrug their shoulders and say that's the way pharmacy is and there's nothing to be done. In fact, managerial decisions have shaped the multi-tasking culture of pharmacy for generations – and managerial choices can change this. While some individuals may claim they 'like to be busy' or 'enjoy all the different things' they get to do, the reality, of course, is that multi-tasking diminishes task focus, attentiveness, and heightens the risk of errors. Managers have significant opportunities to reduce the need for, and risks of, multi-tasking through the use of protected time scheduling practices. While there are cost and resource implications, protected time scheduling simply means that certain crucial tasks requiring concentration (for example, medicines review services, or public health consultations) are specifically scheduled into an individual's workday and all other responsibilities are either deferred or covered by other staff members. Protected time – even if it is only for a few hours can provide an important opportunity to concentrate, focus, and actually accomplish tasks, and it can be incredibly helpful in building morale. In some cases, no additional resources or staff may even be needed – creative scheduling of other staff, or the use of existing technology (e.g. voice mail/email) can provide a buffer zone to allow individuals uninterrupted time to complete certain jobs. As a general principle, all pharmacists and most technicians should have some uninterrupted time each week (4–6 hours) and building this into managerial scheduling practices and organisational policies can make this happen. Finding ways of reducing the necessity to multi-task on a day-in, day-out basis is important for sustainability and mental health of the workforce. It is often not as complex or impossible as it first appears but simply needs to be a managerial choice and priority to implement.

Workload

One of the most controversial issues in workflow management in pharmacy today involves the volume of work, and in particular, the number of prescriptions dispensed in a typical day/shift. Few jurisdictions have regulatory controls over how many prescriptions a pharmacist may 'safely' process/dispense/clinically evaluate over a set period of time, and attempts to introduce such maximums are often derided as being 'unprofessional'. Many other fields – for example, aviation – recognise the impact of workload on safety and quality. Pilots are only allowed to fly a certain maximum number of hours in a row before it is recognised that fatigue will cause errors. For pharmacists however – no such recognition is afforded. Managers need to be very aware of, and respectful of, how excess workload contributes negatively to organisational outcomes and success. Rather than relying on informal mechanisms (e.g. 'if it gets too busy out here, just call me in my office and I'll give you a hand'), actual monitoring and measuring of workload can provide quantitative evidence to support staff expansion/hiring or redeployment to make workload more manageable. Understanding the acceptable, safe, sustainable workload range that enables quality, efficiency, and effectiveness should be a manager's top priority. Defining this range requires input from staff members along with comparisons to other comparator organisations, and will vary depending on the context of practice. For example, a chemotherapy production unit will have a different appropriate workload range than a vaccination clinic. Actually defining the upper and lower bands of acceptable workload range and ensuring staff understand and accept these ranges, is the first step in helping to better manage workload. Failure to acknowledge the real impact of excess and unfair workload will result in decreased morale, employee turnover, increased error and decreased quality and safety.

Technology

Like every field today, technology is integral to success in pharmacy. Amongst health professions, pharmacy has historically been a leader in integrating technology into practice, first with the use of computers and electronic documentation and record storage, and more recently through the use of artificial intelligence and robotics. Simple technologies like fax machines, which were initially purported to save time, have now become time-wasters in many cases. Technology is not inherently always positive and a time-saver, so managers need to be intentional and deliberative in identifying what technologies will support safety, quality, efficiency, effectiveness, and sustainability, and how they need to be implemented and deployed to optimise their benefit. Currently, a general principle guiding technology implementation focuses on the way in which some can help staff control, prioritise, and sequence work as a way of better managing workload. For example, a telephone- or internet-based refill request system allows patients requiring refills on medications to bypass speaking with pharmacy staff members and simply input their request several days in advance of needing it. This allows pharmacy staff greater control in queuing and prioritising, and helps them to manage workflow. Similarly, appointment-based consultations, in which patients schedule time to meet with a pharmacist to undertake a medication review or a vaccination, provides similar benefits. Using technology to facilitate queuing, prioritising and supporting greater control over time has emerged as a particularly important tool for integration in pharmacy. Providing access to email or virtual platforms like Zoom to allow pharmacy staff to virtually consult with patients or speak with other health care professionals, is also a way of helping to manage time more effectively and efficiently. These inexpensive and currently available technologies, when strategically implemented with a view to reducing workload-driven stress, can have significant benefits. Other technologies that facilitate easier access to clinical guidance or clinical/medical/drug information can also reduce the time required to look up important information. One of the most important – though elusive – technologies in pharmacy today are computer systems that fully integrate dispensing, documentation, clinical monitoring and management, and payment/remuneration submissions, rather than requiring four or more separate systems with different software requirements. Technology continues to grow and evolve and will play an increasingly dominant role in workflow design in years ahead; while tools such as robotics and artificial intelligence may have important roles to play, they are typically expensive and difficult to deploy effectively. Managers should focus on existing, widely used and accessible technologies like email, virtual consultation platforms, and integrated documentation systems that can reduce workload related stress in a more immediate manner.

Processes

In both dispensing/compounding intensive and care/service intensive pharmacy practices, managers need to consider processes and protocols that govern day to day work, in an effort to minimise hand-offs, hands involved in work, subjective judgements required, etc. Where intentional and mindful processes are not implemented and monitored, more random and chaotic ones will evolve that compromise safety, quality, and sustainability. For managers to understand processes and how to improve them, they need to actually observe, participate, and innovate. Consider the typical workflow surrounding prescription dispensing in community pharmacy: in many contexts, assistants will receive and do preliminary inputting of data before handing off to a pharmacist for a clinical check, who may hand off to a technician for dispensing, who then hands back to a pharmacist for checking (if required) and educating a patient, who then hands back to an assistant to address inventory/supply or other issues. This process is inefficient, risks error, causes unnecessary bottlenecks and traffic, and delays time to completion for patients. There is no simple, single, or easy solution to process problems in pharmacy as a profession, as each individual pharmacy has its own unique context, circumstances, and constraints. Managers should, however, undertake systematic observations of current processes with an eye to understanding how they can be improved through workflow design principles discussed in this chapter. Comparing current practices to principles outlined above can signpost potential alternatives for further examination and potential process innovation. For example, reversing workflow so it is the pharmacist who both accepts and inputs prescriptions, and simultaneously performs clinical audits and patient education before handing off to a technician for independent dispensing, reduces steps, hand-offs, and hands involved. This may not work in all pharmacies – but some variation of it might be useful to consider. In examining processes, identification of bottlenecks or capacity constraints that slow momentum towards completion is essential. Frequently these bottlenecks occur at hand-offs and in pharmacy it is often the pharmacist that is the most frequent bottleneck. Examining processes through this lens, then considering innovations to address bottlenecks, can be a useful way to enhance quality, efficiency, and effectiveness.

When examining processes and considering improvements, it is often tempting to believe the necessary changes are either too big and impossible to even contemplate, or that small changes won't matter at all, so why bother? Neither of these are true in all cases. The question of whether evolutionary or revolutionary change in processes is needed is complex; there are circumstances where one may be more appropriate than the other. The advantage of evolutionary process innovation, of course, is that it is less disruptive and easier to recover from if it doesn't work, but it also means evolutionary changes may be less impactful. Conversely, revolutionary changes are larger in scope, massively disruptive but can potentially be 'game changers' in supporting better processes. Managing evolutionary change is not necessarily easier: constant small changes can sometimes produce as much stress as a single big change. Process improvements requires sophisticated communication and conflict management skills, keeping people informed and aware, and listening to and authentically responding to concerns. These skills are as essential as identifying bottlenecks and other threats to efficiency, effectiveness, quality, and safety.

Workflow design is the foundation of management success

It is a truism to state that most people spend more time at work than they do at home with their families, and so what happens in the workplace is of significant importance to the personal and professional lives of the workforce. One of the most important and powerful tools managers have is their ability to control workflow. Even in a fast-paced field like pharmacy, managerial decisions around scheduling, multi-tasking, integration of technology, etc. will all have major implications for motivation, engagement, and satisfaction of the workforce. From this perspective, workflow design is actually a form of human resource management, and as such requires sophisticated communication and conflict management skills in addition to analytical, observational, and problem-solving skills. Where organisational malaise exists, workflow is often a part of the problem. Maintaining control over workflow practices can help prevent small problems from spiralling into bigger problems and should be at the top of any manager's agenda. Wherever possible, the best way to understand workflow is to actually participate in it: actually examining workflow through the eyes and experiences of someone who has to live with and succeed within a workflow system, builds not only better understanding of processes but also enhances credibility with team members when change begins.

It can be daunting to even consider tackling a generations long problem like workflow in pharmacy practice. Perhaps unsurprisingly, the typical workflow in prescription processing and compounding has changed very little in over 50 years, despite introduction of new technologies, regulated pharmacy technicians, and other innovations. Problems with bottlenecks, hand-offs, too many hands involved, etc. continue to plague pharmacy workplaces. More vigilant, involved, and innovative managers are needed to improve workflow in all settings. Principles described in this chapter can help managers focus their problem-solving skills in ways that are productive and will enhance safety, quality, efficiency, effectiveness, and sustainability.

References

1. Cain C, Haque S. Organizational workflow and its impact on work quality. In: Hughes R, ed. *Patient Safety and Quality: An Evidence-based Handbook for Nurses, Volume 2*. Rockville: Agency for Healthcare Research and Quality, 2008.

2. So R *et al*. Impact of a 'pharmacist first' innovative workflow plan in patients with hypertension and/or diabetes. *Can Pharm J* 2021; 154(6): 376–380. https://doi.org/10.1177/17151635211016498

3. Karia A *et al*. Community pharmacist workflow: space for pharmacy-based interventions and consultation TimE study protocol. *Int J Pharm Pract* 2020; 28(5): 441–448. https://doi.org/10.1111/ijpp.12625

4. Hohmeier K *et al*. Community pharmacist workflow and medication therapy management delegation: an assessment of preferences and barriers. *J Am Pharm Assoc* 2020; 60(6): 215–223. https://doi.org/10.1016/j.japhy.2020.07.024

5. Hoxsie D *et al*. Analysis of community pharmacy workflow processes in preventing dispensing errors. *J Pharm Pract* 2006; 19(2): 124–130. https://doi.org/10.1177/0897190005285602

6. Jenkins A, Eckel S. Analyzing methods for improved management of workflow in an outpatient pharmacy setting. *Am J Health Syst Pharm* 2012; 69(11): 966–971. https://doi.org/10.2146/ajhp110389

7. Krizner K. Workflow management is critical for everyone. *Drug Topics J* [online] 2019; 163(5).

CHAPTER 16

Policies and procedures

Upon completion of this chapter you should be able to:

- define the terms policy and procedure
- understand how managers can use policies and procedures to build organisational culture and reduce the risk of error
- explain the limitations of policies and procedures
- list the components of an effective policy
- list the components of an effective procedure
- understand the managerial responsibilities for adopting and implementing policies and procedures.

Few people become managers because of an abiding interest in developing and implementing policies and procedures, yet the reality of most managerial roles today is that policies and procedures are an essential component of the role. It is easy to dismiss or disparage them as 'bureaucratic' or 'pointless' but in organisations large and small, policies and procedures are an essential safeguard and a legal requirement. Much of the responsibility for developing, implementing, monitoring, and reporting on policies and procedures falls on managers; learning how to craft and deploy them is an essential skill for management success.

Distinguishing between policy and procedure

In everyday organisational life, the terms policy and procedure are frequently used interchangeably, or simultaneously, negating the fact that they have distinct differences.[1] Policies are used to articulate and put into writing the general parameters or principles that should be used to guide decision making and behaviour within the organisation, but they do not necessarily spell out all details for specific situations.[2] Good policies explain 'why' certain actions are better than others, aligned with organisational mission, vision, and objectives.[3] Procedures focus on the 'how', providing instructions in a methodical step-by-step manner to allow for consistent completion of specific, usually routine, tasks.[2] Procedures frequently include checklists, flowcharts or other mechanisms to help systematise and reduce subjective judgement in day to day work.[3]

Policies are usually developed to help communicate organisational values, philosophies, and commitments, and this is an important tool for understanding organisational culture. Examples of typical topics that should be covered by specific policies include:

- What employees can expect from the employer – important elements related to non-financial benefits (e.g. sick time, parental leave, etc.), vacation/annual leave allocations, sabbatical opportunities, or continuing education practices.
- What employers require of their employees – attendance/punctuality expectations, confidentiality agreements, non-disclosure or non-compete agreements.
- What clients/patients can expect from the organisation – customer service expectations, quality of care standards, turnaround times for delivery of products and services, etc.

Effective and well-written policies establish a strong foundation for a productive workplace culture.[4] Without clear articulation of standards, expectations, and responsibilities, organisations will frequently devolve into chaotic free-for-alls, with each individual assuming their own personal standards and expectations apply at the organisational level. Well-written and effective policies do not simply list rules; instead, they clearly explain the purpose behind the rules that support success in an individual's job.[5] Key attributes of good policies include:[6]

- *Clear, simple, plain, and concise language:* Policies should be written in ways that are easily understood, with minimal reference to jargon or technical terms. Good policies should be easily understood by not only employees, but also clients/patients.
- *Focus on explanation, not implementation:* For policies to work, employees must 'buy-in' and understand their justification. Well-written policies provide a clear rationale for the rules that facilitates buy-in from all stakeholders.
- *Accessibility:* Effective policies are living documents that are consulted on a regular basis as part of routine, day to day work, to ensure consistent application by everyone. Making sure that policies are easily accessible to reduce barriers to retrieval is as important as the written document itself. In many organisations, online versions of policies are available which facilitate computer algorithm driven searches using key terms. In other organisations, binders placed in centralised locations, including a detailed table of contents and a search-term based index, can suffice. For policies to actually work, employees need to know they exist, know where to find them, and be able to consult them quickly to confirm they are conforming to expectations.
- *Be sensible, logical, and practical:* Policies need to be feasible and support day to day work, rather than interfere with it or cause it to become overwhelming. Well-written policies actually make work easier by reducing the need for subjective judgement and specifying how routine tasks should be completed to ensure consistency and reduce unpredictability. They should also represent simple common sense.

In contrast to policies that explain the 'why', procedures explain the 'how', and should provide detailed step-by-step directions on how to complete specific, routine tasks.[6] Checklists or flowcharts are increasingly used to visually depict procedures to minimise the amount of text required.[7] At the minimum, most procedures should include the following:[8]

- Identification of who is responsible for a task, what can be delegated and to whom, and who supervises the person responsible for the task.

- Specific details regarding sequential/logical steps required to complete the task efficiently and effectively, with minimal number of hand-offs, and minimal number of hands involved in the task.
- What 'successful' completion of the task looks like and how it can be assessed by the individual, the supervisor, and the customer.
- Reference to any other supports required.

Example of policy and procedure

To understand the distinction between policies and procedures, consider the common example of annual leave or paid time off (PTO). A vacation policy defines how much PTO an employee is eligible to take, usually based on the number of years of service. It explains why PTO is essential for workplace success and provides support for ensuring all employees take their annual PTO allocation rather than skip or bank it for future use. In contrast, the accompanying procedure would provide a checklist of steps to request and gain approval for PTO, as well as the specific factors that determines who gets priority where multiple individuals request the same time periods for PTO.

Why do policies and procedures matter to an organisation?

Policies and procedures have emerged as one of the most commonly used managerial tactics necessary to build organisational culture and reduce the risk of error and liability.[9] They are important because:

- *They promote consistency across an organisation:* This enhances safety, quality, efficiency, and effectiveness of organisational processes.
- *They build and protect the 'brand' and interests of a business:* Consistent quality in service, care, and products is what helps build a reputation and ultimately drive consumer/patient trust. Policies and procedures are an important way of ensuring consistency that helps build a reputation and brand name for an organisation.
- *They increase compliance:* The existence of policies and procedures, coupled with regular updating and training of all staff, helps to reinforce existing regulations and legal requirements in heavily regulated fields like pharmacy. Pharmacies have statutory obligations to comply with national and regulatory codes and regulations: policies and procedures provide a more detailed and organisation specific road map to ensure individual workers are in compliance with sometimes vague or non-specific legal or regulatory requirements.
- *They are themselves mandated in law:* Many jurisdictions require organisations of all sizes to develop and enforce certain kinds of policies and procedures, for example, related to the prevention of discrimination and promotion of diversity, equity and inclusion, or deterrence of bullying and harassment. Organisations that do not develop and implement these legally mandated policies are out of compliance with employment and other standards/laws, and could face fines and sanctions. Policies and procedures that are required through employment standards acts include, for example, parental and sick leave, vacation time and benefits, termination and discipline, etc.
- *They improve internal efficiencies:* Good policies and procedures eliminate guesswork and subjectivity, and as a result improve managerial and operational efficiencies. They reduce

misunderstanding and prevent disagreement because they are not subject to debate or discussion, but instead they are only subject to implementation and enforcement. This clarity ensures managers are not open to entreaties or appeals from workers, and gives them the ability to rightly claim 'my hands are tied by this policy' which can help reduce conflict and friction.

- *They help navigate critical incidents and crises:* At times of organisational stress, it is easy to become panicked and overwhelmed, and this can interfere with good judgement and principled thinking about a problem. Good policies help organisations and individuals navigate foreseeable crises and reduces guesswork and subjectivity. As such, they help reduce stress associated with the crisis itself as well as how best to manage it. For example, policies related to 'codes' for bomb threats or terrorism usually provide detailed steps to take, phone numbers to call, and instructions for how to shelter. It is extremely comforting during times of stress to simply follow a checklist rather than think, 'do I stay or do I go?'.
- *They act as legal documents that can help reduce risk and conflict:* Policies can have the organisational weight of laws in clearly defining employee–employer relationships and responsibilities. As such, policies have a legal heft that can be intimidating but also comforting in terms of providing clarity and reducing the need for haggling or negotiation.

Limitations of policies and procedures

Despite their near-universal ubiquity in modern organisations, there are important limitations to policies and procedures that need to be acknowledged, including:

- *Limitation on creative problem-solving and thinking:* No policy and procedure can anticipate all possible real world situations, and so some flexibility and creativity will always be required on the part of individual workers. Paradoxically, the predictability and prescriptive nature of policies and procedures may actually hamper creative problem-solving; when employees feel encumbered and cannot 'bend rules', 'follow their gut' or 'take a chance', opportunities might be missed. When a policy or procedure does not actually cover an unanticipated circumstance, employees may become paralysed by indecision and unable to proceed.
- *Variable interpretation is still possible:* Despite all best efforts to craft well-written policies and procedures that limit subjective interpretation, it is very difficult to do consistently. Especially where individuals have nefarious motives or vested interests to try to distort a policy or procedure in ways that are advantageous to them alone, their legalistic nature can be jiu-jitsued and used against managers and organisations in unanticipated ways.
- *Regular reviewing and updating is necessary:* There is considerable time and work required to maintain policies and procedures. As organisational priorities and environmental circumstances evolve, policies and procedures need to be revised and rewritten to keep pace, and this can take hours of time.
- *They can become overwhelming:* Life in modern organisations is complex, and attempts to control complexity through policies and procedures actually introduces its own complications. The sheer number and depth of policies and procedures in many companies today, can be overwhelming and cause employees to disengage and ignore them. It also can set up an antagonistic relationship

between policies and procedures, and employees who may disparage or simply disregard them, claiming 'it's easier to apologise after than try to figure out the right way to do it in the first place'.

Recognising and acknowledging these and other limitations, does not discount the importance and centrality of policies and procedures to modern organisational life or managerial work. It does, however, alert managers to the need to balance these potential limitations with the valuable role they can play in shaping organisational culture and in enhancing safety, quality, efficiency, and effectiveness.

Components of an effective policy

A systematic approach to writing good policies can help managers ensure key elements are addressed. Further, a systematic approach helps increase usability by readers if all policies are written in a consistent manner, using regular topic headings that facilitate greater accessibility to the content. Typical components of a policy should include:[4,5]

1. *Headline:* The headline of a policy is a clear and concise title which succinctly summarises the essence of the policy. Individuals looking for policy guidance will want to look for 'vacation policy', 'sick leave policy', or 'parental leave policy' rather than a complex code number or an unnecessary verbose title that makes indexing and searching difficult.
2. *Policy demographics:* The 'demographics' of a policy refer to technical elements including the official (and usually long-winded) title of the policy, the date it was issued, the date it is effective, the policy number within the organisation, the office or person of origin, and the individual or office that approved the policy.
3. *Purpose of the policy:* A concise and clear statement describing the rationale for the policy is important to include. Such a statement helps readers understand not only the reason for the policy but why it is justified to be written formally as a policy, and not simply handled informally (without a policy).
4. *Detailed policy statement:* A detailed policy statement provides a more in-depth explanation and justification than the purpose, and is usually needed in case legal issues arise or if the policy itself is ever contested. Importantly, the policy should still be comprehensible and useable by readers without a detailed policy statement, but the detailed policy statement is included to provide depth and legal protection as needed.
5. *Applicability:* A clear statement or list of bullet points should indicate who is covered/affected/influenced by the policy as well as consequences for non-compliance with the policy.
6. *Definitions:* In some industries, jargon or technical terminology may be unavoidable in a policy. Wherever possible, clear and plain language should be used, but where not possible, a glossary or list of terms and definitions should be included so as to minimise ambiguity or misunderstanding of language.
7. *Cognisant officers:* This term refers to the specific individual position titles that can be contacted to help with interpretation of the policy, resolve disagreements, or manage questions. The cognisant officer should not be a named individual (since people leave jobs and change phone numbers) but instead be a position title within an organisational chart.

8. *Authorising officers:* The highest administrative officer in the organisation who approves the policy should be listed by position title, not by name.

9. *Related policies:* Often, workplace policies may not be standalone entities but are connected to one another. For example, a 'sick leave' policy and a 'personal days' policy may cover some similar terrain albeit in different ways. Where a policy connects with, duplicates, or somehow is influenced by other policies, it is useful to ensure these are clearly mapped and articulated in both policy documents to minimise confusion.

10. *References:* Policies should provide useful references to help readers understand rationale and justification. For example, an anti-harassment policy may be referenced to prevailing Human Rights Legislation in a jurisdiction, so readers understand how this particular policy fulfils the organisation's legal obligations.

11. *Connection to procedures:* In most cases, policies do not exist in isolation but are linked with specific procedures that explain how to implement or carry out the intent of the policy. While policies and procedures should be separate documents, they need to be linked in order to make sense.

12. *Review, update, modify, and rescind details:* Policies need to be constantly reviewed and updated to meet current and evolving needs. In general, policy documents should never be destroyed in case there is a need to review historical policy decisions for legal or other reasons. Instead, treating a policy as a living document allows it to be updated appropriately in ways that leave a paper trail for readers to understand the various iterations in that evolution.

Components of an effective procedure

Procedure documents should accompany policy documents to explain implementation of policy goals. There are few, if any, circumstances where a procedure document will exist without a policy document. Similar to policies, procedures should be written in a consistent format using plain language so it becomes an easy to use, easily accessible document for training and reference. Key components of an effective procedure will include:[6,7,8]

1. *Headline:* A clear, concise and immediately comprehensible procedure title will help readers understand what the procedure covers and how it connects to the relevant policy or policies. Examples could include 'procedure for requesting vacation' or 'procedure for parental leave'.

2. *Procedure demographic details:* Similar to the policy demographic details, this section refers to technical elements including the official (and usually long) title of the procedure, the date it was issued, the date it is effective, the procedure number within the organisation, the office or person of origin, and the individual or office that approved the procedure.

3. *Procedure description:* This section provides an overview of objectives, functions, and tasks that the procedure is designed to accomplish, as well as providing specific details as to when this particular procedure should – and should not – be used.

4. *Responsibilities:* This section outlines the offices and individual job titles of those who have accountability for coordination and implementation of the procedure, as well as the authority to override or approve exemptions to the procedure, if applicable. It should describe the

responsibility for implementation and set forth the scope of discretionary modification to the procedure that may be available.

5. *Procedural details:* This section is the core of the procedure document, and outlines the specific steps required to complete the procedure effectively, efficiently, safely and to the highest possible degree of quality. Procedural details should be presented in a way that is both readable and immediately transferable to real world work: as a result, checklists, flow charts, diagrams, and other graphics are often used in this section to simply make it more useful. For example, an explanation of how to complete a form can incorporate screen shots of different sections, providing samples to guide readers. Rather than incorporating a separate glossary of terms and definitions, these can be embedded in the procedural details section itself to facilitate more immediate understanding. It can be useful to use multiple methods to provide procedural details (for example, a flow chart diagram and a checklist) as different readers may have different learning styles that benefit from different presentation formats.

6. *Frequently asked questions (FAQs):* FAQs can be a useful tool for clarifying common misconceptions and preventing small misunderstandings about procedures from escalating. This can be an evolving component of the procedure document; as real life users have questions, these can be encapsulated and incorporated in the document to help address issues before they arise.

7. *References:* Where procedures connect to specific policies, other procedures, or relevant laws and regulations, these should be noted in the document itself.

8. *Help information:* The pragmatic orientation of procedures supports inclusion of 'help' information: guidance for users as to what to do if further questions exist, further training is required, or other forms of assistance may be useful.

Developing roadmaps

A roadmap is a useful tool for helping employees navigate large and complex policy and procedure manuals or documents. In general, most individuals find information in such manuals by consulting a table of contents or an index, using key word searching. Roadmaps provide a more practical way of knowing which policies and procedures are relevant to a particular problem or situation, and providing rapid access to them in a linked manner. Particularly where policies and procedures exist to complement existing legislation and regulation that is outside the remit of an employer, roadmaps can make complex decision making more straightforward.

Roadmaps are typically constructed in response to commonly occurring situations that are fraught, complex, and potentially legally difficult. For example, a roadmap to help manage dispensing errors can be useful since policies, procedures, regulations, and laws governing this will come from different places. Another example of a useful roadmap could include purchasing decisions: financial audit, procurement policies, multiple vendor bidding, etc. for large purchases involves different policies and procedures, and a roadmap can help individuals navigate this more seamlessly and confidently.

Roadmaps do not replace or duplicate existing policies and procedures, they simply provide a helpful tool to navigate and access them in a more time efficient way, and to help ensure that nothing relevant is overlooked or forgotten. Managers should consider developing and maintaining useful roadmaps to complement policy and procedure manuals, to support implementation and enhance accessibility. Of course, mechanisms to ensure roadmaps are updated as and when policies and procedures are changed, must also be embedded in the process.

Effective implementation of policies and procedures

Developing policies and procedures is challenging enough, but implementation is crucial to success. Once they have been written, reviewed, revised, and approved, managers have unique responsibilities to ensure successful adoption and implementation. Central to this will be communication, training, monitoring, and follow-up/feedback.

- *Communication:* Well-written policies and procedures should communicate for themselves and require minimal-to-no clarification or additional explanation from the manager. Where clarification is required, it may be an indication that the policy or procedure needs to be updated to address common questions or misconceptions. Beyond this however, effective managerial communication will be required to help a team understand how best to incorporate policies and procedures into daily work and practice. One particularly helpful technique can be for managers to consistently make references to policies and procedures in everyday conversation and guidance, and not simply invoke policies and procedures when problems arise. As team members see and hear managers embedding policies and procedures into everyday work, it establishes a tone and a culture where these documents are real and helpful, rather than abstract and punitive. Using policies and procedures to guide performance appraisals, feedback and coaching, and even in decisions related to promotion and salary increases, sends important signals as to their value in the team and the organisation. Part of communication for implementation also means focusing on ways of making all policies and procedures – but in particular new or revised ones – easily available and accessible for everyone. The traditional 'binder in a centralised location' method has significant limitations as it is paper based, limited to one copy, has no ability to be indexed by key word searches, and tends to simply collect dust on a shelf rather than be used. Managers may want to showcase or review policies and procedures on a regular basis at team or staff meetings, in coaching sessions with individual staff members, or informal discussions. Another element of effective communication involves active solicitation of feedback regarding policies and procedures: asking how current ones are working, what needs to be improved, what's missing, and how can it work better to support practice, are genuine questions that trigger responses that can actually improve implementation and use. As a general principle, avoid weaponising policies and procedures: if the only or main circumstance when staff members hear or think about policies and procedures is when they've made a mistake, it establishes a punitive role for these important and helpful documents.
- *Training:* In the past, new employees were often onboarded into a position by spending a day sitting in a quiet room reading a policy and procedure manual. This is not an effective learning strategy, nor is it a particularly friendly introduction to a team or a workplace. When considering how best to train individuals in policies and procedures, it is first important to create a compelling reason or case for why an employee should be legitimately interested

in them in the first place. Training should first highlight the rationale for use: better quality service, a safer workplace, and consistency in process, all enhance productivity, quality, efficiency, and effectiveness and this is the reason why employees should be self-interested in learning more about policies and procedures. Rather than simply give individuals a manual to read, more sophisticated social-learning techniques may be helpful. For example, use of video-based or online training programs can include games, self-assessment quizzes, simulations, or even 'choose your own adventure' components that help staff members learn about policies and procedures by seeing what happens (virtually or online) when poor choices and decisions are made. Use of video-based simulations and role plays can also be engaging ways of introducing staff to important components of policies and procedures that will affect them directly. If live training options are pursued, use of case-based discussions, after-the-fact analysis, and dissection of errors or problems that arose when policies and procedures were not followed, or testimonials from peers about how helpful these documents are to their work, can be useful teaching techniques. Successful implementation and naturalistic uptake of policies and procedures does not happen automatically, and rarely happens by someone just reading a manual by themselves. Creative teaching and training methods – most likely involving some element of group or social learning including interactive, discussion-based and role-playing focused techniques – will be necessary, but provide a fun and constructive environment to help bring documents to life in practical ways.

- *Monitoring:* Managers need to recognise that policy and procedure documents are never perfect nor unchangeable. Monitoring and modification of these documents is essential for successful implementation. Willingness to accept and incorporate feedback from all stakeholders is important, but so too is a system where managers can objectively monitor the impact, outcomes, and value of their policies and procedures. For example, a policy and procedure focused on error prevention and reporting should also include a monitoring component that actually tracks changes in both the number and nature of errors that occur after training and implementation. This monitored data is essential to help managers adapt to environmental circumstances and ensure their policies and procedures are actually having the expected and desired positive impact. Transparency in how policies and procedures are monitored and how decisions regarding modifications are made is important and needs to be communicated clearly with stakeholders. Monitoring is not a popularity contest; while subjective impressions and feedback can provide useful information, more objective, quantitative monitoring data is essential to judge success. As monitoring data is examined and changes/modifications are made and required, it is essential to communicate these changes and to once again monitor the impact, value, and outcome of the changes themselves.

- *Follow-up and/or feedback:* One of the more challenging but important aspects of successful implementation involves focused follow-up and feedback to ensure compliance with policies and procedures. A clear outline of consequences of non-compliance needs to be communicated effectively with staff – and needs to be enforced. Where there are no or minimal consequences to lack of compliance, policies and procedures will fail, or simply become guidelines instead. Consistency in applying consequences is essential, as is the importance of ensuring such consequences are proportionate, educative, restorative and where appropriate, non-punitive. Understanding reasons for non-compliance is an important managerial responsibility: if non-compliance is due in part to lack of training, it is as much a managerial fault as an employee problem. Feedback on compliance should precede consequences or punishment: mechanisms to allow individuals to know and calibrate the degree to which they are compliant with policies and procedures is important to develop so individuals can self-assess and self-correct prior to managerial intervention being required.

Summary

In most workplaces, policies and procedures are often greeted with polite indifference or groans and eyerolls. The general perception that they are bureaucratic impediments, hoops to jump through, or things to be subverted, diminishes their value to an organisation and are all signs of managerial failure to adequately educate, train, and support implementation. Well crafted policies and procedures are essential to any organisation's success and when implemented well, actually improve the quality of working life for employees by creating consistency, predictability, and reducing the need for subjective judgements. Managers have a central role in developing and implementing policies and procedures and should use this opportunity as a way to enhance operational safety, quality, efficiency, and effectiveness while simultaneously contributing positively to organisational outcomes.

References

1. O'Donnell J, Vogenberg F. Policies and procedures: enhancing pharmacy practice and limiting risk. *Pharmacy and Therapeutics* 2012; 37(6): 341–344.

2. Squires J *et al.* Exploring the role of organizational policies and procedures in promoting research utilization in registered nurses. *Implement Sci* 2007; 2(17). https://doi.org/10.1186/1748-5908-2-17

3. Irving A (2014). *Policies and procedures for healthcare organizations: a risk management perspective.* Middleton: Patient Safety and Quality Healthcare. https://www.psqh.com/analysis/policies-and-procedures-for-healthcare-organizations-a-risk-management-perspective/

4. Strasser P, Randolph S. Developing policies and procedures. *Workplace Health and Safety* 2006; 54(11): 501–504. https://doi.org/10.1177/216507990605401104

5. Stokes M. Evidence-based Policy and Procedure Review System. Michigan: Grand Valley State University, 2020 (dissertation).

6. Amadei L. Why policies and procedures matter. *Risk Management* 2016; 63(9): 12–13.

7. Cousins S *et al.* Healthcare organization policy recommendations for the governance of surgical innovation: review of NHS policies. *British J Surgery* 2022; 109(10): 1004–1012. https://doi.org/10.1093/bjs/znac223

8. Ramdan M (2013). *The skill of policy and procedure writing.* Healthcare Quality Orientation Course/ TQM Aucians Group. https://doi.org/10.13140/RG.2.2.17164.31364

9. Society of Human Resources Management (SHRM). *How to develop and implement a new company policy.* Society of Human Resources Management (SHRM). https://www.shrm.org/resourcesandtools/tools-and-samples/how-to-guides/pages/howtodevelopandimplementanewcompanypolicy.aspx

CHAPTER 17

Inventory management, procurement and the supply chain

Upon completion of this chapter you should be able to:

- understand the inventory goals of pharmacy managers
- detail the major types of inventory management control systems
- explain the important considerations involved in inventory management
- describe the procurement process
- understand how to manage recalls
- explain the processes of counting and organising inventory.

Whether in a hospital, primary care, or community setting, the practice of pharmacy is typically an inventory intensive business. 'Inventory' is an umbrella term encompassing the wide array of goods, supplies, and medications used in the daily practice of pharmacy.[1] Increasingly, regulated pharmacy technicians or specially trained procurement specialists may be integral to inventory management; however, pharmacy managers are also central to the process of inventory management, procurement, and supply chain control, and must understand both general principles and specific techniques for optimising access to medicines and medical supplies.[2,3] It goes without saying that without an adequate stock of medicines and medical supplies, pharmacies cannot serve their patients. Conversely, careless or sub-optimal inventory management and supply chain control is costly, wasteful, and will compromise financial viability of the organisation.[4] Careful management and control of inventory and supply chain can increase profitability, enhance financial sustainability, and provide optimal access to needed medicines and supplies for patients.[4]

Why manage inventory, procurement and supply chains?

Ensuring there are appropriate and adequate supplies of needed medicines so that patients can have timely access to quality, in-date products, is the primary objective of inventory management.[5] Other reasons include minimising the occurrence of out-of-stock situations, limiting the financial burden and inefficiencies associated with carrying too much product that is not being used, and reducing burdens associated with unnecessary ordering of medications and supplies from wholesalers. Pharmacy managers have two primary goals with respect to inventory management[2,3]: the first is to ensure patients have access to products they need as quickly as possible, based on the specific and known needs of the pharmacy's customer/client/patient base. Of course, on occasion, there may be a need to specially order an unusual or rarely used medication or product, or one that is unusually expensive or complex to maintain; regularly used, common medications and products should be in stock, in date, and stored appropriately to minimise the risk of damage or chemical degradation. The second goal of inventory management is to keep medication costs at a minimum by ordering in sufficient quantities to warrant bulk purchase discounts, minimising wastage/spoilage and opportunities for theft, and ensuring inventory moves quickly enough to prevent stale-dating or the medications reaching 'best before' dates – at which point they must be discarded and written off as a financial loss, rather than used to benefit patients.

Inventory management control systems

Across different types of pharmacies, there are three major types of inventory management control systems that are used: manual, periodic, and perpetual. Regardless of the system that is used, inventory management helps managers determine how much of which specific items must be ordered, purchased, delivered, and received in order to fulfil reasonable expectations of patients/customers. Once sold, inventory is transformed into revenue. However, prior to sale, inventory (although generally reported as an asset on a balance sheet, *see* Chapter 6) actually ties up cash flow: too much inventory that is not being sold or used costs an organisation money and reduces cash flow.

Central to understanding effective inventory management is the concept of turnover. Turnover is a way of calculating how often purchased inventory is sold in a given period of time, and often reflects the operational efficiency of a business. There are several accepted ways of calculating turnover. One method involves dividing a business's annual sales by its average inventory balance. A second popular method involves dividing the annual cost of goods sold (COGS) by average inventory. In both cases, 'average inventory balance' is usually estimated as the sum of beginning and ending inventory for the year, and dividing by 2.

The manual, periodic, and perpetual inventory systems are an essential component of this process, as they provide managers with an actual physical count of what is currently on hand and in stock. The manual inventory method is the least sophisticated and least accurate, but it may be sufficient in a services-intensive pharmacy setting where there are relatively few products and supplies purchased or needed. Manual inventory involves a physical counting of products in storage, reconciled against purchases during the year. It is laborious, time-consuming and frequently error-prone because the process of counting pills in bottles, capsules in packages, and all the other things a pharmacy routinely holds, is incredibly challenging to perform accurately. On the other end of the continuum is perpetual inventory, which is only feasible in highly computerised/automated settings. Perpetual inventory provides a running tally of what remains in stock through immediate reconciliation between dispensing and purchasing records. In perpetual inventory models, all purchases are entered into a central computerised database – for example, when 200 capsules of amoxicillin are purchased and received by the pharmacy, this is recorded in the computer system. When a prescription is dispensed for 30 capsules, the prescription processing software automatically connects to the purchasing software and records that 30 capsules have been dispensed, reducing the inventory to 170 capsules available. Running totals are almost instantaneously calculated by linking dispensing and purchasing software programs. While this may sound seamless and elegant, in practice, perpetual inventory still requires manual count confirmation from time to time. In the real world, products get lost or stolen and 'vanish' without being tracked by the dispensing or purchasing software. Further, products are accidentally wasted and will also be uncounted — for example, if an amoxicillin capsule falls on the floor during dispensing, it must be discarded but this won't be recorded in perpetual inventory. Perpetual systems are the most accurate but they rely heavily on automation and technology, complemented by occasional (or 'periodic') manual counts to confirm.

Most pharmacies (large and small) use some variation of periodic/perpetual inventory management. It is most effective when linked with an automatic dispensing system (robotics) to minimise the risk of inventory being miscounted, falling on the floor, or mysteriously disappearing. Point-of-sale technologies that support perpetual inventory can also be programmed to automatically re-order stock once a purchase threshold is reached, minimising the need for human intervention. Alternatively, perpetual inventory systems can generate daily or weekly reports that can be reviewed by the manager who then makes the decision to order (or not) based on trends in the pharmacy. This threshold represents a point at which 'turnover' of inventory is occurring. Though there are disagreements, it is thought that for most pharmacy settings, an annual turnover of approximately 10 is realistic. This means that inventory purchased should be sold every 37 days or less. This 'sweet spot' minimises the risk of expiration, wastage, or theft, but also optimises the frequency of ordering. Of course, individual pharmacies may vary considerably in whether inventory turnover (ITOR) should be higher or lower based on practice specific needs.

Important considerations in inventory management

- *Supply chain constraints:* Since the COVID-19 pandemic, citizens around the world have become conspicuously aware of the concept of a supply chain. The supply chain for goods and products carried by a pharmacy can be exceptionally complicated. Supply chains depict the multiple stages through which raw materials are eventually converted into finished products available for sale and use. For medications, the supply chain can involve multiple steps in multiple countries; for example, raw materials and chemicals needed to produce a medicine may be sourced in one country, which are then shipped to another country for compounding into a medicine, before being sent to a third country for labelling, packaging, and sales. Each of these steps must be carefully monitored to ensure safety and health requirements are met. International organisations including the International Pharmacy Federation (FIP) have published standards for safety, hygiene, and quality for all steps of the pharmaceutical manufacturing process, to safeguard public health and well-being. As the COVID-19 pandemic made clear, these long and complex supply chains have become increasingly vulnerable to disruption – a freak storm, a labour dispute, or a political disagreement (or war) can interfere with countries' abilities to link supply chains. Today, supply chain problems in pharmacy are endemic worldwide and 'drug shortages' are a major public health problem. Tightening turnover ratios (designed to increase profitability and reduce waste) have likely contributed to drug shortages by reducing the buffer of unsold products that can be accessed when supply chains are disrupted. Managers need to be vigilant, adjust turnover expectations, and consider alternative sources (where available) when supply chain constraints occur. A common strategy (utilised in the early months of the pandemic) is to simply reduce the amount individual patients receive to ensure enough medication is available for all. This can be challenging to implement as individual patients may experience considerable anxiety during times of high stress (like a pandemic) if they are only 'allowed' a one month supply of their medicine, when in the past they received two or three months supply at a time. Managers need to carefully and empathetically explain this to patients, should this be necessary, and not just implement without adequate communication.

- *Availability:* Beyond supply chain constraints noted above, there has also been worldwide issues of availability of medications. Reasons for availability constraints include manufacturing equipment breakdowns, recalls issued by manufacturers, decreased access to necessary raw materials, and higher than usual demand. In some cases, hospitals and community pharmacies will be competing against each other to procure medications, further amplifying the problem. Once again, where inventory turnover is too tight, this reduces the capacity of the pharmacy to respond to availability constraints. In some cases, it may be possible to implement 'therapeutic substitution' as a way of dealing with availability (or supply chain) issues. For example, if there is an availability issue with ciprofloxacin, perhaps another quinolone antibiotic that is not suffering availability issues could be automatically substituted instead. Rules governing therapeutic substitution vary considerably: in some jurisdictions, pharmacists can automatically use professional judgement and make substitution decisions independently, quickly, and efficiently. In other jurisdictions, pharmacists must first contact and consult with initial prescribers before this can be done – a time-consuming and laborious process that delays access to the medication for patients. In other jurisdictions, government decrees may be issued that override prescriber autonomy and automatically mandate such substitutions. Managers need to be familiar with the processes in their own jurisdiction and communicate this effectively with staff so they are aware of how to handle availability issues.

- *Expiry dates:* All commercially produced medications and medical products have expiry dates that are based upon the amount of time available to use prior to chemical or physical degradation of the product, lessening efficacy. In most jurisdictions, pharmacies are required to have mechanisms that ensure no outdated/expired products are dispensed, sold, or available for patients to self-select – failure to comply can result in hefty penalties and fines. Some medications – for example, epinephrine – have relatively short expiry dates (typically, about one year). Insufficient turnover of epinephrine stock can lead to wastage, as expired epinephrine must simply be discarded without being used. Ordering the 'right' amount of epinephrine can be challenging – having enough on hand to meet the needs of patients, but not so much that any of it expires. Worse, there is currently a worldwide supply chain and availability issue with epinephrine, making rapid ordering and easy access challenging and leading many managers to stockpile excess inventory of epinephrine. Epinephrine can be a life-saving medication (for example, in the context of a bee sting suffered by an allergic patient). The risk of expiration and wasted inventory is often deemed lower than the risk of not having the medication on hand when a patient needs it. Decisions such as this are extremely important and managers need to have both full information and guiding principles to help them to decide how best to manage inventory in a situation like this. Further, in some jurisdictions where epinephrine supply chain and availability problems have been particularly strong, government officials have, in some cases, advocated for arbitrary extensions of printed expiry dates. This is a very controversial practice since expiry date calculations are premised upon evidence regarding the rate of chemical degradation of a medication that lessens its quality and efficacy. Still – it has been argued – expired epinephrine may be better and more helpful than no epinephrine in situations where these are the only two options. The liability and risk issues of deliberately using, selling, or recommending use of expired inventory is extremely challenging. Managers need to ensure relevant regulatory authorities are consulted and supportive prior to implementing this difficult choice.

- *The 80/20 rule:* This inventory management technique suggests that 80% of a pharmacy's drug costs are spent on only 20% of the total inventory, and thus greater attention needs to be paid to the top 20% of 'fast movers' in the pharmacy. Managing the stock level of this 20% will yield disproportionately positive benefits for both patients and the pharmacy since these are the items most frequently used. Managers need to familiarise themselves with and carefully track/monitor this 20% as these are the items most at risk of supply chain/availability issues or simply running out prior to the next order cycle.

- *ABC:* As an alternative to the 80/20 rule, ABC suggests the entire inventory of a pharmacy can be categorised into three distinct categories based on usage and cost. The 'A' category is typically the 20% of products accounting for 80% of costs, the 'B' category is 15% of products accounting for 15% of costs, while the 'C' category is the 65% of products accounting for 5% of costs. Constant analysis and recalibration of categories is needed to ensure alignment to actual usage and cost. Focusing on the entire inventory but simplifying through use of this kind of three-level classification system, can help managers focus less on low cost products that have minimal impact on profitability and instead emphasise high usage products that are needed by patients.

Procurement

The procurement process describes the steps required to build and maintain an inventory, and order, receive, store, and account for medicines, medical supplies, and other products in the pharmacy. At the core of the procurement process is an invoice. An invoice is an itemised list of goods delivered to the pharmacy with the cost of each product listed, along with the total cost of the order. Invoices are usually linked to purchase orders. In many jurisdictions, large common/bulk buying agents called 'wholesalers' work with multiple pharmacies to negotiate best possible prices for pharmacy specific inventory from individual manufacturers. Rather than ordering directly from the manufacturer, the pharmacy orders from a wholesaler who combines purchases from multiple pharmacies to find cost and process efficiencies. Purchases are then processed using a purchase order – a specialised form with a pre-assigned number or numerical code (the purchase order number) allowing simultaneous tracking of shipping until the order is actually received by the pharmacy. Purchase orders and invoices work together to control costs and reduce the inefficiencies associated with procurement: it allows managers to more accurately track what has been ordered, delivered, and in-process at any given time. Purchasing without a purchase order is usually discouraged because it means those items are now not directly linked to procurement systems and invoicing practices, and such purchases can easily become lost in perpetual inventory.

Wholesalers are amongst the most common ways pharmacies order medications, medical supplies and other products stored in inventory. Because there are literally thousands of different individual manufacturers of products and goods used by pharmacies, it would be extremely cumbersome and inefficient to have pharmacies order from each manufacturer separately and individually. Wholesalers simplify the ordering process considerably and usually negotiate bulk discounts, meaning even small pharmacies enjoy best possible prices for products purchased. Wholesalers usually use computerised or electronic ordering systems that integrate purchase orders and invoices, and feed directly into perpetual inventory systems to facilitate better inventory control. Larger pharmacy groups (for example a multiple or chain pharmacy, or group of hospitals or clinics) may order from wholesalers but still maintain their own warehouse to receive deliveries prior to shipping to individual pharmacies. This system can allow for even greater bulk purchasing discounts as well as reducing risks of supply chain or availability issues causing drug shortages.

Ordering is part of the procurement process and is essential to ensure that the pharmacy remains adequately stocked. Perpetual inventory systems can facilitate automated ordering or generate suggestions of what needs to be ordered, but in general the final placement of an order still requires some form of human approval. Even when perpetual inventory systems exist, some form of manual confirmation system linked to a periodic inventory process is often used to provide confirmation. Common methods include the use of stickers: wholesalers provide pre-printed stickers with each product they supply with the item number and price listed; once the stock is seen to be running low, the sticker is simply removed and affixed to an ordering sheet, or a bar code reader is used to upload the information to an electronic order form sent directly to the wholesaler. Alternatively – and especially for smaller pharmacy operations, a card system can be used which allows staff to simply place a pre-printed card with ordering information in a central location, that is subsequently used by the manager to generate purchase orders. This involves the use of periodic automatic replacement (PAR) level inventory, a system that defines minimal or optimal levels of inventory for each item that should be on hand in the pharmacy at all times. Defining these PAR levels is a managerial responsibility in consultation with staff and other stakeholders.

Once purchased orders are produced and sent, products are assembled at the wholesaler and delivered to the pharmacy. This leads to the next stage of procurement, simply called 'receiving'. A systematic process is required to ensure that all delivered products are fully and properly accounted for, and recorded and stored appropriately and safely. The manager generally designates an individual (usually a technician or assistant) to act as a receiving clerk; this individual receives the delivery from a driver/courier, then must first manually and visually verify that the quantity of boxes/carriers received corresponds to the expected quantity and what is listed on the purchasing order. Packages should then be visually inspected prior to opening to ensure they have not been damaged or tampered with. The receiving clerk then opens packages and inspects for damaged, outdated/expired, or wrong products that have been included in the delivery. Any of these products must be immediately separated from the rest for processing to return to the wholesaler. Most wholesalers provide only a small window of opportunity to undertake this process; failure to identify and return problem products in this window of time effectively means the pharmacy is now 'stuck' with this product and will be required to pay for it. Delivery packages will also contain invoices which serve as an important double check and reconciliation with the purchase order. Invoices should list name, strength, and dosage form of all medications shipped, along with costs, quantities, and other information. In some cases, if the full amount of the purchase order is not available, the invoice will indicate how much more is 'owing' with future deliveries. The receiving clerk must carefully match up the invoice to verify that everything listed has actually been shipped as indicated. Once verified, the invoice is then signed and dated and can be used to set up perpetual inventory in a computerised system.

Storage is an integral part of the procurement process, since some medications have unique storage requirements including refrigeration or freezing, flammable containment, or other hazardous substance storage guidelines. These products should be stored first to avoid damage, harm, or decreased potency of the product. Each jurisdiction has legal requirements for handling and storage of hazardous or toxic materials (for example, chemotherapy in the context of a pharmacy) and all staff need to be fully trained and confident in how to handle and store these products as part of the procurement process. This is an essential management function with significant legal and regulatory implications, and managers must be attentive and fully comply with legal requirements.

The final stage of procurement involves payment back to the wholesaler or vendor for products received. Often, the signature of the receiving clerk is all that is needed to allow accounting departments to pay for products received. As a cash flow management technique, some organisations have policies governing how long they may delay payment to the wholesaler/vendor before incurring a late-fee penalty. The objective is to pay invoices in full ('accounts payable') at the last possible moment prior to a fee being charged, in order to optimise availability of cash flow. Managers rarely have decision making authority in this area, but need to be aware of organisational or corporate policies and practices with respect to the payment of invoices, in case any issues arise.

In some cases, procurement may also include the process of returns. Returns refers to products that have expired or are no longer used by the pharmacy; in some cases these can be returned to wholesalers and manufacturers, and a partial refund may be available. In other cases, returns are shipped back to the wholesaler who then destroys them with no rebate available. Jurisdiction specific regulations govern return policies, and managers need to become familiar with this process to minimise clutter and storage costs associated with expired or underused products in the pharmacy.

Managing recalls

Periodically, a manufacturing flaw or defect is discovered only after products are ordered, shipped, and received by pharmacies around the world. Recalls are issued by manufacturers when they are made aware of problems with their products, including unanticipated adverse drug events or reactions, or manufacturing flaws that could compromise safety, quality, or efficacy. Manufacturers may be compelled to recall products by governments (for example, the Food and Drug Administration (FDA) in the United States) due to problems such as improper/inaccurate labelling, production errors resulting in problems with the medication, contamination during the manufacturing or shipping process, or (in rare cases) government mandated removal of products from the marketplace due to safety reasons. In some cases, manufacturers may choose to voluntarily recall products due to minor issues of labelling, branding, or appearance, without being forced to by government. There are three broad categories of recalls affecting pharmacies:

1. Class I recalls occur when a product may cause serious harm to a patient, up to and including death.
2. Class II recalls occur because of temporary or reversible health related effects.
3. Class III recalls are issued when the product has a very low possibility of causing actual health consequences, despite other problems including appearance, abnormal colouring, container defects, or unusual odours.

Whether voluntary or mandated recalls are issued, manufacturers and wholesalers have statutory obligations to follow up with purchasers of their products and inform them of the situation. This recall notice provides details on what products are being recalled, identification information (e.g. drug name, expiration date, lot number, etc.) and clear information on why the recall is being issued. Details on what to do with this product will also be included. In some cases, especially for Class I and Class 2 recalls, the recall may extend to products that patients have received through dispensing or bought over-the-counter. In this case, the pharmacy has a legal obligation to make reasonable efforts to contact all patients who have been affected by the recall and follow up carefully. In the event the recalled product has been used, a detailed history needs to be taken to determine if the patient is at risk of any safety or health consequences. Unused product should be immediately recovered from the patient and a strategy for managing its replacement should be determined to minimise inconvenience or health related effects. If no product was used/consumed, the product must still be swiftly recovered and a strategy for replacing with an alternative, unaffected product needs to be developed.

Perpetual inventory systems allow pharmacies to confirm they have not received a recalled product within a reasonable period of time. In the event the recalled product was ever a part of the pharmacy's inventory, processes for recovery must be prioritised. In general, recalls should be completed the same day they are received, and all steps should be taken carefully and fully documented by the manager.

Counting inventory

Despite advances in technology that support perpetual inventory, it is almost inevitable that physical verification of expected inventory will be necessary, at least once a year. Annual inventory counts are often unpleasant and painful for staff; in some jurisdictions, professional inventory counters can be hired and paid to do this work. In most cases, annual inventory counts will be done at a time when the pharmacy is completely closed or has very little business to conduct, in order to ensure that all medications are counted at the same time to provide the most accurate reflection of true inventory. Given the central role of accurate inventory to financial statements and budgets, and ultimately to the profitability and viability of the pharmacy, this work must be taken seriously.

Cycle counts provide an alternative method for auditing particular/specific products in an inventory at a specified time. They should be undertaken on a periodic but regular basis to ensure what is on the pharmacy's shelf matches what the perpetual inventory predicts. Cycle counts are usually done on both high-risk medications that may be particularly vulnerable to shrinkage (theft) or wastage, or on medications that are particularly expensive. For example, in hospitals, nurses are often required to undertake daily narcotic/controlled substance cycle counts to ensure any narcotic medications stored on the unit are fully accounted for on a daily basis. The value of the cycle count is to identify inventory management and control problems early, and well before an annual count happens and major damage may have occurred. Cycle counts allow managers to continually monitor inventory levels without stopping business or interrupting operations; when completed correctly they allow greater and tighter control over inventory. However since cycle counts typically occur while business is ongoing, there is a higher risk for error than with annual counts and any errors in cycle counts could cascade further through the perpetual inventory system over time. Great caution must be exercised with cycle counts, most frequently involving at least two different independent counters working separately, then comparing data.

Organising inventory

One of the most important aspects of inventory control relates to decisions made by managers as to how best to organise products. In most pharmacies, there will be thousands of different products including prescription, non-prescription and over-the-counter medications, as well as a plethora of other medical supplies and products. Within the pharmacy, decisions need to be made as to how to best organise medications to facilitate efficient and safe access, particularly given the large number of sound-alike and look-alike medications that risk dispensing errors. Traditionally, most pharmacies have organised medications alphabetically by generic medication name, so medications for completely different indications will be stored adjacent to one another, simply because of the first letter of their generic name. In other cases, 'fast movers' or the 20% of products that account for 80% of sales, will be stored separately in a more convenient area for staff to access. In some jurisdictions, the tradition exists to file products alphabetically based on manufacturers' or trade names rather than generic names. In many pharmacies, certain kinds of products are separated based on packaging: for example, all birth control pills are kept in a specific separate area and not filed alphabetically with other medications. Similarly, eye drops, liquid formulations, etc. are all stored together based on dosage form.

Regardless of the type of inventory organisation system the manager decides to use, other error prevention strategies also need to be incorporated. For example, separation of products with similar looking packaging, or separation of different dosages of the same medication using physical dividers, can help prevent accidental selection of the wrong product during the dispensing process. Many managers use stickers or other alert systems for high-risk medications that are the most prone to dispensing error.

Part of this process also involves steps to ensure regular rotation of inventory stock throughout the pharmacy. New products should be placed at the back of the queue for use, ensuring that products received first are used up/dispensed/purchased first. Careful attention to expiry dates is also needed: products with the shortest expiration date need to be put at the front of the queue so they are more likely to be used up before they must be wasted. Care must also be taken to ensure shelving is not overcrowded or unnecessarily cluttered: visual clutter increases the risk of selecting the wrong product and potentially becoming a patient safety issue.

Summary

The inventory management and control process in pharmacy is complex but essential for operational efficiency and organisational success. Managers have significant opportunities to enhance efficiency and effectiveness of the pharmacy by developing strong procurement and inventory control policies and procedures, and ensuring these are followed by all staff. It is sometimes said that inventory is the lifeblood of most pharmacies: despite the shift towards more service and care delivery, most pharmacies still rely heavily on dispensing and the sale of products in order to generate business and revenue. Stewardship of this inventory is critical and an important opportunity for managers to have a direct and positive impact on business operations.

References

1. Ali A. Inventory management in pharmacy practice: a review of literature. *Arch Pharmacy Pract* 2011; 2(4): 151–156.
2. Villalobos-Madriz J *et al.* Implementation of supply management strategies by the Pharmacy Service in a general hospital during the COVID-19 pandemic. *Exploratory Res Clin and Social Pharmacy* 2022; 7: 100161. https://doi.org/10.1016/j.rcsop.2022.100161
3. Okeagu C *et al.* Principles of supply chain management in time of crisis. *Best Pract Res Clin Anaesthesiol* 2021; 35(3): 369–376. https://doi.org/10.1016/j.bpa.2020.11.007
4. Bialas C *et al.* Improving hospital pharmacy inventory management using data segmentation. *Am J Health-Syst Pharm* 2020; 77(5): 371–377. https://doi.org/10.1093/ajhp/zxz264
5. Association of Healthcare Internal Auditors/Deloitte PLC (2015). *Evaluating hospital pharmacy inventory management and revenue cycle processes: white paper guidance for healthcare internal auditors.* Costa Messa: Association of Healthcare Internal Auditors/Deloitte PLC. https://www.rxscan.com/wp-content/uploads/2019/06/EvaluatingHospitalPharmacyInventoryManagementandRevenueCycleProcesses.pdf

Further reading

Kaylor A. *Fundamentals of the pharmaceutical supply chain.* Massachusetts: Pharma news intelligence. https://pharmanewsintel.com/news/fundamentals-of-the-pharmaceutical-supply-chain

Ingersoll K (2015). *Inventory management for the pharmacy technician.* Florida: Elite learning. https://s3.amazonaws.com/EliteCME_WebSite_2013/f/pdf/RPTFL04IMI14.pdf

Sciacco A, Strömberg J (2022). *Drug inventory management (Part 1): Ensuring availability to stay competitive.* Relex solutions. https://www.relexsolutions.com/resources/drug-inventory-management-ensuring-availability-to-stay-competitive/

SOS Inventory. *Pharmaceutical inventory management.* Texas: SOS Inventory. https://www.sosinventory.com/pharmaceutical-inventory-management

CHAPTER 18

Patient safety

Upon completion of this chapter you should be able to:

- explain a pharmacist's role in patient safety
- understand the management of patient safety in pharmacy
- recognise the importance of public health surveillance and how it should be implemented by a manager.

Arguably, the single most important managerial function in pharmacy is patient safety.[1] Medicines are common but very powerful agents – used appropriately, they can prevent and treat disease and enhance quality of life and life expectancy. However, when used incorrectly, medicines have tremendous potential to trigger harm, impair functioning and even cause death. Medication errors are pervasive across primary, secondary, and tertiary care, with hundreds of thousands of medication errors reported each year – and many hundreds of thousands more occurring but not being reported.[2,3,4] Beyond actual errors, preventable adverse drug events, suboptimal therapeutic choices, and other forms of medicines induced harm are a significant cause of hospitalisation around the globe, and are emerging as a major public health concern.[5,6]

As the health care profession focused on stewardship of medicines, pharmacists have long been identified as pivotal in ensuring the safe and effective use of medicines.[1] Given the expanding scope of practice of pharmacists in many jurisdictions, pharmacists are assuming greater responsibilities for patient safety beyond medicines use, including public health activities and safe and effective use of medical devices and diagnostic tests. In all pharmacy settings, patient safety should be an organisational priority. As a result, managerial roles and responsibilities to promote, ensure, and monitor for patient safety, have emerged as critical activities requiring dedicated time, attention, and focus.

Pharmacists' roles in patient safety

Ensuring the safe and appropriate use of medicines is the core function of the profession.[7] In their day to day work of assessing and/or initiating prescriptions, pharmacists follow systematic processes to ensure patients are receiving the most appropriate medication, dosing, and formulation, and that these patients have the knowledge, skills, and confidence to use them safely and effectively. Traditionally, this role has been implemented through screening/audit activities of new and refilled prescriptions involving detailed analysis of potential drug–drug, drug–food, drug–medical conditions and other forms of interactions that could cause adverse drug events. This form of safety work emphasised reduction in potential harm caused by medications, and, of course, continues to be important. More recently, as pharmacists' clinical knowledge and skills have evolved, there has been increasing recognition that 'safety' is not simply about reducing the risk of harmful events, but also ensuring optimal prescribing and use of medicines based on patient-specific factors. This shift in recognition, that the 'right' medicine is not simply the one that is least likely to cause harm but the one that is most likely to produce beneficial responses with minimal adverse consequences, has amplified the importance of pharmacists in the health care team.[8]

In many jurisdictions, pharmacists have received greater and more expansive prescribing authorities than ever before, meaning that pharmacists now independently assess patients and initiate/prescribe medication treatments as part of a multidisciplinary care team.[9] In this context, 'safety' has evolved even further from simply medicines used but to the overall physical and psychological health and well-being of the person who is taking the medicines.[9] Safety considerations are not simply biochemical calculations but instead they consider issues of daily functioning/activities of daily living, quality of life, mobility, and lucidity.[10] As the pharmacist's role in safety has evolved, so has the integration of pharmacists into multidisciplinary teams consisting of multiple health care professionals. In many cases, these professionals are not co-located within the same building or practice, but instead must work collaboratively and communicate virtually or through electronic means to safeguard patients' interests and safety.

It is difficult to calculate the positive impact of this evolution in the pharmacist's role in patient safety, but there is broad recognition that greater integration of pharmacists in the health care system has resulted in improved quality care and health outcomes.[11] Despite this, however, there have been significant and extremely distressing failures of patient safety that underscore the need for further work in this area. Perhaps the most startling recent failure has been the 'opioid crisis', the recognition of society-wide harm inflicted upon diverse communities globally, entirely triggered by health care professionals.[12,13] Initially described in the United States, subsequently in Canada, Australia, New Zealand and now more recently in the United Kingdom and Europe, inappropriate and unsafe prescribing of opioid analgesics has led to devastating consequences, particularly in more vulnerable socio-economic communities. Inappropriate opioid prescribing and dispensing practices has led to medical, social, criminal, and other problems that we are only now starting to grapple with – without necessarily understanding the failure of patient safety systems that allowed it to perpetuate in the first place. Potential future patient safety alarms have been sounded with respect to antibiotic stewardship and the problems of antimicrobial resistance that are linked to poor prescribing, dispensing, and usage patterns of common antibiotics.[14] Mental health professionals have noted how patient safety failures in respect to the use of antidepressants and other psychoactive medications has been damaging; in this context, 'safety' is not simply about prescribing a medication then abandoning a patient, but instead recognising that psychiatric medications are part of a system of care that needs to be robust and continue after medications are prescribed.[15]

While central to the work of pharmacists and the goals of the health care system, patient safety is a complex issue requiring intentional management to support its success. Some pharmacy managers may be tempted to think 'safety' is another professional's job, or something individual pharmacists are responsible for on their own. The reality is that managerial direction and decisions are essential in creating a workplace that not simply values patient safety but integrates proactive patient safety measures in day to day practice.

Management of patient safety in pharmacy

A management plan to support patient safety needs to begin with a clear understanding of processes and potential points in the care continuum where risk of harm may be greatest. While each manager will need to consider its own unique patient population and practice context, there are common points that most, if not all, pharmacists and practices will emphasise in enhancing safety protocols and practices.

Provision of daily patient care and services

In most practices, pharmacists provide two broad categories of service to patients: compounding/dispensing and technical services, and patient care activities. The line between these two broad categories is not necessarily clear or stark; for example, the act of reviewing a prescription from another health care professional for therapeutic safety and appropriateness prior to dispensing, is a patient care activity.

Creating safe practices involves examination of current activities and the application of best practice exemplars that are widely available for review. For the category of dispensing activities, managers need to consider the whole of the process and how problems in any one step can heighten the risk of errors of omission or commission. Central to this is an examination of workflow in the pharmacy: as noted in Chapter 15, a general principle of patient safety is to minimise the number of hand-offs and hands involved in a process to enhance efficiency and reduce the risk of errors.[16] Managerial decisions around staffing, workflow, composition of the workforce (e.g. regulated versus unregulated technicians) all directly influence workflow. While managers have interests in this with respect to efficiency and cost-effectiveness for profitability, there are also important impacts regarding safety. A workflow that permits (or in many cases, inadvertently encourages) interruptions will increase the risk of errors. The foundation of safe practice is an efficient, effective, and safe workflow and workplace environment (see Chapter 15). Managers have the ability to design workplaces in alignment with these principles and should do so in order to enhance patient safety.

The manager's role extends beyond workplace design and workflow, and should also provide support to the practice of pharmacists and technicians involved in dispensing activities. It is unhelpful to simply assume that qualified, registered professionals 'know' how to do their work safely and efficiently. It is essential that tools be provided to help individuals follow standardised, methodical systems of checks and balances to ensure safe practice occurs. This can include development of policies and procedures as well as deployment of checklists that itemise steps required to safely dispense prescriptions. Many organisations have generated algorithms or lists that serve as reminders of good dispensing practice, and that can serve as an audit and verification tool for managers to ensure adherence. Such algorithms can also be used by managers as part of ongoing performance management, feedback, and coaching systems, as well as for more systematic training and on-boarding of newly hired individuals. From a safety perspective, the value of a consistent process, that occurs regardless of who happens to show up at work on a given day, is important, and managerial control of this is essential.

Some managers may have difficulty conceptualising how similar checklists and algorithms can be created and implemented for 'care' and 'service' activities, as by their nature they may be less routinised and more individualised to patient needs. Activities ranging from patient education to motivational interviewing, new medicines review services, vaccination provision, public health screening, etc. can also benefit from a similar algorithmic or checklist-driven managerial philosophy to ensure systematic and safe step-wise approaches are routinely used. Simply relying on 'professionalism', 'judgement', or 'common sense' on the part of the workforce will lead to inconsistencies, missed steps, and potential errors.

In summary, from a managerial perspective, patient safety is enhanced through development, implementation, and ongoing monitoring of the use of checklists and algorithms for routine and important uncommon technical and care/service activities undertaken in the pharmacy. The art of management, in this case, is to ensure this does not become a sterile bureaucratic exercise that is simply ignored by the workforce, but truly helpful guidance that is appreciated and relied upon by staff because they understand its value and impact on keeping patients safe.

Longitudinal and multi-disciplinary relationships

The risk of error increases as hand-offs and multiple hands become more involved in patient care work. The reality of health care today is that it is a team sport: intra- and inter-professional collaboration are not only necessary but contribute positively to outcomes as the complexity of health care delivery has increased. This necessitates hand-offs, multiple hands, and the development of longitudinal and multi-disciplinary relationships with both patients and other health care providers. Managers need to implement techniques to leverage this reality in ways that actually enhance, rather than risk, patient safety.

A fundamental strength of multi-disciplinary relationships is the opportunity to have checks and double checks for both decisions made and tasks completed. Historically, pharmacists have served as a 'second check' on prescribers of medicines and this is a useful precedent to consider as health care practices have evolved. Developing processes that embed 'second checks' in both decision making and task completion is an important safety measure. For example, as pharmacists become independent prescribers – who is double checking their work? Other pharmacists involved in dispensing, physicians or nurses could all play this important role, but managers need to ensure it is proceduralised in a way that ensures the double check is simply part of the process, not something the prescribing pharmacist needs to consciously remember to do. A system approach to 'baking in' double checks of decisions and processes can be an important safety measure, even if on the surface it appears to impede efficiency or increase costs. An important management job in this area involves communication systems that facilitate this double checking and that support timely delivery of feedback from the 'checker' in the event issues are identified. This has been facilitated considerably through the use of technologies, ranging from fax machines to email to computerised order entry systems requiring verification. In designing workplaces, multi-disciplinary double checks are an important safeguard.

A relatively underdeveloped additional safeguard is the development of workflow practices that encourage longitudinal relationships. Historically, general practitioners (GPs) have claimed to be the primary entry point to health care for patients, and have prided themselves on 'knowing' and 'walking' with patients for decades together. Longitudinal relationships with patients have helped GPs observe and more ably respond to subtle changes in health status, and help create the rapport, trust, and empathy that supports better and safer health care. As other professionals, like pharmacists, now have expanded scopes of practice, this valuable longitudinal approach should be considered as well. Historically, pharmacists have had transactional relationships with patients, focused on simply answering a question or filling a prescription at a single point in time. From a safety perspective, it would be preferable to create practice schedules and workflows that facilitate longer-term relationship building – for example, through the use of an appointment-based, rather than walk-in based model for pharmacy practice. Longitudinal patient care is a patient safety activity and managerial decisions can help pharmacy evolve towards this in a more direct manner. Beyond implementing appointment time slots, other options for longitudinal patient care include more stable/predictable scheduling and shift rotations for staff, creation of a customer service model that provides pharmacists with sufficient time with each individual patient, and a practice of introducing oneself by name and role to patients so they know the pharmacist as a person, not just a job title. These relatively incremental changes can encourage the evolution of longitudinal relationships that will enhance safety, improve health outcomes, and actually enhance job satisfaction of pharmacists.

Better integration of technology into practice

Amongst health care professions, pharmacy has always been at the forefront of technological innovation. Today, a variety of technologies exist to support practice, ranging from robotics and automated dispensing systems, to artificial intelligence to support clinical decision making, and telecommunications options like email and Zoom to facilitate contact with patients and other health care professionals. While many different technologies exist, their implementation into pharmacy practice has often been haphazard and somewhat random, which actually has increased the risk of harm and decreased patient safety.[17] A more intentional approach to the integration of technology into practice should have the opposite result: when mindfully and strategically deployed, technologies ranging from telephone based refill request services to video conferencing that allows pharmacists to participate in multidisciplinary team meetings, should all have the potential to enhance the quality and safety of care provided.

The key, of course, will be managerial decisions related to implementation, and to provide sufficient support and time for training and use. A clear rationale for a new technology needs to connect to the strategic objectives of the organisation before it is actually implemented: too often new technologies are simply dumped into a workplace without a clear understanding of what they are supposed to accomplish. Prior to the implementation of a new technology, fundamental workflow redesign should also be undertaken, led by the manager with full staff input. Often, a new machine, computer, or technology is simply placed in a pharmacy with the expectation that staff will figure out how to incorporate it into daily workflow. Physical placement of new devices is a crucial issue for managers to manage: plunking video conference hardware in a room distant and separate from the dispensary will reduce its daily usage, while enabling existing computers or providing portable laptops/tablets for video conferencing may encourage use, providing acoustic privacy concerns can be addressed. Requiring individuals to change computers, log out of programs, or interfere with the dispensing software process to consult decision support systems, decreases the likelihood that decision support will be used and actually increases risks to patient safety.

Technology can be an important asset for enhancing patient safety by reducing subjectivity and the need for individual judgement, being more technically accurate at certain activities (such as dispensing) than human beings, and by rapidly accessing information to support evidence-based decision making. Managerial planning is required to unleash this potential by decreasing barriers and inefficiencies for staff to access and use technology on a daily basis, and by ensuring sufficient time is provided for training and rehearsal to build skills and confidence. As a general principle, every new technology that is implemented will require the manager to re-examine current workflow practices and workplace design to determine optimal methods for implementation: this should be an expected and anticipated managerial responsibility. When implemented well, technology has strong potential to enhance patient safety; when implemented poorly it is likely that technology will actually increase the risk of error and harm.

Reporting and organisational learning

Much of the patient safety literature in pharmacy has focused on the central role of reporting and the capacity of individuals and organisations to learn from such reports.[18] Reporting is the process of documenting issues, problems, or concerns, then analysing this data for the purpose of quality improvement and prevention of problems in the future. From a safety perspective, there are two broad categories of reports that are important: error, incident, or 'near-miss' reports and adverse drug event reports.

Error, incident and near-miss reports

This category of reporting is essential to developing a safety culture within a pharmacy, as it allows all staff to reflect upon and learn from their colleagues' own experiences and to consider the ways in which the system (i.e. the workplace, the organisation, or the health care setting) contributes to the possibilities of errors.

A medication error is defined as a situation where '...there has been an error in the process of prescribing, preparing, dispensing, administering, monitoring or providing advice on medicines'.[19] In contrast, medication incidents are described as situations where the expected course of events in the support of and/or administration of medication is not followed, whether or not actual harm occurs. Examples of medication incidents include dispensing medications to the wrong patient, or an incorrect dose or dosage form being given. Finally, near-misses are events where the potential for harm was real, but the problem did not actually reach the patient because of a timely intervention by health care providers, family members or patients themselves. Sometimes described as 'close calls' or 'good catches', near-misses are often simply a result of good luck rather than planning.

Pharmacists – like all human beings – can and do make mistakes. Whether the consequences of the mistake are catastrophic or not, the simple fact a mistake has been made can be psychologically and professionally difficult to manage. While the outcome of an error from a patient care perspective is, of course, essential to know, all errors – whether they cause direct harm or not – should be documented and analysed to prevent future errors from occurring. It is, of course, human nature to not want to admit one's errors, and in a professional or workplace context there may be additional pressure to hide or overlook errors, particularly if no direct harm resulted. Managers have an important role in creating a culture of awareness, understanding, and transparency with respect to errors that views them as learning and improvement opportunities rather than moments to administer punishment.

Error reporting is the cornerstone of safe professional practice. Willingness to disclose, investigate, analyse and learn from previous errors is essential to prevent them from occurring in the future. Managers have a critical role to play in creating a workplace environment where error reporting is not viewed as punitive but educational; where staff members fear consequences associated with admitting to errors, incidents, or near-misses, they are unlikely to disclose them and even less likely to report them in a written format that facilitates analysis and sharing. Managers need to develop supportive policies and procedures, but more importantly, develop workplace cultures that recognise that errors are system issues, not individual deficiencies. This begins with explicit acknowledgement that professionals do not go to work to make errors – and when errors do occur there is a system of workplace practices, checks, balances, and communication that need to be examined to understand how and why it happened.

A system-level perspective on errors also means managers need to provide support to reduce impact and manage consequences associated with errors. In some circumstances, managers themselves may need to step in and directly intervene – for example, directly contact a patient affected by an error to apologise, discuss next steps, and monitor to ensure harm is minimised, rather than punitively require the staff member involved to manage this.

Learning from previous errors is crucial and involves careful, constructive, and objective analysis of the sequence of events leading up to and following the error. There are many resources available that can be used to help guide a review and analysis of error reports, and can help managers identify the most salient information to gather and focus on as part of the analysis process.[20,21,22]

From a managerial perspective, it is important to expect that errors, incidents, and near-misses will happen. Policies and procedures can be useful tools to provide staff with clear guidance on how to manage these when they occur, including the kinds of documentation and reports that should be completed. Further, identification of situations where managers should lead and take on a more direct role in communication (particularly with patients or other external stakeholders, including prescribers) should be made explicit. Processes for reviewing, analysing, and learning from error reports should also be formalised to reduce the likelihood of similar errors occurring in the future. Beyond these important procedural points, managers need to support a culture of honest disclosure of error, one that emphasises system enablers rather than individual deficits. A 'blame and shame' culture with respect to errors simply causes individuals to hide and deny, rather than manage responsibly and learn from mistakes. Building this culture and workplace environment needs to be done intentionally and consistently modelled for it to be believable; simply stating 'we don't blame and shame' will not work if behaviours and communication patterns do not reinforce this ideal.

Adverse drug events

As medication stewards, pharmacists are closest to the day to day experiences patients have with medications, medical devices, vaccines, and other health related products. Part of this stewardship also involves responsibility for contributing to public health surveillance regarding ongoing safety, efficacy, quality, and value of these expensive technologies.

Adverse drug events are inevitable consequences of population-wide use of pharmaceuticals and health care technologies. Despite years of clinical trials, testing, and evaluation, not all adverse drug events can be known until products are widely available for use. Pharmacies are central to the post-marketing surveillance process, and pharmacy staff have unique responsibilities to monitor and report adverse drug events and other adverse consequences experienced by patients.

Literature suggests there is significant under-reporting of adverse events of all sorts.[23] Where catastrophic, life-threatening adverse events occur, there is a strong likelihood that it will be documented and reported to authorities by a health care professional. However, where adverse events are mild, innocuous, or where a full and rapid recovery occurs, intentions to complete reports often get forgotten. As a result, early warning indicators of product issues go unreported and the likelihood of a serious adverse event occurring in the future may increase.

Managers need to reinforce the importance of adverse event reporting and highlight professional responsibilities of pharmacists and regulated pharmacy technicians to support public health surveillance. Beyond simple reinforcement, however, it is important for managers to consider how to make it easier, more convenient, and more likely that all (or at least the vast majority) of actual and suspected adverse events do indeed get reported. At its simplest, this may mean making necessary forms readily available in paper format or through a quick online link on a convenient computer. If individuals need to search for the correct form, this presents a barrier that may result in non-reporting. Structural incentives to promote adverse event reporting could also be considered: for example, sharing recent adverse event reports with other staff members and showcasing the individual who completed the report. Using performance appraisals as an opportunity to review processes with staff and review actual completed reports, can highlight the importance the manager places on timely and full reporting. Following up with staff who have not filed adverse event reports for a period of time and reminding them of their professional responsibilities can also be useful.

Unfortunately, adverse event reporting is often perceived as a bureaucratic nuisance or as a make-work project – 'no one reads these anyway, so what's the point in wasting my time?'. In reality, adverse event reporting is a significant public health safeguard and one of the most important data sources relied upon for post-marketing surveillance. Managers should not rely on some imagined, internalised sense of professionalism on the part of staff to report; instead, looking at logistical barriers to reporting, and considering ways of motivating and incentivising staff to report, will be necessary to ensure this important activity is undertaken.

Public health surveillance

In May 2000, in the rural community of Walkerton Ontario, Canada's worst public health disaster involving drinking water occurred.[24] At least 7 people died and over 2300 became ill due to contamination of the water supply. This tragedy could have been significantly worse and resulted in even more deaths and illness were it not for the sharp eyes and foresight of community pharmacists in this town, who noted a sudden and sharp increase in the number of customers seeking over-the-counter (OTC) anti-diarrheal products. This observation was reported to public health officials who in turn were able to respond more quickly and contain the contamination, sparing the community the worst possible consequences.

As this case illustrates, pharmacies are uniquely well placed to be the eyes and ears of public health in their communities. Monitoring sales of over-the-counter products or other trends involving goods and services provided through pharmacies, gives pharmacists and regulated technicians unique opportunities to prevent small problems from becoming larger problems. The lesson of Walkerton Canada is instructive for pharmacies worldwide: rather than simply observe and anecdotally or casually comment on an unusually large volume of sales of OTC anti-diarrheal products, these pharmacists went the extra step of alerting public health officials and proving the data they had for analysis.

Managerial support for this type of public health surveillance activity is essential. The first individuals to notice how quickly anti-diarrheal products were selling may not be dispensary staff, but check-out clerks, or those who stock shelves. Many individuals purchasing anti-diarrheal products may feel some embarrassment and so will buy them without speaking to a pharmacist or staff member directly. Importantly, the pharmacists who reported their observations had no idea at the time that there was any problem with the water supply: they did not need to have 'an answer' for their observation, and instead allowed public health officers to do their job in analysing this trend.

Creating a culture that promotes public health surveillance within the pharmacy, involving the entire staff (not just regulated professionals) is an important managerial job. While community pharmacies are, of course, businesses, they are also health care centres, relied upon by their neighbourhoods and plugged into broader primary care systems. Training and a clear process for reporting seemingly random observations is an important part of creating this culture.

Public health surveillance extends to not simply considering sales of OTC products, but to tighter connections to the neighbourhood and community. Other public health concerns that may be identified in pharmacies include domestic, spousal, elder, or child abuse. While many jurisdictions have compulsory reporting requirements for suspected child abuse, other forms of abuse are not necessarily covered. Managers have important opportunities to safeguard public well-being by using the role of 'eyes and ears of public health' in a productive way. As with adverse event reporting, clear policies, a culture of honest disclosure, and processes for communicating suspected problems or simply even unusual observations, need to be developed.

Summary

Patient safety should be the central concern of every health and care professional: as noted in the Hippocratic oath, 'first, do no harm'. When considering their roles and responsibilities, creating a 'safety culture' should be central to a manager's work and philosophy. A safety culture is an amalgam of values and beliefs, policies/procedures/processes, and communication techniques focused on clarity and transparency.[25] A safety culture is not simply lofty rhetoric but a pattern of behaviour that is modelled and enacted on a daily basis. Central to safety culture is the recognition that 'blame and shame' of individuals is rarely productive or helpful: instead, documentation, analysis and learning is the way to prevent small problems from becoming large, and preventing problems from repeating in the future.

Arguably one of the most important responsibilities – and opportunities – managers have is to contribute to the creation of a safety culture to ensure the health and well-being of staff. Pharmacy is a physically, cognitively, and emotionally intensive field, and professional and non-professional staff alike are vulnerable to occupational stress. Much of a manager's role is to minimise cognitive and emotional load contributing to errors through managerial decisions related to workplace design, workflow, scheduling, technology implementation, etc. While it is impossible to remove all sources of stress, working to minimise the impact and effect of stress on morale, health, and motivation is important. Occupational stress can be corrosive and will – if unchecked or poorly managed – lead to burnout. Research has highlighted the corrosive effects of excessive occupational stress and burnout on patient safety, pharmacy operations, and profitability. Burned out employees make more errors and the ones they do make are more consequential and dealt with less effectively. Careful monitoring of staff for signs and symptoms of burnout is an important element of safety culture. This includes regular check-ins regarding well-being, investigating changes in behaviour related to attendance, motivation, punctuality, dress, eating habits, etc. and creating a team culture where colleagues look out for each other and caringly enquire when small problems start to arise. As patterns of worrisome behaviour emerge that could be linked to burnout, it is essential to follow up professionally, efficiently, and respectfully. Encouraging or requiring staff members to take earned vacation/leave, scheduling mandatory breaks and lunch periods, and other managerial interventions are important tools for supporting staff well-being.

From a manager's perspective, the best way to ensure patient safety in the pharmacy is to support the morale and physical and emotional health of the workforce: it is not only effective in reducing the risk of errors and patient harm, but also a way of enhancing retention of staff. A culture of patient safety requires multiple approaches and constant vigilance to maintain. Managers should carefully consider the array of options available (policies, procedures, checklists, technology, training, workflow and scheduling, workplace design and techniques to reduce occupational stress and mitigate burnout) and deploy these effectively to keep patients, staff, and the practice itself, safe.

References

1. Aboneh E *et al*. Evaluation of patient safety culture in community pharmacies. *J Patient Saf* 2020; 16(1): e18–e24. https://doi.org/10.1097/pts.0000000000000245

2. Knudsen P *et al*. Preventing medication errors in community pharmacy: frequency and seriousness of medication errors. *BMJ Quality and Safety* 2007; 16: 291–296. https://doi.org/10.1136/qshc.2006.018770

3. Pervanas H *et al*. Evaluation of medication errors in community pharmacy settings: a retrospective report. *J Pharmacy Technology* 2015; 32(2): 71–74. https://doi.org/10.1177/8755122515617199

4. Rogers E *et al*. A just culture approach to managing medication errors. *Hosp Pharm* 2017; 52(4): 308–315. https://doi.org/10.1310/hpj5204-308

5. Aronson J. Medication errors: what they are, how they happen, and how to avoid them. *Int J Medicine* 2009; 102(8): 513–521. https://doi.org/10.1093/qjmed/hcp052

6. Alrabadi N *et al*. Medication errors: a focus on nursing practice. *J Pharmaceutical Health Services Research* 2021; 12(1): 78–86. https://doi.org/10.1093/jphsr/rmaa025

7. Luchen G *et al*. (2021). *The role of community pharmacists in patient safety*. Rockville: Agency for Healthcare Research and Quality. https://psnet.ahrq.gov/perspective/role-community-pharmacists-patient-safety

8. McFarland M *et al*. Medication optimization: integration of comprehensive medication management into practice. *Am Health Drug Benefits* 2021; 14(3): 111–114.

9. Yuksel N *et al*. Prescribing by pharmacists in Alberta. *Am J Health Syst Pharm* 2008; 65(22): 2126–2132. https://doi.org/10.2146/ajhp080247

10. Guirguis L *et al*. Survey of pharmacist prescribing practices in Alberta. *Am J Health Syst Pharm* 2017; 74(2): 62–69. https://doi.org/10.2146/ajhp150349

11. Macgregor P. Pharmacists for patient safety. *Can J Hosp Pharm* 2015; 68(3): 270. https://doi.org/10.4212%2Fcjhp.v68i3.1464

12. Chisholm-Burns M *et al*. The opioid crisis: origins, trends, policies and the roles of pharmacists. *Am J Health Syst Pharm* 2019; 76(7): 424–435. https://doi.org/10.1093/ajhp/zxy089

13. Bratberg J *et al*. Pharmacists and the opioid crisis: a narrative review of pharmacists' practice roles. *J Am Coll Clinical Pharm* 2020; 3(2): 478–484. https://doi.org/10.1002/jac5.1171

14. Monmaturapoj T *et al*. What influences the implementation and sustainability of antibiotic stewardship programmes in hospitals? A qualitative study of antibiotic pharmacists' perspectives across South West England. *Eur J Hosp Pharm* 2022; 29: e46–e51. https://doi.org/10.1136/ejhpharm-2020-002540

15. Farag M *et al*. Impact of a clinical pharmacist on medication safety in mental health Hospital-in-the-Home: a retrospective analysis. *Int J Clin Pharm* 2022; 44(4): 947–955. https://doi.org/10.1007/s11096-022-01409-4

16. Fudge N, Swinglehurst D. It's all about patient safety: an ethnographic study of how pharmacy staff construct medicines safety in the context of polypharmacy. *BMJ Open* 2021; 11: e042504. https://doi.org/10.1136/bmjopen-2020-042504

17. Schneider P. The impact of technology on safe medicines use and pharmacy practice in the US. *Front Pharmacol* 2018; 9. https://doi.org/10.3389/fphar.2018.01361

18. Hall N *et al*. Exploration of prescribing error reporting across primary care: a qualitative study. *BMJ Open* 2022; 12: e050283. https://doi.org/10.1136/bmjopen-2021-050283

19. Aronson J. Medication errors: definitions and classification. *Br J Clin Pharmacol* 2009; 67(6): 599–604. https://doi.org/10.1111/j.1365-2125.2009.03415x

20. Aronson J. Medication errors: what they are, how they happen and how to avoid them. *QJM Int J Medicine* 2009; 102(8): 513–521. https://doi.org/10.1093/qjmed/hcp052

21. Maxwell S. Clinical therapeutics and good prescribing. In: Ralston S *et al*. eds. *Davidson's Principles and Practice of Medicine,* 23rd edn. London: Elsevier, 2018: 13–36.

22. Kapaki V. The anatomy of medication errors. In: Stawicki S, Firstenberg M, eds. *Vignettes in Patient Safety*. London: Intech Open, 2018: 77–92.

23. World Health Organization (WHO)(2017). *Medication without harm: WHO global patient safety challenge*. Geneva: World Health Organization. https://www.who.int/publications/i/item/WHO-HIS-SDS-2017.6

24. Edge V *et al*. Syndromic surveillance of gastrointestinal illness using pharmacy over the counter sales: a retrospective study of waterborne outbreaks in Saskatchewan and Ontario. *Can J Public Health* 2004; 95(6): 446–450. https://doi.org/10.1007/BF03403991

25. Ashcroft D *et al*. Safety culture assessment in community pharmacy: development, face validity, and feasibility of the Manchester Patient Safety Assessment Framework. BMJ *Qual & Saf* 2005; 14: 417–421. https://dx.doi.org/10.1136/qshc.2005.014332

Further reading

American Pharmacists Association. *Pharmacists' impact on patient safety*. Washington DC: American Pharmacists Association. https://pharmacist.com/Portals/0/PDFS/Practice/PharmacistsImpactonPatientSafety_Web.pdf?ver=dYeAzw1N3-PG9eSkMMsV-a%3D%3D

Centre for pharmacy postgraduate education (CPPE). *Patient safety*. Manchester: Centre for pharmacy postgraduate education (CPPE). https://www.cppe.ac.uk/gateway/patientsaf

College of Pharmacists of Manitoba. *Community pharmacy safety culture toolkit*. Winnipeg: College of Pharmacists of Manitoba. https://cphm.ca/wp-content/uploads/Resource-Library/SafetyIQ/CPSC-Toolkit-FINAL.pdf

Dopp A *et al* (2020). *Pharmacist role in patient safety*. Rockville: Agency for Healthcare Research and Quality. https://psnet.ahrq.gov/perspective/pharmacist-role-patient-safety

CHAPTER 19

Strategic thinking, behaviour and planning

Upon completion of this chapter you should be able to:

- understand the importance of strategy in effective leadership
- define the term strategy
- list the pillars of effective strategy
- detail the methods for strategic planning
- understand how a leader should implement strategic behaviour.

It is sometimes said that 'if you think you can't…you're right'. This saying reflects one of the most important elements of effective leadership, the ability to think, act, and plan in a strategic, rather than tactical, manner. While there are many different approaches and philosophies of leadership, most of them share a common foundation: the capacity to understand and capitalise on unpredictable environments in ways that optimise returns and maximise potential for success.

What is strategy?

The term strategy can have different meanings in different contexts, but usually it refers to the ability to plan and mobilise resources (including people) to achieve specific short-, mid-, and long-term goals.[1] Strategic thinking involves a thoughtful, evidence-informed selection of goals and mindful resilient actions taken to achieve them. In daily life, all human beings have experience of strategic thinking: whatever has been accomplished in life, individuals need to select goals (e.g. in careers and relationships) then consider the best, most efficient and effective pathway, or series of steps, required to achieve these goals.[2,3] Success in strategy refers to the qualities associated with choosing the right (most appropriate or best) goals, and the right (most effective and efficient) actions to achieve these goals.[4] Unrealistically ambitious – or lazily underwhelming – goals are a sign of poor strategic thinking. Ambitious but achievable goals are essential. Such goals alone do not guarantee success: a clear-eyed plan and a level of organisation and attentiveness to systems and time, are all required to achieve these goals.[5] Along the way, individuals need to be resolute but flexible: open to the ever-changing environment but steady, focused, and resilient in pursuing well-considered goals.

For leaders, this process of strategic thinking is amplified considerably because it involves the reputation and 'brand' of a business, the working lives of staff, the day to day operations of an organisation, and the finances and resources that keep it all functioning. The risks and rewards of strategic thinking and planning are many, but the process can be complicated. One particular complication of note, is the tendency for some leaders to confuse or conflate 'strategy' with 'tactics'.

In daily conversation, there may be little or no consideration paid to the differences between strategies and tactics but for leaders the differences are significant, and confusion between the two can lead to disastrous outcomes.[6] While strategy refers to the specific goals and selection of actions required to achieve them, tactics are the more detailed steps involved in undertaking those actions. Tactical thinking is crucial for success, especially for managers who must consider implementation and operational details[7]; however tactical thinking without a strategic orientation may result in random, disjointed, and disorganised activities that actually interfere with the attainment of goals.[8]

Consider the distinction between strategy and tactics with respect to personal financial planning. Personal financial 'success' is not simply about who has the most money at a specific point in time; instead, for most people, success involves stability, the ability to weather ups and downs in the economy, and predictability as to how much money will be available to fund daily life, now and in the future. Strategic financial thinking requires individuals to set goals such as: how much money do I need each month in retirement, how much risk am I willing to take to get that money, and what is the right balance between stocks, bonds, real estate, and other potential actions I could take? A strategic financial plan takes answers to these questions and provides a structure for investing over a person's working life to achieve the goals that were established within the parameters of risk that were defined. If successful, a stable, predictable, and resilient pool of investments will fund retirement in a comfortable way that allows an individual to sleep easily at night. In contrast, a tactical approach to personal finances may not involve long-term goals and may not consider risks and rewards fully. A tactical approach would likely focus on the immediate, short-term gyrations of the market. A strategic approach to personal finances may involve careful research of high-quality companies, purchases of their stock, and the resilience to 'buy and hold' despite short-term economic ups and downs...because the long-term dominates short-term volatility. In contrast, a tactical approach may mean constantly buying and selling stocks, with a view to never losing money...get in and get out quickly and focus on day to day momentum. While tactical approaches to the stock market can, and have, resulted in financial success for some, it comes at an enormous price in terms of anxiety, daily attentiveness to stock market changes, and the ability to dedicate significant time to constantly monitoring individual company shares. In reality, the vast majority of individuals who take this tactical approach to finances actually lose considerable amounts of money in the mid- and long-term, in addition to experiencing anxiety and not having stability and predictability. In contrast, a longer term, plan-based strategic approach will likely not produce the same short-term market highs but will also likely avoid the mid-term market lows...and provide a more predictable, safer, and less anxiety-producing pathway to achieving goals.

As a leader, it can sometimes be easy to confuse strategy with tactics, or to focus on short-term wins at the expense of longer term success. It can also be easy to 'get lost in the weeds' and focus too intently on detailed operational decisions that managers should be trusted to make. These risks distract leaders from their more important responsibilities and opportunities, to focus on the longer game and to build incrementally and sustainably, rather than be a firecracker that shines brightly for a moment, then burns itself out. Good leaders understand that strategy and tactics are both necessary and essential for success: they are flip sides of the same coin. Trying to achieve goals only with strategy won't work because attentiveness to details of the concrete steps and action items are needed to bring these to life. When leaders only focus on strategy, they end up spending too much time planning and talking, with insufficient attention to doing the actual work and implementing the actions needed to really achieve goals. Conversely, goals cannot be met through tactics – or actions – alone. Tactics without a strategic backbone will quickly turn into random activities disconnected from one another, producing much work but no meaningful or sustainable progress, because no overall goals were articulated. Where tactics alone are used, individuals take arbitrary actions and knee-jerk responses to maximise short-term success, compromising longer term opportunities, and this frequently leads to frustration and burnout.

The pillars of effective strategy

Evidence-informed decision making

Decisions should be well considered and well researched. Gathering data from reliable sources, confirming it, and rechecking assumptions and calculations, is essential. In some cases, leaders can become intoxicated by their own role and self-perceived power, and wilfully disregard or ignore evidence that points to problems or concerns; developing and learning to rely upon credible and useful evidence sources to guide strategic thinking is an important counterweight to this tendency.

Have a vision statement

As noted above, there is a crucial distinction between strategy and tactics. While both are essential, they play different roles in an organisation. At the core of strategy is a clear vision, most frequently written and articulated in the form of a vision statement. The vision statement provides all stakeholders with an understanding of 'why' the organisation exists, and should inspire and excite managers, staff, and clients. It provides an opportunity to define an organisation within a broader complex environment, and what makes that organisation unique, important, and special. A vision is often aspirational but still provides the psychological fuel needed by managers and staff to work to their fullest potential. Examples of exemplary vision statements include:

- Amazon: To build a place where people can come to find and discover anything they might want to buy – online.
- Google: To provide access to the world's information in one click.
- Ben and Jerry's: Making the best ice cream in the nicest possible way.

Crafting a bold vision and articulating it in the form of a statement is a collaborative process but one that requires leadership. While it may, sometimes, come across as lofty and unrealistic, vision statements play an important role in strategy because they define a goal, inspire interest, and help clients and staff connect to one another. Clarity and concision are essential for successful vision statements: the central idea embodied in the vision must resonate with readers and be instantly understood. Formalising vision statements can be supported by:[9]

1. Project 5, 10 or 15 years into the future...do not concentrate on today's mundane realities and problems, but instead on a future-oriented, aspirational ideal.
2. Be big, be bold: Vision statements need to inspire, and as a result they need to rise 'out of the weeds' and not be concerned with operational details. While a vision may never be fully realised, even partial attainment of a bold vision can be a major success.
3. Use the present tense: Using action oriented verbs in the present tense conveys a sense of possibility and immediacy to the vision statement. Future tense and arbitrary deadlines create the possibility of delay and deferral which can frustrate the attainment of a vision.
4. Don't use jargon, don't use complex terminology: The vision statement is a single, concise sentence that makes sense to every stakeholder – including staff, managers, shareholders, clients, competitors, and innocent bystanders. Technical terminology or jargon interferes with understanding and reduces excitement – it should be avoided.
5. Be authentic: A vision statement needs to embody the actual beliefs, values, and sentiments of a leader and an organisation. Where leaders are inauthentic or feel they need to fake enthusiasm, vision statements will fall flat and not be believable. Aligning vision with actual beliefs, values, and goals is essential for success.

Create a mission

Similar to a vision statement, a mission statement is an essential component of strategic thinking and planning. While the vision outlines the 'why', the mission outlines the 'what' and 'how' of an organisation. It should outline core functions performed by the organisation and how they are done better and differently than anyone else. A good mission statement should be no more than two sentences long but still be concise, catchy, focused on actions, and inspirational. Examples of powerful mission statements include:

- Tesla: To accelerate the world's transition to sustainable energy. Tesla believes the faster the world stops relying on fossil fuels and moves towards a zero-emission future, the better.
- Patagonia: We're in business to save our home planet. We will build the best products, cause no unnecessary harm, use business to inspire, and implement solutions to the environmental crisis.
- Google: Our company mission is to organise the world's information and make it universally accessible and useful.

While similarly lofty and aspirational, mission statements are more specific, plausible, and clear than vision statements. For example, Google's vision speaks to generic 'access', while it's mission makes this more actionable by focusing on organising and making information accessible and useful. Both the mission and the vision reflect values and beliefs around free access to information: the mission, however, helps readers understand that the way free access is gained is through organisation, universal accessibility, and usefulness of the information.

Effective mission statements typically consist of four key elements:[10]

1. *Value:* What is the underlying importance or necessity of the organisation to both clients and employees? This can be drawn from the vision statement but needs to be clarified and specified in the mission.

2. *Inspiration:* Why would anyone want to work for this organisation? Or buy their products/services? Or be associated with them in any way? What is the 'feel-good' proposition that will lead any stakeholder to want to be connected to this organisation?

3. *Plausibility:* Actionable, realistic, and reasonable mission statements are important, to reduce the risk of eye-rolling cynicism. It can be a challenge to balance the need to be inspirational with the necessity of being plausible, but a mission statement needs to make sense to readers as something that could actually be accomplished.

4. *Specificity:* While vision statements can be lofty, mission statements need to make these aspirations more concrete by specifically connecting activities that are relevant to achieving a vision. It should be clear how these activities in the mission actually help an organisation achieve its vision.

The mission statement is an essential companion to a vision statement – and vice-versa. One without the other cannot succeed alone. Understanding the crucial distinctions between the two, and aligning the vision and the mission in an authentic way that is consistent with organisational values, beliefs, and behaviours, is an essential leadership role.

Focus

Leadership is inherently complex, involving multiple simultaneous pressures, opportunities, risks, and rewards. It is inaccurate to believe that leaders are simply charismatic cheerleaders who can channel positive energy in a mindless, emotion-laden manner. Instead, success in strategic thinking, planning, and behaviour requires a high degree of focus and organisation. Focus means leaders need to recognise when they are 'in the weeds' and acting as managers (or worse, micromanagers). Unfocused leadership often results in a shift towards managerial activities such as direct supervision or operational control. Nervous or inexperienced leaders may prefer these managerial roles since they seem 'safer' and more concrete than the somewhat nebulous job of establishing vision and mission. Leaders need to focus on leadership, and not simultaneously try to insert managerial responsibilities into their already busy schedules. Failure to focus on leadership often means leadership will be absent. This can result in a shift away from strategy and into tactics, with a resultant lack of clarity and direction on organisation needs. Focusing on strategy, and trusting managers or others with tactical decisions, can allow leaders the time and cognitive/emotional capacity necessary to truly excel in this essential role.

Coupled with the need to focus, is the requirement to be organised and efficient. Strategic work requires a high degree of organisation but also the ability to be flexible and reflective with sufficient time to simply imagine and speculate. Visions and missions do not write themselves, nor do they spontaneously emerge from thin air: they arise through a creative and reflective process that is introspective and open, and leaders need sufficient time and space to be inventive, rather than being mired in daily operational decisions and activities. Often, it is up to leaders themselves to find and ringfence the time and space necessary for this kind of blue-sky imagining. The cognitive and emotional work associated with leadership is significant and the most effective leaders organise their time in ways that provides periods of unscheduled, unprogrammed quiet time to allow for speculation, reading, and reflection. Leadership should not be equated with being a headless chicken running to and fro, filling every waking hour with meetings or interactions with others. Organising a schedule and protecting time on a regular basis to encourage reflection and creativity, is essential.

Communication and collaboration

Leadership is often described as a team sport and in the context of strategic planning, thinking, and behaving, communication and collaboration with others is central to success. While leaders may begin the process of articulating visions and missions, these cannot be dictated from above, particularly in a field like pharmacy that will be filled with strong and independently-minded professionals. Leaders may propose, but staff will dispose of ideas or concepts that are inauthentic and do not resonate. Crafting effective strategies, visions, and missions requires authentic and engaged communication, effective listening, and true collaboration. Starting this process does not mean leaders have a monopoly on the outcome: instead, the best outcomes arise when leaders find ways of truly engaging managers, staff, clients, and other stakeholders in the process through transparent communication and authentic engagement.

The strategic plan

One of the essential responsibilities of leadership is the development of a strategic plan. Every organisation (large, small, public-sector or private-sector) should have a process for regular strategic planning and steps in place for monitoring and course corrections as needed. A strategic plan builds upon the initial strategic thinking leaders undertake and provides an essential structure for understanding how an organisation will grow, thrive and succeed.

There are different models and methods for developing and documenting a strategic plan, but most plans describe an organisation's current state, its desired future state, and the process of how it plans to shift from the current state to that desired future state. While specific formats may vary, most strategic plans should include:[11]

1. *Vision:* A clear description of where the organisation wants to go.
2. *Mission:* A broad outline of how the organisation will get there.
3. *Values:* A description of how the organisation 'behaves' on the journey and what rules and culture will define the voyage.
4. *Focus:* Specific areas of emphasis or topics that will be the concentrated attention and effort of the organisation, its leaders, its managers and its staff.
5. *Goals:* Achievable, realistic, and specific outcomes the organisation needs to achieve in order to succeed in its vision, mission and focus, in a manner that is aligned with its values.
6. *Objectives:* Shorter-term, measurable, activity or task-oriented work that is required in order to help achieve a goal; often multiple objectives are needed for each goal as there are different stepping stones or building-blocks that are required.
7. *Key performance indicators(KPIs):* Quantitative or qualitative measurements that are reliable and valid that help all stakeholders understand whether, and how completely and successfully, objectives and goals have been achieved, and how these achievements help the organisation meet its mission and vision.

An effective strategic plan must be rooted in clear-eyed, real world evidence and a comprehensive understanding of the environment within which the organisation itself operates: a vision or mission that is detached from reality, ignores competitors, and overlooks significant political, social, or economic changes in the environment, will be untethered from reality and consequently will not succeed. As part of the strategic thinking and planning process, it is important to undertake systematic examination of these environmental risks and opportunities, and integrate this into strategic thinking, articulation of vision and mission, and the elements of the strategic plan itself.

One of the most commonly used tools and approaches to understand how the organisation intersects with its broader environment is the SWOT analysis.[12] SWOT is an acronym meaning strengths, weaknesses, opportunities and threats, and is a method for analysing and identifying an organisation's internal strengths and weaknesses, as well as external/environmental/political/social/ economic opportunities and threats. Strengths and weaknesses are internally focused reflections, examining day to day functions and operations within the organisation. In contrast, opportunities and threats focus on an external analysis of the industry within which the organisation operates, whether that is a for-profit business or non-profit/governmental agency.

- *Strengths:* What does the organisation do well, better than others, and best in its field? What are the advantages the organisation has over others in the field? What do clients/customers/ patients perceive as the unique and important value added element the organisation brings?
- *Weaknesses:* Where does the organisation need to improve, in areas related to human resources, financial planning/stability/sustainability, resource utilisation and productivity? Where have there been problems in the past that continue to exist in the present and may persist into the future? What have been the consequences of these problems?
- *Opportunities:* Identifying and quantifying areas of potential growth (including increasing a customer/patient base, introducing new products and services, expanding into new geographic markets, moving into virtual/online spaces, etc.) requires both speculation and creativity, as well as data or evidence to support novel ideas.
- *Threats:* What are the broader environmental and societal issues facing not only this organisation but the industry within which the organisation operates? What are the political issues (e.g. increased regulatory scrutiny, change in government funding of programs, evolution of protected scopes of practice)? What are the economic issues (e.g. inflation, deflation, supply chain constraints)? What are the technological issues (e.g. shift to virtual delivery of goods and services, work-from-home pressures)? What are the social issues (e.g. rise of misinformation, decreased trust in professional expertise)? What are the climate breakdown issues (e.g. heat stress, flooding, etc.)? Comprehensive threats assessment can sometimes actually uncover potential opportunities for organisations who are quick to recognise the impact of threats and are able to mobilise resources to respond to them effectively and efficiently.

The SWOT process requires systematic gathering of high-quality data and evidence, not simply opinion and conjecture. For example, it may be facile to claim a strength of an organisation is its workforce: while this may be a temporary feel-good statement, it is important to accurately assess this claim by (for example) comparing rates of employee turnover to other competitors, or comparing qualifications/credentials to other peer organisations, or measuring productivity per employee and contrasting with other employers in the field. When undertaking a SWOT analysis, it is essential that it is done in an honest, transparent, and evidence-based way in order to be sufficiently accurate to form the foundation of a strategic plan. Every claim of strength, weakness, opportunity, and threat needs to be substantiated by data in some way; where claims are unsubstantiated, they should be regarded with skepticism and not relied upon for strategic planning purposes.

The end result of a SWOT analysis should be an opportunity to examine what differentiates an organisation from others in the field, what opportunities for growth exist, and what risks exist (both within the company and externally from competitors or from other environmental changes). SWOT analysis is not a formula that produces a single answer, but it is a process of filtering complex information in a systematic way that can help leaders identify and leverage options. Most importantly, it can provide leaders with an opportunity to prioritise and focus their energy and attention on the most impactful future options that will help an organisation to thrive.

Despite its ubiquity, there have been criticisms of the SWOT approach to strategic planning, since it is somewhat detached from action and requires significant additional work to translate strengths, weaknesses, opportunities, and threats into real and meaningful activities. In some cases, the SOAR model may be more appropriate.[13] SOAR maintains the strengths and opportunities elements of SWOT, but replaces weaknesses and threats with aspirations and results:

- *Aspirations:* These focus on what the organisation wants to do, who they want to serve, and where and how they wish to operate. These aspirations must be practical, actionable, and specific, and require leaders to move from simple lofty rhetoric into more pragmatic activities that have meaning and value to the organisation and its stakeholders.
- *Results:* This section should address how the organisation can identify, monitor, and evaluate progress towards aspirations and opportunities that have been identified using defensible, reliable, and valid qualitative and quantitative measurements. It provides an important way of preventing strategic planning from becoming unrealistically lofty by reminding leaders of the need to actually prove they have achieved what they have set out to do, and provides a transparent way of monitoring progress towards strategic goals.

The SOAR approach is generally considered to be more action oriented and pragmatic than the SWOT approach (which is typically seen as more analytical and reflective); as a result, SOAR is more frequently favoured by newer, less well-established organisations who are in a growth or development phase, while SWOT may be more appropriate for more established organisations concerned with consolidating their position, identity, or brand. Importantly, SOAR provides an option for organisations that do not actually know what their weaknesses are because they are too new; instead it is more forward looking and positive, while SWOT tends to be useful where established opposing forces or competition are well-known and understood.

Beyond SWOT and SOAR, other methods for strategic planning include the PESTEL analysis, which examines six broader societal factors (political, economic, social, technological, environmental, and legal/regulatory) and how these may influence mission and vision.[14] The PESTEL analysis can be a useful preliminary step in identifying threats and weaknesses in the SWOT model, and provides an in depth examination of the external realities facing an organisation. Popularised by Harvard Business Professor Michael Porter, the Five Forces model of planning is widely used in highly competitive for-profit industry settings that helps leaders define the intensity of competition and the attractiveness (or lack of attractiveness) of the industry itself in terms of profitability. This model includes three 'horizontal forces': threats from substitute products and services, threats from established competitors, and threats from those who may come into the industry group. Industry groups that have high barriers to entry (for example, a highly regulated field like pharmacy) typically have greater opportunities to manage these horizontal forces. In contrast, there are two 'vertical forces': the bargaining power of suppliers and of customers/patients. In the Five Forces model, the ability of customers/patients to simply take their business elsewhere unless they are satisfied is a significant point of interest, and strategic planning strongly emphasises vision, mission, goals, and objectives to reduce this risk to the organisation.

There is no single or perfect model for strategic planning and analysis but understanding the variety of approaches available and used can be helpful for leaders in identifying how best to proceed given the specific context of their organisation. The selection of SWOT versus SOAR versus PESTEL versus Five Forces or any other model will be based on organisation specific characteristics as well as simple preferences. There are advantages and disadvantages to each of these models; more important than selecting the 'perfect' option is simply selecting one and getting on with the important work of strategic analysis and planning.

Strategic behaviour

Thinking, analysing, and planning in a strategic manner requires work, organisation, and commitment. For leaders, the process does not end with production of a strategic plan; instead, once a plan is produced, a new phase of strategic behaviour unfolds. Strategic behaviour describes the constellation of actions required to bring a strategic plan to life and embed it within the day to day activities and operations of an organisation. Too often, strategic plans simply gather dust on shelves, or remain unrealistically lofty documents that do not resonate with managers, staff, clients, or other stakeholders. Strategic behaviours are those that help organisations ensure strategic plans are enacted and that vision, mission, goals, and objectives are realised.

With the widespread use of strategic thinking and planning processes across organisations big and small, there is an unfortunately widespread rise in cynicism and distrust associated with strategy. In part, this may reflect 'strategy burnout', in which individual managers, workers (and some leaders) lose faith in the ability of strategic planning to actually produce meaningful or sustainable improvements. This can be a result of overly ambitious targets, poorly conceived plans, or faulty environmental analyses not rooted in data. Where cynicism about strategic planning and its potential exists within an organisation, it is likely to undermine the possibility of successful implementation.

Leaders have a crucial role to play in countering, addressing, and dealing with cynicism or distrust of the strategic planning process. A first crucial step is to enhance transparency and communication so that all those affected by the strategic plan have not only opportunities to participate but incentive and motivation to truly engage in the process. This is a crucial distinction for leaders to understand: simply dictating strategy to staff means they are not invested and consequently have little incentive to do anything differently than they've always done before. Simply providing opportunities for people to show up and provide feedback is too passive an approach and generally results in only 'squeaky wheels' (i.e. those with a strong opinion) to actually participate. Inventive ways of having as many stakeholders as possible be engaged – not simply participate – in the strategic thinking, analysis, and planning process is a strategic behaviour that should be a priority.

One method for this may be to make more people leaders in the process and find organisational mechanisms to help individual staff and managers feel greater responsibility and ownership for strategic plans, goals, and objectives. This can be challenging for some leaders as it means relinquishing control, but it is an important tool for building buy-in across an organisation for strategic planning. Linking budgets and control over money to strategic planning – and avoiding the temptation of micromanaging by leaders! – is a useful approach to consider. Using annual performance appraisal processes linked to specific strategic priorities, goals, and objectives can help by tying annual salary increases to success in achieving strategic plan outcomes. Celebrating individual's successes and creativity/initiatives in a public way can also generate more positive impressions of the strategic planning process.

Regardless of the method selected, leaders must be aware of the importance of finding ways of engaging all stakeholders in strategic thinking, analysis, and planning throughout the life cycle of the strategic plan itself. Cultivating nascent leadership interests and skills of individuals across an organisation can be a powerful strategic behaviour that can enhance the likelihood of successful implementation of a strategic plan.

Summary

The responsibilities of leadership are many, but perhaps the most important function leaders have is to provide strategic direction for an organisation. 'Providing' direction does not mean dictating and forcing it upon everyone else: instead, it means using a series of thinking, analytical, planning, and behavioural tools and techniques to create an organisational culture that is engaged in its vision and mission, and focused on the goals and objectives necessary to achieve success in a manner that is aligned and consistent with its values. Transparent communication, effective listening, and collaborative processes are essential. In addition, authenticity in leadership style and approach are necessary to make strategic planning possible and successful.

References

1. Huebner C, Flessa S. Strategic management in healthcare: a call for long-term and systems-thinking in an uncertain system. *Int J Environ Res Public Health* 2022; 19(14): 8617. https://doi.org/10.3390/ijerph19148617

2. JCO Oncology Practice. Strategic planning: why it makes a difference and how to do it. *J Oncol Pract* 2009; 5(3): 139–143. https://doi.org/10.1200/JOP.0936501

3. Donev D *et al.* Strategic Planning in Health Care – General Approach. In: Kragelj L, Bozikov J, eds. *Methods and Tools in Public Health*, 1st edn. Skopje: Hans Jacobs Publishing, 2010: 849–872.

4. Harrison D, Ortmeier B. Strategic planning in the community pharmacy: strategic planning is crucial in today's dynamic health care environment, but a surprisingly small number of pharmacies actually use the process. *J Am Pharm Assoc* 1996; 36(9): 583–588. https://doi.org/10.1016/s1086-5802(16)30120-6

5. Harrison D. Strategic planning by independent community pharmacies. *J Am Pharm Assoc* 2005; 45(6): 726–733. https://doi.org/10.1331/154434505774909652

6. Mackay D, Zundel M. Recovering the divide: a review of strategy and tactics in business and management. *Int J Management Reviews* 2017; 19(2): 175–194. https://doi.org/10.1111/ijmr.12091

7. Casadesus-Masanell R, Ricart J (2009). *From strategy to business models to tactics*. Boston: Harvard Business School. https://www.hbs.edu/ris/Publication%20Files/10-036.pdf

8. Society for Human Resource Management (SHRM). *What is the difference between a strategic plan and a tactical plan?* Society for Human Resource Management (SHRM). https://www.shrm.org/resourcesandtools/tools-and-samples/hr-qa/pages/couldyouexplainthedifferencebetweenstrategicandtacticalplansandgiveexamplesofeach.aspx

9. Kirkpatrick S. How to build a better vision statement. *Academic Leadership: The online journal* 2008; 6(4). https://doi.org/10.58809/KLTT3796

10. Alegre I *et al*. The real mission of the mission statement: a systematic review of the literature. *J Management and Organization* 2018; 24(4): 456–473. https://doi.org/10.1017jmo.2017.82

11. Martin R. The Big Lie of strategic planning. *Harvard Business Review* [online] 2014. https://hbr.org/2014/01/the-big-lie-of-strategic-planning

12. Gurel E. SWOT analysis: a theoretical review. *J Int Social Research* 2017; 10(51): 994–1006.

13. Cole M *et al*. Measuring strengths, opportunities, aspirations, and results: psychometric properties of the 12-item SOAR Scale. *Front Psychol* 2022; 13. https://doi.org/10.3389/fpsyg.2022.854406

14. Siddiqui A. The use of PESTEL analysis tool of quality management in health care business and its advantages. *Am J Biomed Sci and Res* 2021; 14(6): 507–512. https://doi.org.10.34297ajbsr.2021.14.002046

CHAPTER 20

Understanding and leveraging power as a leader

Upon completion of this chapter you should be able to:

- define the terms power and conformity
- detail the seven sources of power
- outline the processes for leaders to understand their personal sources of power.

It is sometimes said there is a 'leadership crisis' in professions such as pharmacy, with too few members of the profession electing to take on complex and demanding managerial or leadership roles.[1] When members of a profession refuse to lead it, others who are not part of that profession will step in their place.[2] Leaders (for example, accountants, business people, physicians or nurses) who are not pharmacists do not understand the culture of the profession, have not experienced day to day practice, and may lack the networks to understand the reality and nuances of practitioners' experiences.[2] As a result, these leaders may make decisions that are misaligned with the profession's aspirations and culture and this can produce friction, demoralisation and distrust.[3] Further, when people from outside the profession lead that profession, they may not have the same allegiance, interests, or pride in the profession that is necessary to support continuing growth and aspiration.

The value and importance of having pharmacists step up to be leaders in their own profession has not unleashed great interest by pharmacists in assuming these roles. Studies suggest part of the reason for this may be the psychology and temperament of many pharmacists themselves (*see* Chapter 2), as the dominant emotional intelligence of pharmacists is Assimilator. Assimilators typically value structure and organisation but may not have the self-confidence and interest in competitive success that has historically characterised leadership in most fields. Pharmacists themselves may perceive a lack of personal power they feel is a prerequisite for leadership, imagining others are more powerful and persuasive and therefore should be better leaders.

Understanding and leveraging one's power is important for all human beings, whether they have leadership roles or not. For some, the word 'power' has a pejorative or negative connotation, as though a bludgeon is being wielded unfairly over others. Some pharmacists may even go out of their way to deny or hide personal power as a way of feeling 'nice' or avoiding confrontation. Reflecting on one's assumptions about power, one's relationship with one's own power, and how responding to other's power influences our thinking and behaviour is crucial for leaders...and for those being lead.

What is power?

Power is not an inherently positive or negative aspect of daily life, but simply the ability to influence the thinking and behaviour of others, or the ability to get things done in a way that one wants them to be done.[4] Power is an instrument or tool that is part of every day social interactions. All human beings have power: consider a tiny baby whose cry can jolt adults into action or whose smile can cause the hearts of even the most serious-minded people to melt. Consciously or unconsciously, we are constantly leveraging our own power, assessing the powers of others, and calibrating our thinking and behaviours accordingly. For leaders, it is essential to understand core concepts associated with power, honestly self-appraise one's own powers, and mindfully leverage power in ways that are fair, appropriate, proportionate and ultimately aligned with professional and organisational (rather than simply personal) objectives.[5]

Negative connotations associated with power frequently arise because certain kinds of powers are used as a weapon of sorts, to compel others to do things they do not wish to do. The well-known phrase 'absolute power corrupts absolutely', reflects the generally negative view of power and the desire to hide it from plain sight as a way of appearing modest and humble. When human beings do not reflect upon power and understand how it works, they are more likely to be manipulated and power is more likely to become a tool for abuse than a productive and important instrument for accomplishing valuable outcomes.

What is conformity?

The flip-side of power is conformity, the tendency for human beings to think and behave in ways that are consistent with specific norms and expectations.[6] Where individuals do not reflect and understand power, they are more susceptible to the influence of other's powers (as malign politicians of yesterday and today have learned). Conformity works because of the emotional discomfort and cognitive dissonance that is triggered when one member of a group does not align behaviours with group expectations.[7] Consider, for example, how queuing for a bus highlights both power and conformity in action. Historically in the United Kingdom, individuals waiting for a bus have conformed to the social power of others and long-standing tradition, and simply know they should stand in a line, one after another, approximately one metre apart, to signify who arrived at the stop first and who – in fairness – should have first priority to board the bus when it arrives. In contrast, in most of North America, there is a tradition of 'clumping' at bus stops, rather than queuing in an orderly fashion, and non-verbal negotiation mechanisms are used by the clumpers to acknowledge that whoever arrived first gets to board first. A North American visiting Manchester may be seen as rude and uncivilised, while a British person visiting Cleveland may be seen as snobby and stand-offish. The power of social judgment is impressively clear in the way that it shapes individual's behaviours in public spaces. This power may not be expressed in specific verbal comments (e.g. 'get to the back of the line, you bloody fool!') but in a variety of subtle, non-verbal cues that allow individuals in the queue (or clump) to collectively exert power to drive conformity.

The ways in which different kinds of power trigger conformity has been a source of fascination and significant research in social psychology. The Asch study was one of the first to demonstrate how average people can be easily convinced to completely ignore objective reality simply because of the presence of others and the power of peer pressure.[8] In his experiments, he showed research subjects two straight lines: one was clearly and objectively shorter than the other. When research subjects were placed into groups of three, four, or five other people – all of whom were actors pretending to be research participants – a fascinating (and disturbing) result emerged. When asked to indicate which line was longer, the actors, confidently and boldly, claimed the shorter line was longer – before the real participant had a chance to express their answer. As the experiment progressed, the actors became more belligerent, aggressive, and confident in their wrong answer, saying things like 'of course this line is shorter, any idiot can see that!'. The more aggressively wrong the actors were, and the larger the number of actors were, the more likely it became that the actual research participant would yield to the wrong opinion. In follow-up interviews with the actual research participants, they indicated that they wilfully complied with the wrong statement simply because they felt they must be missing something if other 'average' participants were all in agreement. The implications of the Asch study for understanding human behaviour are interesting – and somewhat chilling given the ways in which misinformation, political polarisation, and other contemporary issues have come to dominate daily life.

Other conformity studies by researchers such as Zimbardo[9] and Milgram[10] have highlighted the ways in which different forms of authority, power, social pressure, and a desire to be liked by others influences human behaviour. Studies such as these point to the importance of what Milgram described as 'Agentic State theory':

> *"The essence of obedience consists in the fact that a person comes to view themselves as the instrument for carrying out another person's wishes, and they therefore no longer see themselves as responsible for their actions. Once this critical shift in viewpoint has occurred in the person, all essential features of obedience follow".*[10]

As one considers recent history (and even contemporary reality), these chilling thoughts regarding compliance, conformity, power, and control should serve as a sobering reminder to all leaders of how easily leadership can run astray.

The seven sources of power

Understanding conformity provides us with an important tool for understanding how power influences the behaviour of others. The model of power described by Raven and French is amongst the most widely used ways of highlighting different kinds of powers individuals have.[11] This model does not prioritise or privilege one kind of power over another, nor does it suggest some forms of power are more effective or better than others. Rather, it highlights different sources or kinds of power as a tool for self-reflection and building self-awareness. Once an individual understands where their sources of power reside, they are then better able to leverage this power in ways that are authentic, comfortable, and appropriate for a context. For example, many people instinctively believe the most effective form of power is punishment (the ability to penalise others for not conforming). Most of us have experienced the harsh emotional consequences of being punished and this makes us believe it is the strongest or best form of power to wield over others. Conversely, that emotional memory also makes many of us uncomfortable thinking about power at all, since we cannot reconcile an image of ourselves as decent, kind, fair-minded individuals who also may wield punishment power. Indeed, fear of exerting punishment power may be an important reason why pharmacists decide not to pursue leadership roles: they fear they cannot wield it effectively or well – or perhaps they fear the consequences if it turns out they can and do wield it well. There is nothing magical about punishment power...and indeed, in the Raven and French model, it is only one source of power that may or may not be an important factor for a specific individual's self-understanding. Where punishment power is not a prominent source of an individual's power – other powers will exist and will compensate.

A central premise for leaders to understand the seven sources of power is for them to gain self-awareness as to what works best for them in terms of persuading other people. Recognising and being able to articulate one's personal sources of powers provides important clues as to how to behave when persuasion is necessary. Each individual will leverage a different constellation of powers in a specific situation, suggesting there is no single or best way to be a leader. What is more important, is that each leader understands and is authentic to their true sources of power, and use those in a responsible, fair, and proportionate way.

The seven sources of power are: positional, charismatic, relational, informational, expertise, rewards, and punishment.

Positional power

Positional power is the type of influence and authority that stems from a formal role and title, such as 'President', 'Queen', 'Mum', 'Professor', 'Doctor', or 'Supervisor'. The conferred authority that comes with a title, degree, role, vote, or election has a kind of social power. For example, the fact that someone has won a popular vote in an election and has been selected by the country as a President, should convey legitimacy on that individual to have certain authority, power, and ability to persuade others. Positional power is built on a foundation of a social expectation and norms: for example, the more education a person has, the higher they will typically be in an organisational hierarchy; this usually translates into higher levels of competency, greater trust in their judgement, and ultimately greater responsibility. Much of the power of health care professionals stems from their education, title, and status, which ultimately translates into legal powers (such as prescribing or dispensing) that are not available to everyone else in society.

Positional power can often be quite ruthlessly hierarchical: for example, within a health care team setting, the more education an individual has, the higher their rank in the hierarchy, and the more positional power they can wield. Thus, the positional power of physicians (who will typically undertake 12 or more years of post-secondary education to qualify) will be generally higher than for nurses, pharmacists, or others. Importantly, this positional power is independent of actual experience, expertise, a proven track record of success, etc.; it simply flows to the individual because of their title and degree, and therefore it can be a cause of resentment from others in some cases. In many organisations, positional power is reinforced through the visual depiction of hierarchy in an organisational chart: a president is literally, and metaphorically, higher on the chart than a vice president, a supervisor, or an administrative assistant and this higher position reinforces the power they have.

Positional power works because social norms and pressure exist to reinforce conformity: most individuals will confer respect and are more likely to be persuaded by someone with the title of 'Doctor' or 'Professor' than simply their first name. The value of positional power may be in decline as honorific titles and degrees are no longer as prestigious or awe-inspiring as they were a generation ago. There is a risk that individuals who believe they have positional power simply will do what they are told – behaving in this way breeds contempt and cynicism of leadership, degrees, and titles. Leveraged appropriately, positional power can provide individuals with a starting point for persuasion that is based on socially conferred privileges that must be responsibly managed.

Charismatic power

The power of charisma and its ability to persuade others involves the use of charm, personality, style or even physical attractiveness. The word 'charisma' derives from a Greek term used to refer to specific gifts of divine origin bestowed on certain individuals as a favour from the gods. These gifts represented certain kinds of talents, physical beauty, or social charm that set individuals apart from everyone else and signified they should have specific powers within a society. Today, the term charisma applies to individuals with a magnetic personality, a unique and enviable style, or a quick wit and sense of humour that makes them interesting and compelling speakers.

Charismatic power functions by creating a kind of positive psychological energy. Charismatic individuals radiate energy that is attractive to others. Most people want to please and be liked by charismatic individuals and this is the root of the power they have over others. Charismatic power is strongly connected to local culture and social norms: what passes as charismatic in one place may be viewed as appalling in another place. For example, many political leaders rely on charismatic power as a prelude to gaining positional power through an election. They radiate an energy that says they are 'strong', 'decisive', and 'put the people first': however, to outsiders who did not vote for them, this same charisma can be viewed as 'pig-headed', 'short-sighted', and 'xenophobic'. Charismatic power can be quite fickle: it relies strongly on a relationship between leaders and followers that must be constantly replenished.

Charismatic power can be risky in other ways, especially when it starts to become no more than a 'cult of personality'. Increasingly, politicians in many Western countries have come to rely, uncomfortably, on charismatic power as the source of their appeal to voters, in the hope that if voters 'like' them as a person, they are more likely to elect them into office...regardless of their policies, positions, credentials, expertise, or experience. Charismatic power appears to be increasing in its importance for many leaders: in a world where there is more and easier access to information, people appear to be more susceptible than ever to a strong and compelling personality, rather than to the substance of what that individual is saying or doing. Charismatic power of this sort oversimplifies complex realities, overpromises and under-delivers, and can have a significant role to play on the spread and amplification of misinformation. When leveraged proportionately and appropriately, charismatic power is a useful tool for building emotional connections and social networks that can support persuasive approaches to behavioural change.

Relational power

Also called 'network power', relational power highlights the way in which an individual's personal, familial, social, and professional connections and contacts can play an important role in leadership and persuasion. It is sometimes said, 'it's not what you know – it's who you know', and this describes the ways in which relational power can be useful – or potentially abused. Relational power understands that everyone is part of complex webs of social relationships; the power of these webs can be greater than the power of any individual within that web, and relational power allows individuals to maximise the impact of the webs within which they operate. Relational power opens doors for some individuals – doors that are simply not openable for others. For example, an individual from a privileged, upper middle-class neighbourhood and family background, may simply have greater opportunities to observe professional work, attend better schools, participate in extracurricular enrichment activities, etc. compared to an individual who comes from a less affluent background who may need to start working part-time after school from the age of 15. Relational power is reflected in the somewhat homogenous academic and social backgrounds of many political leaders: for example, in the UK, 20 of Britain's Prime Ministers were all educated at the same school (Eton). While the quality of education at Eton is no doubt very strong, the relational power of Etonians also played an important role in these individual's leadership success.

The uncomfortable flip-side of relational power, of course, is that it tends to reinforce and amplify success for people of 'a certain kind': those from traditionally disadvantaged groups – including recent immigrants, members of the LGBTQ2S+ communities, BAME (Black, Asian Minority Ethnic) or BIPOC (Black, Indigenous or People of Colour) individuals – may not have the kinds of relational powers that are recognised and rewarded in certain social, political or economic contexts. Further, relational power can sometimes mean that individuals that have it tend to hoard it – for themselves and their own children – rather than using it to open doors for others. The concept of 'privilege' describes the ways in which relational power can be leveraged as both a useful tool for persuasion and as a weapon to exclude others. Recently, there has been increasing understanding of the fundamental unfairness associated with the misuse or abuse of relational powers, and attempts to redress it – through, for example, affirmative action or preferential hiring practices – have generated controversy.

All human beings have some form of relational power because all human beings exist within complex social networks and webs. Understanding one's own relational power as a function of these webs and understanding the contexts and circumstances in which this relational power can be advantageous and nobly leveraged, is essential. Equally essential however, is recognising when – through unearned privileges that are accidents of birth – relational power is being used inappropriately and unfairly, hoarding opportunities for some at the expense of others.

Informational power

For a generation, the expression 'information is power' has denoted the central role of knowledge in predicting success in professional life. Informational power focuses on the knowledge, data, facts, and understanding an individual has and the way this differentiates them from others and generates opportunities to leverage influence. In general, those with more education, more professional experience, and more opportunities to gather data have greater amounts of informational power than others.

The nature of informational power has evolved significantly with the rise of the internet and social media. In the not-too-distant past, informational power was simply the ability to access and understand complex information that was beyond the comprehension of 'average' people. For example, in the past, one of the major sources of physicians' powers was their understanding of human biology. Until the mid 20th century, it was common for newly married couples to visit their family doctor to learn 'how to have a baby' (i.e. how to engage in sexual intercourse); until the 1950s, access to sexual health information was extremely limited and it was only socially acceptable for doctors (and priests) to explain the mechanics of procreation to young people. Of course, today, this information is easily and freely available and this source of informational power for doctors is no longer relevant.

This example highlights the waning importance of informational power in the modern world. As everything becomes accessible online to everyone, power rooted in information and facts has less significance. This, coupled with a generally higher overall level of literacy and education in the population, means the gap between professionals and the public has narrowed, further straining the power of information. Today, informational power may be more important in technological fields, or in business (where advanced knowledge of important information can result in competitive advantages and huge profits). The decline of the importance of informational power has special resonance for a profession like pharmacy where 'knowledge' has historically been more important than a particular clinical skill; this is perhaps one reason why pharmacy has, in the early 21st century, had to reinvent itself as a more hands-on, clinically-oriented profession rather than one that was rooted in simply 'knowing' things about medicines.

Expertise power

Expertise power is the power associated with the ability to perform a specific and valuable skill that is rare and necessary. It focuses on being able to perform a concrete task, activity or skill, rather than simply 'knowing' what should be done. For example, many people might 'know' they need to change a washer on a leaky tap, but very few people can actually perform this activity. Knowing versus doing is at the heart of expertise power.

The expertise of a 15-year-old effortlessly navigating technology, the internet, and social media may contrast with the skills of a 57-year-old who gets flummoxed easily by the ever-changing world of computers. Expertise power is at its most impactful when specific skills are demonstrated with effortless self-confidence which allows for creative and self-assured problem-solving. Today, expertise power is amongst the most valued kinds of power, particularly as day to day life becomes more complicated and anxiety-provoking for many individuals. However, expertise power that is decoupled or disconnected from information power may be problematic: knowing how to do something impressive today does not guarantee that skill will be relevant tomorrow. Knowledge, while somewhat devalued in the current era, still has the advantage of providing a foundation for learning of new skills as things evolve, whilst only focusing on the skill itself can result in short-term, unsustainable success. For example, an expert Facebook user may struggle as more video-based and story-based platforms like TikTok and Instagram emerge since the text, photo, and conversational foundation of Facebook is quite different than other (now more popular) social media platforms. There is a strong seductive appeal to the value of expert power rooted in effortless demonstration of a valued skill; however, skill that is not built on a foundation of knowledge (informational power) may not be long-lived or able to evolve as the environment changes.

Reward power

The ability to control and administer rewards is one of the most important ways of persuading others to do things. Leaders with reward power can leverage desired, valuable and scarce rewards (such as salary increases, vacation benefits, perquisites such as conference attendance, or even social praise and admiration) as a tool to incentivise certain behaviours and to dis-incentivise others. In some cases, reward power builds upon positional power – those with named leadership or managerial roles often have the responsibility for deciding other people's salaries. It is important to note, however, that reward power is not simply about tangible benefits: some of the most meaningful and powerful rewards that shape people's behaviour include respect and admiration from others.

Novice leaders tend to overestimate the value and importance of reward power and may tend to overemphasise it in their day to day work as leaders. While rewards are an important and useful tool, care needs to be taken to not over-rely upon or overindulge in reward power, for fear of creating a workplace or organisational culture where the reward itself – rather than the desired behaviour – becomes the objective for staff. A well-known example of this occurs in education settings, where teachers have the reward power associated with assigning grades and selecting students for prestigious awards and honours. From the earliest years of education, students learn that if they behave in ways desired by the teacher (e.g. come to class every day, do your homework, be nice to others, perform well on tests, etc.) they will be rewarded (e.g. good grades, becoming the 'teacher's pet', awards, etc). Unfortunately, this culture of over-reliance on reward power in education has now produced an educational culture where the reward – not the actual learning – is the endpoint itself. For example, today there are many students – including pharmacy students! – who do not actually 'learn' and do not truly acquire deep, sustainable knowledge through their education. Instead, they simply cram details to do well on an exam then promptly forget them...yet in the process, still get rewarded by getting a high grade or even an academic achievement award. The grade itself has replaced the desired behaviour of actual learning, and the fundamental nature of the academic experience has been changed. Reward power works in the short-term and can be effective – but care must be taken to not over-rely upon it to the point where (as in the case of education) the reward dominates the desired behaviour.

Punishment power

The ability to assign sanctions and penalties on other people who are not behaving in a desired way, describes punishment power. Punishment and reward power often co-exist (i.e. a leader with reward power often has punishment power as well, and both may be connected to positional power). Importantly, leaders make conscious and unconscious decisions as to whether to prioritise and privilege the use of rewards or punishments as a way of persuading and incentivising desired behaviours.

Punishment power is one of the most challenging forms of power to wield effectively and many individuals express discomfort, or even outright denial, when told they possess this kind of power. Even when leaders know they possess the ultimate power (e.g. the ability to fire someone from their job), they may experience psychological discomfort in actually leveraging it. The use of punishment power in leadership and organisations has historically been limited and volatile, and there is always risk of subversion, hostility, disagreement, and 'blowback' when punishment power is leveraged. Conversely, failure of leaders to actually use their punishment power in a way that is proportionate, fair, and transparent – when it is necessary – can also produce problematic outcomes and increase the risk of bad behaviour.

Unfortunately, there is no simple formula as to how punishment power can be best leveraged to optimise success. General principles for the effective and proportionate use of punishment power include:

- if you have it, accept it – do not run away, deny, hide, or avoid it
- acknowledge that punishments – like rewards – have their place in the toolkit of powers leveraged by leaders and accept that they will be necessary and used
- use a principles-based approach to punishment that emphasises predictability, fairness, transparency and proportionality
- consistency is essential
- learn to manage personal discomfort associated with punishment power rather than avoiding its use altogether.

Now what?

Raven and French's model of power helps leaders reflect upon and understand their personal sources of power. While there is no definitive diagnostic test that can define an individual's unique sources of power, reflection on the general principles discussed in this chapter can help leaders articulate and better understand where their powers, their comfort, and their strengths with respect to leveraging power, exist. Everyone will have their own preferences for how power should be leveraged; as a result, in leadership there are rarely one-size-fits-all answers to problems. Instead, leveraging one's most formidable powers most effectively can produce the most impactful outcomes. An example scenario is detailed below.

Box 1: An example scenario of the need for leaders to self-understand their powers

Sam is an award winning, popular pharmacist in your practice, in a small town. Recently Sam wrote an article in the local newspaper complaining about same-sex marriage, claiming homosexuality is 'an illness', that it was 'ruining society', and that Sam supported those who would 'get violent' about it. No customers have complained to you, and you have heard some customers actually congratulating Sam on this article. You have not observed any patient-specific performance issues with Sam in the pharmacy.

How – as a leader – should this situation be addressed? There may be a range of answers: some may believe nothing should be done because it's a free country and Sam has a right to an opinion. Others may believe that Sam is actually right and would be supportive. It is hoped that the majority of pharmacists, leaders, and reasonable individuals would not think in these terms: Sam's call for violence is disturbing and the claim that homosexuality is an illness is simply factually wrong – and the kind of misinformation that a health care professional should never be spreading or supporting. Based on these points, a leader should recognise both an opportunity and a responsibility to intervene. But what – specifically – should be done?

The answer will depend on the leader's own self-understanding of their powers. For example, some leaders who are more comfortable with punishment power may sanction Sam – perhaps even dismissing Sam for views that are contrary to the health care professionals' code of ethics and for spreading misinformation in the community. A leader who is less comfortable with punishment power may instead use informational power and require Sam to review recent literature highlighting the normalcy of homosexuality and building knowledge and awareness of the impact of homophobia on patients and families. A leader who is comfortable with relational power may choose to leverage professional networks to influence Sam; for example, rather than dealing with Sam one-on-one, contact the regulatory body to investigate the matter as one of professional misconduct. A leader with charismatic power may wish to invite Sam for a cup of tea and a chat, and use positive psychology, conversation, and personal charm to try to change Sam's opinions and behaviours.

All of these options are possible, but they will all depend on the leader's self-awareness and understanding of where their power resides and how confident they feel in leveraging one type of power over another. As can be seen, leadership and power are complex because there are rarely single right answers to complex problems, and the best possible option is often a function of the individual leader's own psychology, temperament, and self-awareness. Reflecting upon this case can help individual's think about how they would handle Sam, in the context of where their confidence lies with respect to effective, proportionate, fair, and consistent leveraging of power.

Summary

Fear of power may be one reason why some pharmacists avoid leadership roles. Arguably, the simple fact of being a health care professional means that all pharmacists will need to be leaders at some point: in the example of Sam above, the case was specifically written in a way to not define whether 'you' were a manager, a leader, a colleague, or a subordinate. Instead, the situation itself called for leadership and a response, regardless of position, title, or role. Fearing one's own power does not make it go away, nor does it diminish the responsibility for action in certain situations. Instead, it can be more productive to pro-actively reflect on one's powers, identify and articulate where one's dominant powers reside, and learn to leverage power more effectively, confidently, and proportionately in situations where it is necessary.

References

1. White S, Enright S. Is there still a pharmacy leadership crisis? A seven-year follow-up assessment. *Am J Health Syst Pharm* 2013; 70(5): 443–447. https://doi.org/10.2146/ajhp120258

2. Shikaze D *et al*. Community pharmacists' attitudes, opinions, and beliefs about leadership in the profession: an exploratory study. *Can Pharm J* 2018; 151(3): 315–321. https://doi.org/10.1177/1715163518790984

3. Bachynsky J, Tindall W. It's time for more pharmacy leadership from within. *Can Pharm J* 2018; 151(6): 388–394. https://doi.org/10.1177/1715163518803875

4. Gregory P *et al*. Community pharmacists' perceptions of leadership. *Res Social Adm Pharm* 2020; 16(12): 1737–1745. https://doi.org/10.1016/j.sapharm.2020.02.001

5. Peyton T *et al*. Examining the relationship between leaders' power use, followers' motivational outlooks, and followers' work intentions. *Front Psychol* 2018; 9: 2620. https://doi.org/10.3389%2Ffpsyg.2018.02620

6. Feldman S. Enforcing social conformity: a theory of authoritarianism. *Political Psychology* 2003; 24(1): 41–74. https://doi.org/10.1111/0162-895X.00316

7. Sowden S *et al*. Quantifying compliance and acceptance through public and private social conformity. *Conscious Cogn* 2018; 65: 359–367. https://doi.org/10.1016/j.concog.2018.08.009

8. Larsen K. Conformity in the Asch experiment. *J Social Psychology* 1974; 94(2): 303–304. https://doi.org/10.1080/00224545.1974.9923224

9. Haslam S, Reicher S. Contesting the nature of conformity: what Milgram and Zimbardo's studies really show. *PLoS Biol* [online] 2012; 10(11): e1001426. https://doi.org/10.1371/journal.pbio.1001426

10. Griggs R. Milgram's obedience study: a contentious classic reinterpreted. *Teaching of Psychology* 2016; 44(1): 32–37. https://doi.org/10.1177/0098628316677644

11. French J, Raven B. The Bases of Social Power. In: Cartwright D, ed. *Studies in Social Power*. Ann Arbor: Institute for Social Research, 1959: 150–167.

CHAPTER 21

Hard talk

> **Upon completion of this chapter you should be able to:**
> - define the term conversational dynamics
> - understand the principles and applications of effective communication
> - explain the importance of rapport
> - list hard talk techniques
> - outline persuasive techniques
> - understand the limits of hard talk.

One of the most challenging elements of leadership – and one of the most frequently cited reasons pharmacists give for not wanting to become leaders – is the necessity of having difficult conversations.[1] Fear of having to support unpopular positions, break bad news, or tackle controversial topics is often connected to a lack of self-confidence in being able to manage interpersonal situations and challenges. Importantly, whether one is in a named or formal leadership position or not, difficult conversations are part of everyday life and day to day activities as a pharmacist. They are simply unavoidable if one is to be part of any kind of social grouping. Understanding the principles of effective communication and applying these to sensitive and difficult conversations can help build skills and confidence, and ultimately support greater opportunities to assume leadership roles.

Understanding conversational dynamics

It is sometimes said that 'conversation is the lifeblood of leadership'. It is the main vehicle through which leaders persuade, nudge, convince, compel, and lead.[2] The responsibilities of leadership sometimes means recognising that many conversations need to occur simultaneously, and that the same conversation may be necessary to have multiple times with different individuals in different contexts.[3] Conversational dynamics describes the social and psychological characteristics of interpersonal communication that allow individuals to effectively interact with one another to share information.[4] Importantly, 'information' is not simply facts, data, and words: it also includes the emotional state of mind of the individuals involved in the conversation and the unique social context of the interaction itself.[2,3,4] Communication – the way we observe and listen, then in turn respond and speak with others – is crucial for leadership. Communication is more than simply knowing how to speak: it is a complex and nuanced dynamic between two people that relies upon noticing, emotional intelligence, checking in, and empathy. It is often defined as a reciprocal dynamic between receivers and senders involving verbal and non-verbal cues and messages.[5]

- *Reciprocal:* Communication is a two-way interaction, not a one-way lecture. Each person in a conversation should be giving and taking equally. Even when one person may appear quiet (i.e. not saying anything) they still may be communicating through their body language, their eye contact, or their facial expressions, and this form of communication can be just as (if not more) important than words that are spoken.
- *Dynamic:* Communication is rarely a static or predictable event; instead, it is a process that constantly evolves moment to moment. Partners in any conversation are constantly changing roles (e.g. one person speaks, the other listens, or one person displays emotions while the other notices). The rules governing conversations vary from pair to pair and can change rapidly in the middle of the conversation itself: a small grimace or a raised eyebrow can rapidly change the tone and the significance of a conversation. This ever-changing dynamic means that both partners in a conversation must constantly be interpreting what the other is saying...and not saying.
- *Receivers:* During a conversation, both partners are constantly receiving information from one another. Most obviously, this information is in the form of the words and verbal messages being conveyed, but at other times it will involve certain behaviours or non-verbal cues such as eye contact, body posture, hand gestures, and facial expressions. The volume of information that is received can sometimes be overwhelming, causing some individuals to simply shut down or wilfully disregard/overlook non-verbal cues.
- *Senders:* During a conversation, both partners are also constantly sending information to one another. At times, one of the partners may be consciously aware of the information they are sending (e.g. when carefully selecting a word or calibrating a gesture). At other times, a partner may not be aware of the unconscious verbal or non-verbal information that is being sent (e.g. when an inadvertent or accidental smile crops or, or when one does a double-take in response to something that is startling).
- *Verbal cues:* The words we select when we speak are an important part of communication, but probably not as important as we sometimes think. Words and word choice are of course significant: think of the difference when someone gives a 'reason' as opposed to an 'excuse' for being late. Selecting the correct word can make all the difference between a tense stand-off and an amicable conversation – but conversation is about much more than simple word choices.
- *Non-verbal cues:* When leaders communicate (as opposed to lecture), they are simultaneously sending and receiving both verbal and non-verbal cues. Non-verbal cues are all those forms of communication that do not involve words – everything from the way we carry ourselves (posture) to the distance we leave between each other while speaking, to the facial gestures we use, to the eye contact we maintain, and the deliberate and unconscious tics and movements we make in response to what we are seeing and hearing from another person.

Leaders recognise the inherent complexity of interpersonal communication but also its centrality to human interactions. The nuanced interplay between verbal and non-verbal communication means that the real, underlying meaning or intention of each partner may be clouded. The term 'mixed messaging' refers to situations where verbal and non-verbal messages are at odds with one another: for example, if someone asks 'how are you doing?' and the response is 'great!', the accompanying non-verbal communication with each statement will be crucial for deciphering meaning. A genuine concern around the well-being of another person can be communicated verbally by saying 'how are you doing', but it requires accompanying genuine non-verbal messaging involving eye contact, appropriate facial gestures and the correct tone of voice. We all have experience of someone asking 'how are you doing' but not doing so in a genuine manner and we recognise this as fake. Similarly, the response of 'great!' will be interpreted differently if the tone of voice is sarcastic or the pitch of the spoken word goes down (rather than up).

Conversational dynamics can be viewed as a process of receivers and senders sussing one another out to decide how authentic and genuine they both are, through determining how many mixed messages are sent and how well-aligned each other's verbal and non-verbal cues actually are. When honest, genuine, aligned verbal and non-verbal messaging occurs in a reliable and predictable manner between individuals, the communication is usually considered to be effective.

Effective communication establishes rapport

Rapport can be described as a feeling of comfort between two people. When rapport exists, each person looks forward to spending time with the other, anticipating good communication and a sense of comfort in the presence of the other person. Rapport is not established instantly – it takes time, repeated exposure, and predictable positive experiences before individuals feel the emotional connection that signals rapport. As rapport builds, individuals move from formal to informal communication patters that are more time-efficient, effortless, comfortable, and ultimately more rewarding for both.

Rapport is the foundation for trust

Trust is one of the most important and essential attributes of human interaction – without trust between individuals, life as we know it would not be possible. As communication grows into rapport, trust may (or may not) emerge as the reliability of each partner in a dynamic is evaluated. Trust requires time and testing to confirm it. Difficult situations or conversations are amongst the most effective ways in which trust is tested, confirmed, and amplified over time.

As leaders, it is sometimes tempting to assume that everyone immediately trusts what we say, simply because we are leaders. While a degree, a professional title, or a lab coat may be an external symbol of someone who is trustworthy, the reality is that for many people the emotional feeling of trusting someone requires more. Trust does not mean simply not telling lies. It involves a genuine belief by the patient that the leader truly has their best interests at heart. Trust develops when leaders are able to prove to others that they genuinely are interested in them and their well-being, and are willing to take the time and provide the attention needed to prove it.

From trust comes empathy

Empathy is an invisible, almost chemical, connection between individuals who have proven themselves to one another in a way that no longer requires on-going testing. Empathy is both a way of describing a highly-evolved interaction between individuals and a concrete communication technique signalled by appropriate and well-timed verbal and non-verbal responses to what another person is saying. When empathy between individuals occurs, it provides both parties with a sense of comfort, confidence, and security.

Why does empathy matter so much in leadership? It is sometimes said that 'others will only care about what you say if they know you care about what they feel'. If we are genuinely interested in helping others rather than promoting our own self-interest, then they will be genuinely interested in our suggestions, our advice, and what we say. Simply telling or lecturing a person isn't helpful. They may smile, nod and politely agree, but in the absence of empathy – or trust, rapport, or true communication – we are possibly wasting our breath if we really think other people will listen to us and follow our good advice. When others feel empathy with their leader, they are in a primed emotional state. They are actually more attuned and more interested in conversations because they now have an emotional investment in a shared relationship. With empathy, everyone literally hears more, listens more attentively, can recall more details, and is more likely to understand what was said. Without empathy, the message can be 'in one ear and out the other'.

As can be seen, effective communication by itself is necessary but insufficient: it is the first step in a sequence leading to rapport, trust, and ultimately empathy. The difficult but important conversations of leadership are not simply about skilled communication but rely upon empathy that is built over time and through rapport and trust. Leaders who expect individuals will simply listen to them because they are leaders, or who lack authenticity in conversation, cannot build the kind of rapport, trust, and empathy needed to facilitate success in difficult conversations. Conversely, empathic relationships between leaders and others does not automatically guarantee success in difficult situations – but without empathy, success is unlikely. Thinking of communication and interpersonal interactions as a process rather than a single event in time, and recognising that each conversation, interaction, and discussion is a time where receivers and senders will test each other's authenticity and empathy, allows leaders to recognise that it takes time, patience, and attention to build the foundation necessary to have difficult conversations. Success with 'hard talk' is not instantaneous, but instead the result of mindful investments in empathic relationship building over time.

For some potential leaders, this realisation can be daunting and exhausting, leading them to question whether leadership is even worth it and whether they have the time or interest to invest in all of this. This is an important question to consider and requires genuine introspection and authentic self-awareness. Leadership that is untethered from relationships and not grounded in empathy will rarely succeed or be rewarding to the leader. Willingness to dedicate time, attention, and genuine interest in others is essential for leadership success.

Hard talk techniques

Empathy is the foundation of successful communication in difficult situations; attempting to deal with a situational or communication challenge without having an empathic relationship rooted in rapport and trust will often lead to unsuccessful outcomes. Having an empathic relationship prior to engaging in 'hard talk' does not necessarily guarantee success, but it significantly increases the likelihood of a positive outcome. Empathy cannot be rushed, faked, or forced, especially in difficult situations. Belatedly attempting to form rapport and trust with an individual after years of ignoring or overlooking them can actually worsen relationships and should be avoided.

Even with a foundation of a strong relationship with an individual, there are still important communication and persuasion techniques that can be useful for leaders to consider;

these are most effective when they are utilised in the context of an already established relationship but can still be of some limited use in other situations. These techniques include: summarising, reflecting, paraphrasing, and empathising.

- *Summarising:* Summarising involves the use of listening and speaking to accurately synopsise or sum up the factual content of what has been said by another person. Summarising is a useful communication technique in situations where multiple facts or a complex sequence of events are being discussed, to establish an agreed upon and consistent framing of what is being said. Summarising focuses on technical and factual issues and details, but typically does not engage with emotional issues, beliefs, or interpretations. Summarising provides the receiver of communication with an opportunity to demonstrate to the sender that they have been listened to. For example, in a situation where an individual expresses strong disagreement about an organisation's decision to support a local LGBTQ2S+ event, a summarising response may be 'I've listened to what you've said; you are opposed to us supporting this event because it may affect our own staff morale.' Summarising provides opportunities to clarify individual's positions, establish a common and respectful vocabulary for discussion, and provide a springboard for higher and more impactful forms of communication.
- *Reflecting:* Reflecting represents a higher form of communication and involves the use of speaking, listening, and observing. Reflecting includes synopsising of factual content but then further extends this to include the receiver's observations of verbal and non-verbal cues and messages that have been sent. When reflecting, the receiver of communication demonstrates to the sender that they have been listened to and heard. The distinction between 'listening' and 'hearing' is important: when we hear another person, we are incorporating more than simple facts and details and are moving to the point where we explicitly acknowledge that there are emotions, beliefs, and opinions that are important and influencing what is being said. For example, in the situation described previously, where an individual expresses strong disagreement about an organisation's decision to support a local LGBTQ2S+ event, a reflecting statement may be 'okay, I hear that you are opposed to us supporting this event because it may affect our own staff morale. I'm not sure I understand why, but it's clear you have a strong feeling about this – can you tell me more?' By indicating that the leader has observed a 'strong feeling' and inviting the individual to 'tell me more', the leader is engaging in a more complex form of communication but one that may ultimately produce a more meaningful conversation and outcome.
- *Paraphrasing:* The next higher level of communication involves speaking, listening, observing, and understanding. Paraphrasing includes synopsising factual content, the receiver's observations of verbal and non-verbal cues and messages, as well as the receiver's interpretation of the hidden meaning behind all of this. Recognising that 'mixed messages' or misaligned verbal and non-verbal cues can be difficult to decipher, paraphrasing represents a higher form of communication where the receiver attempts to integrate multiple forms of communication and meaning, and provide an encapsulation of this back to the sender for confirmation and as a springboard for further discussion. When paraphrasing a conversation, leaders indicate that they have listened, heard, and understood (but not necessarily fully accept) what is being said. In the example of the situation of the LBGTQ2S+ event sponsorship, a paraphrasing response may be, 'I am getting the sense that your feeling of

discomfort in the organisation supporting this event isn't so much about what the rest of the staff is saying or believing, but more about your own beliefs and opinions. Can we discuss this further?' Paraphrasing of this sort attempts to be respectful of diverse (even offensive) opinions, avoids labelling or name-calling, attempts to keep conversations going rather than shutting them down by giving an order, and represents a genuine attempt at conversation and understanding rather than judgement.

- *Empathising:* The highest level of communication involves speaking, listening, observing, understanding, and acknowledging. Importantly, acknowledging does not necessarily mean simply accepting – in some cases it can mean respectfully disagreeing while still recognising that a person who holds a different opinion may change over time. Empathising includes synopsising of factual content, the receiver's observations of verbal and non-verbal cues/messages, interpretation of hidden meanings, and honest and respectful consideration. It can be a challenge empathising with another person, especially when the topic is something the leader finds offensive or personally difficult themselves. For example, in the situation described in the previous sections, most leaders would likely expect their staff to be supportive of all patients regardless of race, culture or sexual orientation. Empathising in this case can be difficult if an instinctive emotional response from the leader is to judge the person opposed to supporting the LGBTQ2S+ event as 'homophobic' or 'bigoted'. Labelling words such as these can interfere with conversation and lead to situations where leaders simply exert punishment power. In this situation, the exertion of punishment power may set the stage for further disagreement, conflict, and unhappiness in the long run. Instead, an empathising response might be 'I understand you have personal difficulty accepting our decision to support this event, and I'm sorry this decision is causing you such concern. I know how much you've contributed to our organisation, and I'm hoping you'll be able to contribute to this event. We all have gay and lesbian family, friends and coworkers, and our business has many loyal and great clients we want to support. This is important for our business but really important for me – I want us to have an organisation that includes everyone, where everyone feels comfortable to be themselves...including you. Let's both think about how we can make this happen and talk more?'

A leader who contents themselves with only summarising would never get to the level of connectivity represented by the empathising statement, and this represents a lost opportunity to demonstrate leadership. A leader who attempts to leap to an empathising statement without establishing a foundation of empathy in a relationship is unlikely to be successful. In between, reflecting and paraphrasing statements can provide a more incremental or gradual way of building towards empathy but will not have the same potential for successful outcomes.

Admittedly – this is difficult. 'Hard talk' is hard for a reason: situations such as this are awkward and difficult and, in many cases, even experienced leaders would prefer to simply avoid or ignore them to minimise the risk of conflict, aggravation or irritation. Of course, leadership means not wilfully overlooking situations simply because they are difficult. Gaining confidence in using empathising statements where they are appropriate and warranted is a skill that can be rehearsed and developed over time. Recognising that empathising works when there is a foundation built upon rapport and trust means leaders need to invest today in relationships with others so that when difficult conversations are needed tomorrow, there will be a greater likelihood of success.

Persuasive techniques

Beyond empathising, there are other techniques successful leaders can consider in helping to persuade individuals to do things they'd rather not do. These techniques are also most effective in the context of relationships built on rapport, trust, and empathy, but are specific options to consider when hard talk is needed.[5]

- *The foot-in-the-door:* This persuasion technique is used as a way to nudge individuals towards specific behaviours or actions when they express resistance. Rather than force individuals to do things they don't wish to do, a nudge of this sort can provide an incremental and face-saving way for leaders to create more positive conditions for change. The foot-in-the-door technique is based on the notion that a small, incremental behavioural change will – over time – lead to more change. While an individual may not be able or willing to agree to a large behavioural change right now, the foot-in-the-door gives them an opportunity to test drive or use 'baby steps' that can eventually support more wholesale change. In the example of the LGBTQ2S+ event described above, a foot-in-the-door technique may be to ask the resistant individual to support the event in a small but meaningful way: rather than 'march at the front of the parade', perhaps this individual could help with behind-the-scenes logistics to bring them into contact with others who are supportive of this event. Over time, seeing how positive the experience of being involved can be, the resistant individual may start to have a change of mind, or heart.
- *The door-in-the-face:* This technique of persuasion derives its impact in opposite ways to the foot-in-the-door. While the foot-in-the-door approach focuses on small, incremental, acceptable behavioural changes that may eventually lead to larger, more sustainable ones, the door-in-the-face begins with a request for an entirely unacceptable change, followed quickly by a request for something smaller and more acceptable. This works because of the tendency of individuals to want to find ways of avoiding being seen as someone who is negative or says 'no': by following up a large, unacceptable request with a smaller, more acceptable one, the likelihood of acceptance is greater than by simply starting with the small request in the first place. In the example of the LGBTQ2S+ event described above, a door-in-the-face approach might be to ask the individual to wear a t-shirt and march in a parade, but when the individual feels forced to say no to that, follow up by asking them to simply hand out pride t-shirts to others who will march in the parade. By providing a face-saving way for this individual to participate without being conspicuous, it may eventually lead to more positive changes in the future.
- *Low-balling:* This persuasive technique involves sequencing behavioural changes in a way that involves smaller more acceptable requests followed by larger more difficult requests. Rather than ask for everything at once, low-balling works on the principle that, having agreed to one part of a compound request, an individual is more likely to agree to the second part if it is asked in sequence, rather than asking for both at the same time. For example, asking a reluctant individual to hand out pride t-shirts at a pride parade may be a step too far for some people; however, asking an individual, 'would you at least be willing to hand out t-shirts?', gaining agreement to this request, then following it up with 'great, we'll be handing them out at the pride parade!' is more likely to result in acceptance of both propositions than asking 'would you be willing to hand out t-shirts at the pride parade?'

- *Ingratiation:* One of the most widely used persuasive techniques, ingratiation is a way of leveraging charismatic power to change behaviour. Ingratiation relies on an individual liking the person making a request and wanting to please them. When using ingratiation as a persuasive technique, it is often premised with a statement such as 'do me a favour?' as a way of suggesting a difficult behavioural choice can be more easily made if a person believes they will be liked. Ingratiation can be successfully used in the context of long-standing warm relationships between individuals, but it is often a high-risk strategy: if despite appealing to a person's desire to be liked, the request is refused, this may be interpreted as a personal failure rather than as a philosophical objection. Ingratiation as a leadership technique should be rarely and cautiously used, if at all: while it may appear easy and may yield some success, over time, repeated use of ingratiation is simply irritating and actually starts to diminish rather than build relationships.
- *Fear:* The use of punishment power (*see* Chapter 20) is a persuasive technique that can be leveraged in difficult situations. The use of threats as a way of encouraging individuals to behave in certain ways has been relied upon by some leaders in the past. For example, an impatient and imprudent leader may simply say, 'I don't care if you're homophobic or don't like gay people, that's not my concern. But you're an employee and unless you come to the parade, you won't have a job tomorrow.' Such a draconian approach may produce a short-term behavioural change, but in all likelihood will not be conducive to longer term relationships and behaviours. Fear, threats, intimidation, and direct orders may have some place in the leader's toolkit but should be very cautiously and judiciously used, with a clear understanding of the long-term consequences and costs associated with using them – even once. Fearing a leader's power or judgement does result in behavioural change – in the very short or immediate term only. Over time, leaders who rely upon this technique will find they are simply creating conditions where everyone else subverts their intentions, works around them, and this ultimately leads to dissatisfaction or open hostility.

The use of persuasive techniques such as these are important tools for leaders to consider and use appropriately, proportionately, and judiciously. Hard talk requires careful selection of words and approaches, particularly where behavioural change is a crucial element.

The limits of hard talk

It is, of course, unrealistic to expect that conversation and persuasion will always solve the difficult situations leaders must face. While it is tempting to believe empathy, trust, rapport, and relationships carefully built over time, will always yield positive results and outcomes, hard talk is hard precisely because it defies easy solutions. Still, effective leaders must invest sufficient time and energy into conversations and attempt to persuade others, leveraging and building relationships and using techniques, such as those discussed in this chapter, to the best of their ability.

There will, however, be circumstances where leadership requires more than simply hard talk, and where conversation and relationships prove ineffective at achieving desired outcomes. Some of the most difficult – but important – work of leadership is in recognising those situations where hard talk is insufficient. In the case described above, there may be situations where no amount of cajoling, persuasion or conversation may be effective in addressing strongly held beliefs of others. In such situations, leaders need to develop their own philosophy of action to ensure their behaviours align with their values, organisational expectations, and societal norms.

What should a leader, who has tried everything to persuade individuals to support their organisation's commitment to LGBTQ2S+ events and causes, do when faced with intractable resistance? The reality may be that at a certain point, leaders will have to shift from hard talk to hard action, and this can be a wrenching decision and process. Girding oneself for this can be difficult but it is part of leadership and requires clarity of mind, attentiveness to one's emotional state, and a principled, values-based approach that is consistent, coherent, and clear to everyone.

In a case such as this, ambivalence or inauthenticity of the leader's views and beliefs on the issue will be a significant problem. Half-hearted support for the LGBTQ2S+ community will be transparent to both opponents and advocates alike and will lead to ineffective leadership. Where persuasion and communication are no longer effective, then clear and principled action may be necessary to demonstrate alignment with the leader's values and the organisation's mission and vision. In some cases, this may require unpopular and controversial decisions, but it is important to recognise that doing nothing – or worse, reversing – will produce its own consequences and controversy. In such cases, leaders need to consider ways of supporting themselves through difficult situations. This can include assembling a team of advisors, finding coaches or mentors to help work through difficult conversations and decision making, and being very closely attuned to their own personal psychological state and health during difficult times. Leaders need to recognise that they are not islands, alone and apart from everyone else: like all human beings, leaders need their own supportive community in order to be effective leaders, especially when difficult decisions and situations occur. An infrastructure of support that includes family, friends, professional colleagues, health and mental health professionals and others is necessary for all leaders facing difficult situations. Having this infrastructure in place and knowing how to navigate it effectively before it is actually needed is most helpful: the time to build a supporting infrastructure for leadership is before it needs to be mobilised.

Summary

Difficult conversations and decisions are a part of leadership. While there is an art to effective conversation and persuasion, there are techniques and approaches that can be useful in supporting best possible outcomes in challenging situations. Most of these will rely upon pre-existing strong relationships based on trust, rapport, and empathy. Effective use of communication techniques such as paraphrasing and empathising are important for leaders to master and leverage frequently. Building expertise in the use of persuasive techniques can also be helpful in managing difficult conversations.

It is also important to anticipate there will be circumstances where even the best communication and strongest relationships are still insufficient at breaking impasses and producing positive outcomes. In such cases, leaders have choices: in some of these cases, compromises may be possible that can at least placate most individuals. In some cases, however, especially those involving strongly held beliefs, compromise may not be possible. In these cases, leaders need to consider their own values and principles, their organisation's mission and vision, and broader societal impacts. Developing a support team or infrastructure around the leader to help them manage such difficult situations is essential, and should include both personal, professional, and health/mental health related supports. While it is impossible to fully anticipate all possible kinds of difficult situations and conversations a leader may face, it is imperative to plan in advance, prepare for the worst, but aim for the best possible outcomes.

References

1. Shikaze D *et al*. Community pharmacists' attitudes, opinions, and beliefs about leadership in the profession: an exploratory study. *Can Pharm J* 2018; 151(5): 315–321. https://doi.org/10.1177/1715163518790984

2. Farrell M. Difficult conversations – leadership reflections. *J Library Administration* 2015; 55(4): 302–311. https://doi.org/10.1080/01930826.2015.1038931

3. Prober C *et al*. Managing difficult conversations: an essential communication skill for all professionals and leaders. *Academic Medicine* 2022; 97(7): 973–976. https://doi.org/10.1097/acm.0000000000004692

4. Knight R. How to handle difficult conversations at work. *Harvard Business Review* [online] 2015. https://hbr.org/2015/01/how-to-handle-difficult-conversations-at-work

5. Austin Z. *Communication in Interprofessional Care: Theory and Applications*, 1st edn. Washington DC: American Pharmacists' Association, 2020.

CHAPTER 22

Leading change

Upon completion of this chapter you should be able to:

- understand why change and change resistance is inevitable
- recognise subversive behaviour
- explain how change leadership can be enhanced
- outline how to lead change in pharmacy.

It is sometimes said that the real work of leaders is to drag people kicking and screaming into a future they can't imagine and don't particularly want. Change leadership is an integral part of any leader's role; while there are circumstances where maintaining the status quo may be the path of least resistance and the most popular option, the reality, of course, is that technological, societal, and scientific evolution have a direct influence on the day to day lives of individuals and daily practice of professionals.

Change is difficult, particularly for those who feel rewarded by and comfortable with the way things are currently done. Change is also inevitable: the rapidity with which innovations become part of everyday life is a testimony to not only human ingenuity, but to the unavoidable reality that leaders, managers, workers, and citizens must accept. From a change leadership perspective, the objective is not to deny change or to force it on unwilling people, but instead to create an environment where change is expected and embraced rather than resisted and feared.

Why are change and change resistance inevitable?

One of the most frequent questions leaders are asked may be 'why do we have to change?'. The sense that 'if it's not broken, why do we need to fix it?' is a natural human response to situations where we feel we will lose confidence, control, and mastery over our environment. Resistance to change is – for most individuals – not only a natural state but it may also be a protective one.[1] Resistance to change represents support for continuity, for current conditions, and an endorsement of previous decisions and practices. Some measure of resistance to change is also healthy, forcing proponents of change to actively and clearly articulate their rationale and proposals. Labelling those who are change resistant as 'dinosaurs', or other forms of name-calling, does little to address the fundamental reasons why leaders need to anticipate and embrace change resistance.

Change resistance is usually rooted in strong, primordial emotions such as fear and anger.[2] These foundational emotions have, in some situations, a strong, protective influence, shielding individuals from potential harm and alerting them to possible danger. As primordial emotions, they are notoriously resistant to logic: trying to use reason and sense to argue against fear and anger is rarely successful on its own. Responding to change resistance with further emotional escalation – for example, a tit-for-tat fear and anger retaliation – will generally only escalate problems and further harden positions and feelings.[3]

Recognising that both change and change resistance are unavoidable realities that can be managed, is important for leaders.[4] Responding to change resistance with strong emotions is as unproductive as responding to it with only logic and reasoning. Change resistance may not always be overt, articulate, and clear; instead, it often appears in the form of foot-dragging, petty sabotage, or 'quiet quitting' (inertia). Understanding the psychology of change resistance can provide leaders with potential insights into how to better manage it, and move forward balancing both emotional and rational elements. Key drivers of change resistance include:[5,6]

- *Loss of control:* Over time, most individuals become comfortable with their roles, responsibilities and organisational territory. The sense of control over even a very small or limited scope of work provides important psychological comfort, including a sense of mastery and a feeling of autonomy. Fearing loss of control is one of the most important drivers of change resistance because it feels psychologically threatening. Loss of control connects to loss of autonomy, which in turn leads to questions of identity, purpose, and self-worth. By anticipating this issue, leaders can consider techniques to provide individuals with a greater sense of control over the change process itself, for example, by providing them with options (rather than a single pathway) for change or integrating people into planning processes earlier rather than later.
- *Uncertainty:* While no one can predict the future, the need for stability and certainty in professional life is a commonly held value. The expression, 'better the devil you know than the one you don't know' highlights the belief that, no matter how bad the status quo may be, at least people know it, and understand how to work within and around it. Uncertainty triggers fear because it disrupts the carefully calibrated understanding of predictability, stability, and certainty. Human beings will often prefer to remain stuck in miserable but predictable situations rather than risk an unknown but potentially better future. Uncertainty tolerance is likely connected to emotional intelligence; recalling that most pharmacists are Assimilators, and that Assimilators have amongst the strongest needs for predictability, leaders need to accept this reality and consider ways of managing uncertainty. One technique that can be helpful is to consider smaller, incremental changes rather than 'big bang' dramatic ones. Giving individuals time to learn to cope with uncertainty and opportunities to learn that the anxiety of small changes can be overcome, can help set the stage for more productive change dynamics in the future.
- *Shock:* In situations where leaders do not communicate clearly, consistently, and transparently, change can come as a surprise or shock, further amplifying strong emotional responses like fear and anger. When individuals have little or no time to prepare themselves for change – to imagine how their lives will evolve and how they will cope/adapt – this lays the foundation for change resistance. Effective change leaders should avoid this by being as open and transparent in the change process as possible: planting seeds early and keeping people informed along the way can reduce the impact of shock and surprise, which in turn can lessen the intensity of fear and anger associated with change.
- *Shame:* One of the often overlooked causes for change resistance is the issue of shame. The belief that 'we are changing because what I did in the past wasn't good enough' triggers strong

emotional feelings of defensiveness and anger. Those responsible for and who benefited from the previous way of doing things, may feel unfairly maligned or blamed as change occurs and this builds resistance. Change leadership must find ways of helping those associated with the past and current ways of doing things feel honoured and appreciated even though things will evolve. Allowing those from the 'old guard' to maintain prestige, honour, and dignity and not experience shame or derision is essential; it makes it easier for everyone to let go of the past and embrace the future.

- *Self-confidence:* Rapid change of any sort triggers fear of competence drift: the concern that individuals may not be able to learn new technologies, adapt to new processes, or keep up with new trends. Where change implementation is too quick, individuals may experience stress and exhaustion in simply learning how new systems operate. Leaders need to anticipate a learning curve for any kind of change process and provide abundant support for education, training, mentorship, coaching, and supports during the process. Where possible, overlapping periods where different systems run simultaneously to provide individuals with sufficient time to learn and rehearse, can be helpful.

- *Knock-on effects:* Organisational change can be difficult because organisations are complex entities with many different co-dependencies and relationships. Change in one part of an organisation or with one team will undoubtedly produce unintended consequences or knock-on effects in other areas, which can amplify change resistance. Leaders need to think broadly and engage multiple stakeholders in change processes to ensure that what seems like a small, local, and delimited change does not cascade into problems across an organisation.

- *It's work:* Ultimately, change resistance is a universal phenomenon because it requires people to do more work and invest more of their scarce and precious cognitive and emotional resources, often at a time and in a way that may be inconvenient or difficult. Leaders need to avoid mindless cheerleading about the benefits of change and instead recognise that change requires work and commitment: where possible, allocating additional and sufficient resources to minimise the amount of individual additional work required can be helpful and a strong positive signal to those affected by the change. Where additional resources are not possible, adjustments to workplace expectations and reductions in workload can also be helpful. Failure to admit, acknowledge, and actually deal with the fact that change will inevitably mean more work for individuals, will likely heighten change resistance.

Understanding subversion

Subversion describes the deliberate undermining of power and authority of a leader, system or institution, and is one of the most commonly encountered forms of change resistance. Subversion is a process used to resist change that generally carries less risk, cost, or difficulty than outright disagreement or belligerence. Subversion is sometimes referred to as 'passive aggressive' behaviour because it is a form of disagreement that is often communicated through very nuanced, indirect language and subtle forms of behaviour. The key to understanding subversion is to recognise that it is usually a tool that is used by individuals who have perceived they have little or no power to actually express and have their views heard or acknowledged, and who simultaneously are afraid that if they were to be honest with their views, punishment would follow. The objective of subversion is often to indirectly undermine authority without being obvious and therefore subject to formal discipline.

Subversive behaviour in organisations can sometimes be difficult to pinpoint or detect – and that is exactly why it is so frequently used. Fear of punishment limits what overt actions or words can be used, so subversion manifests itself in quieter ways, including:[7]

- *Gossip and innuendo:* A frequently used tool of subversion is to spread vaguely believable but factually inaccurate claims about individuals, as a way of reducing their authority and undermining their claims to leadership. Frequently, demographic characteristics may be the root of this innuendo – as a result, individuals such as women, members of racialised minority groups (Black, Asian, Minority Ethnic (BAME) or Black, Indigenous, or People of Colour (BIPOC)), those with minority sexual orientations, etc. are at highest risk of this form of subversion. The objective of the subverter is to actually reduce the social standing and diminish the status of the individual as a way of resisting change.
- *Information hoarding:* An often overlooked subversive behaviour associated with change resistance, is unwillingness to transparently share information with others (including leaders). Hoarding of information and unwillingness to share openly makes informed decision making difficult and creates a negative workplace environment. It usually occurs in the context of fear of loss of control and can be difficult to detect and manage effectively. Where individual team members have particular control over important components of a process, or unique skills not generally seen across a team, information hoarding may be more commonplace. Leaders should ensure there is sufficient redundancy of knowledge and skills across an organisation, to reduce the likelihood a single individual can have a stranglehold on information or processes that can threaten a change process.
- *Taking it out on others:* Where individuals feel powerless or afraid to directly address leaders, they may be tempted to exert their own more limited power on those they have more control over, including their own subordinates. Presenting one face to leaders and another face to those in lower power positions is a common subversive technique that provides individuals with some sense of control and autonomy, but also helps them manage the potential shame associated with change.
- *Quiet quitting:* In some cases, individuals who resist change feel they do not have an option to resign or quit. Their strong emotional response to potential change may lead to a systematic pattern of underperformance in which they are physically present at work but motivationally absent and disinterested. So-called quiet quitting means organisations are not benefiting from peak or optimal performance, and individuals become 'deadwood'. Also termed 'psychological presenteeism', quiet quitting is a frustrating but common subversive behaviour, since the individual is doing enough to avoid outright discipline or performance management, but clearly is capable of doing more. There is often a tendency for leaders to be frustrated but simply ignore quiet quitting subversion for fear of triggering or escalating conflict, and instead simply work around the quiet quitter as best as possible. Unfortunately, ignoring quiet quitting may inadvertently encourage other change resisters to follow suit. As a result, it is important to address undermotivation, disengagement, and similar behaviours, most often through respectful, empathic discussion and dialogue in ways that are designed to find mutually acceptable compromises that will advance the change process.

- *Sycophancy:* An intriguing form of subversion is counterintuitive – the use of charm and flattery in a manipulative manner. Sycophancy refers to the deliberate use of obsequious behaviour as a way to gain advantage. In a change resistant individual, sycophancy can sometimes be an effective way of avoiding certain elements of change by coddling favouritism with the leader. This, of course, can build resentment and hostility from others. Sycophancy as a change resistance strategy can be particularly effective where leaders themselves feel uncertain and vulnerable, or if the leader has a strong need to be liked by others. Often, sycophancy will not be identified or detected by the leader; those around the leader (including peers of the sycophant) are often better placed to identify and call out this behaviour. Resisting the ego flattery associated with sycophancy can be difficult but is essential to ensure this form of subversion does not amplify.
- *Avoidance:* The most common form of subversion is simple avoidance, for example, by absenteeism, making excuses for missing meetings or deadlines, and simply not showing up... but always with a reason and a smile. Avoidance as subversion relies on the perception that leaders are unwilling to risk confrontation or expend time and energy dealing with behaviour that is not hostile or aggressive, and the avoider will simply be ignored. Of course, avoidance is an infectious disease: if the avoider succeeds in resisting change through this behaviour it will encourage others to pursue a similar strategy. Further, where avoidance is successful, it breeds resentment amongst others due to the perception of unfair treatment. Leaders need to avoid the temptation to simply overlook avoidance: it needs to be managed proportionately and directly to send a signal that it is neither acceptable nor a successful tactic to use.

Subversion of change initiatives is an all too common phenomenon faced by leaders. Relying on personal charisma, charm, or leadership title alone will not prevent subversion from occurring and derailing change leadership efforts. Recognising common forms of subversion and addressing them in a timely fashion is important and should be supported by an understanding of the psychological reasons behind change resistance.

How can change leadership be enhanced?

Across virtually all sectors, change leadership has emerged as a major issue and an important skill. A variety of different theories and models have emerged to guide leaders in advancing change within organisations. One of the best known and most widely used change leadership models was developed by John Kotter who researched and described eight steps for leading change:[8]

- Step 1: *Create a sense of urgency*
  Motivating, inspiring, and creating an environment where all stakeholders understand and accept the pressing need for change is an important leadership task. Where stakeholders believe the status quo is sufficient, or where they believe 'if it ain't broke, why fix it?', change resistance will be amplified. A sense of urgency is often created due to impending threats from competitors, environmental events that affect a business or organisation (for example, a change in government or shifts in remuneration policies), or societal transitions (for example, the COVID-19 pandemic). Leaders need to harness the events in their environment to create

and transmit a sense of need and urgency, to motivate, build momentum and create conditions that will support positive attitudes towards change.

- Step 2: *Build a guiding coalition*
  Savvy leaders recognise that change leadership is a team sport: leaders by themselves have limited influence and success in overcoming change resistance and actually producing positive outcomes. Instead, leaders recognise that a carefully selected team or network of allies – a guiding coalition – is needed. This coalition should represent different stakeholder groups and interests and be representative of the diversity of the workforce and those affected by the change. Limiting the guiding coalition to other leaders is a mistake: this form of top-down change leadership is rarely successful as it generally only encourages subversion rather than engagement with the change process.

- Step 3: *Form a strategic vision*
  Strategic planning is crucial to change leadership. Change cannot be simply dictated from above, it needs to be part of an overarching process that connects to a vision, mission, goals and objectives. Leaders need to clearly explain how the future will be different – and better – than the past as a result of the change, as a way to generate buy-in and commitment from others. Beyond simply an aspirational vision, clarity around how that vision will be operationalised is also important to enhance confidence that this is more than simply lofty rhetoric.

- Step 4: *Enlist and mobilise*
  True change can only occur and be sustained when the vast majority of individuals actually accept, embrace, and rally around it. Individuals must want the change initiative to succeed for it to actually work; where indifference, apathy, or negativity exist in large numbers, change is unlikely to be successful or sustainable. The first three steps of this change leadership process speak to the importance of creating an environment and psychological conditions conducive to having individuals actually connect with, and engage with, the change process itself. In step 4, leaders must undertake active work to enlist and mobilise as many – ideally all – stakeholders to their cause. This is most often done in the context of strong pre-existing relationships with individuals, at all levels, that are built upon effective communication, rapport, trust, and empathy.

- Step 5: *Enable action by removing barriers*
  In many cases, one of the most impactful roles of a leader is to remove the obstacles that slow down progress, create roadblocks, or prevent change from occurring. Examples of these obstacles/barriers could include arcane policies and procedures from a different era, or bureaucratic requirements that demotivate or produce inefficiencies. Rather than first focusing on making change within existing environmental constraints, change leadership involves identifying and removing the barriers that prevented evolution and change in the first place. By removing these barriers, it creates conditions for the enlisted and mobilised stakeholders to quickly innovate and effectively work across silos, generate impact, and ultimately see the results of investing their psychological energy in productive/positive ways aligned with the strategic vision for change.

- Step 6: *Generate short-term wins*
  The expression 'pick low-hanging fruit first', describes a change leadership technique that recognises the positive psychological effects of early success in implementing change. Where individual's and stakeholder's first experience with change involves difficulty or failure, they

may sour on the whole change enterprise; change leadership requires leaders to carefully select and orchestrate conditions to support short-term success and early wins as a way of building momentum and trust. Individuals are likely to be more persistent, energetic, and tenacious in the face of obstacles if those obstacles occur later in the change process.

- Step 7: *Sustain momentum and acceleration*
  Change leadership recognises that change is a process, not an event. It does not happen at a single moment in time but involves ongoing investment and dedication. Short-term wins can be helpful, but over time, mindful techniques to sustain enthusiasm and energy are needed to overcome the inevitable exhaustion that occurs with change. Change is work – hard work. Sustaining momentum typically involves celebrating and recognising accomplishments, rewarding success, and finding ways of supporting and mitigating the worst elements of failures. Perseverance and grit are necessary in change, and this must be modelled in change leadership.
- Step 8: *Institutionalise change*
  Sustainability over the long-term is an important expectation of change leadership; time, energy, and resources dedicated to change should have long-term impacts and 'staying power', and this means ensuring that change is not simply focused on some individuals (who may leave an organisation) or some processes (which might become outdated with the next software update), but instead are entrenched in the culture of the organisation. Institutionalising change has both a leadership and a managerial element to it: for example, adapting policies, procedures, and reward schemes to align with the change may be a manager's responsibility but will require leadership and close monitoring.

The Kotter change leadership model is one of many approaches to consider; it has been used in a variety of pharmacy and health care settings as well as in private sector organisations. While others may vary in the specifics, most change leadership models emphasise similar facets, including finding ways of generating psychological energy and positivity amongst stakeholders, recognising that top-down imposed change is rarely successful, and focusing on the sustainability of change in the long-term. The value of any change leadership model is the step-wise approach to the complex psychological, organisational, administrative, and practical elements of change. Systematic and mindful approaches to the connections between these elements is essential for success.

Leading change in pharmacy

Most of the leadership literature focused on change has been researched and written outside the context of pharmacy and the health care workforce. While many leadership change issues will be similar regardless of the workplace context, the unique concerns and needs of the pharmacy workforce has highlighted the value of a bespoke change leadership model that recognises the unique stressors, emotional intelligence, and workplace pattern of pharmacists. In customising a change leadership model for the pharmacy profession, it is hoped that leaders will have a more specific set of tools to support, manage, and lead change within a profession that is often resistant to it.

The '9Ps of practice change' model was researched and developed based on interviews with community pharmacists in Canada.[9] Of course, the focus on one subset of the profession (community pharmacy) in one country (Canada) may limit its applicability broadly, but it still represents a unique pharmacy-specific perspective on how best to mobilise change and motivate pharmacists. At the core of this model is the recognition that the emotional intelligence of most pharmacists (Assimilator) introduces important opportunities for change leadership that more generic change models may not consider fully.

The 9Ps model highlights the value of a methodical, systematic, and proceduralised approach to change leadership that is particularly resonant for Assimilators. While some leaders may decry the 'spoon feeding' implicit in this stepwise approach, it is worth considering its potential value in leading change. Similar to Kotter's model, each of the steps in the 9Ps has specific objectives and focused tactics to enhance the likelihood of successful implementation. Figure 1 illustrates the process.

- Step 1: *Permission*
  Pharmacists are generally highly conscientious, rule bound, and are resistant to risk or activities that go beyond generally allowable or expected actions. Particularly in the context of practice expansion involving new tasks historically undertaken by others (such as physicians), an important first step in leading change is to ensure and clearly communicate that appropriate permissions from others have been received. In some cases, this might require legislative or regulatory change (for example, to allow pharmacists to prescribe). In other cases, permission may be needed from other professionals to take over roles that were traditionally theirs. Pharmacists generally resist change if they feel or fear it is stepping on other's toes or would be regarded as outside their role: ensuring that pharmacists know and accept that they have permission to change (not just from the leader but from the involved stakeholders) is an important first step in leading change.

- Step 2: *Process pointers*
  As Assimilators, most pharmacists tend to be very detail oriented, and a major component of change resistance can relate to paralysis associated with understanding how the change itself is supposed to be enacted in the workplace. Process pointers or details regarding implementation of change are an important next step. While some leaders may feel that professionals like pharmacists should 'just be able to figure it out and do it', the reality is that most pharmacists will resist change unless step by step details regarding logistics and implementation are provided. This may seem to be more of a managerial rather than leadership task, but it points to the importance of leaders and managers working closely through a change process to support pharmacists' needs.

- Step 3: *Practice*
  Rehearsal in a safe, simulated setting prior to 'going live' with a change is an important way of addressing change resistance. Finding ways of allowing pharmacists to 'test drive' a major change in a way that doesn't actually involve real world consequences can help provide reassurance, boost self-confidence, and reduce the risk of change resistance. In many cases, techniques such as clinical simulation involving actors (rather than patients) can be a useful teaching tool to help support more positive opinions to change.

- Step 4: *Positive reinforcement*
  It is essential for leaders of pharmacists to recognise their perfectionist tendencies may sometimes be an overwhelming barrier to change. Most pharmacists have strong psychological needs for accuracy, safety, and risk avoidance; coupled with this is a strong need to be liked

and respected by others. One element of change resistance for pharmacists is the fear that a mistake will lead to individuals becoming angry with or disliking them. Throughout a change process, positive reinforcement, praise, and emotional support are important elements to leverage frequently to reduce change resistance and to enhance successful implementation.

- Step 5: *Personalised attention*
  One of the most overlooked but important elements of change leadership is the recognition that each individual must undertake change within a team, a large group, an organisation, and even a whole profession. There is a tendency (in the name of efficiency) for leaders to issue blanket statements and group messages that treat every member of a group or profession as the same. Leaders who find ways of providing personalised attention to individuals, as they are moving through a change process, will find this to be a very productive and helpful approach for reducing change resistance and enhancing confidence. Though it is time-consuming, interpersonally exhausting, and (in some ways) inefficient and cost-ineffective, in the longer term a focus on personalised attention throughout the change process will likely make that process smoother and more successful. Importantly, personalised attention need not come directly from leaders; managers, peers, or others can also provide the kind of personalised attention that is necessary. It will be up to the leader, however, to ensure this occurs and that resources and time are provided to allow for personalised attention in some way.

- Step 6: *Peer referencing*
  A powerful driver for overcoming change resistance has nothing to do with leaders and managers: it is the response of peers and colleagues that can enhance the likelihood of successful implementation. Importantly, peer referencing specifically does not involve leaders: the presence or direct hand of leadership in the process will diminish the authenticity of peer referencing and will be discounted by individuals, inadvertently increasing change resistance. Leaders need to develop nuanced approaches to showcasing change champions who are truly peers, without interfering with or engineering this process in an overt or obvious way.

- Step 7: *Physician acceptance*
  Research has highlighted a somewhat fraught relationship between many pharmacists and their physician colleagues. The need for physician approval and acceptance is of psychological importance to most pharmacists. Particularly in the context of a change initiative that involves scope of practice expansion or activities that impinge upon physicians' traditional roles, acceptance of this change by individual physicians appears to be particularly important. There may be less of a need for acceptance from other professionals (such as nurses), but this too should be considered. In this model, physician acceptance is different from permission: permission focuses on a more system wide, regulatory, or legislative level, while acceptance involves the actual individuals the pharmacist works with on a regular basis.

- Step 8: *Patients' expectations*
  An interesting insight from this research relates to the important roles patients have in helping pharmacists overcome change resistance. Where patients have faith in, and expectations of, pharmacists, these pharmacists are more likely to overcome internalised psychological barriers and generate faith in themselves to successfully implement change. Leaders who are able to mobilise patients as part of the change leadership process will find more successful outcomes, lessened resistance, and enhanced motivation of pharmacists to fully engage in the process.

- Step 9: *Professional identity*

  Perhaps the most important – and challenging – element of the 9Ps of practice change, is
  the need for leaders to directly address the issue of professional identity (*see* Chapter 4).
  A significant, internalised, psychological barrier to change for pharmacists is their understanding
  of their own professional selves: many pharmacists see themselves as helpers, followers of
  orders, and advisors, rather than as decision makers, responsibility-takers, and true colleagues/
  peers of physicians. Where professional identity is limited and narrow, change resistance will be
  heightened. Techniques for supporting a more expansive professional identity are challenging
  and time-consuming to implement, and there are limited examples of how leaders might
  accomplish this. Further research in this particular area is ongoing and needed to truly address
  change resistance. Recognising that professional identity can be a barrier to change is important:
  creative interventions by leaders to support expansion of professional identity will likely be
  individual and context specific and will continue to evolve.

Figure 1: *The 9Ps of the practice change model.*

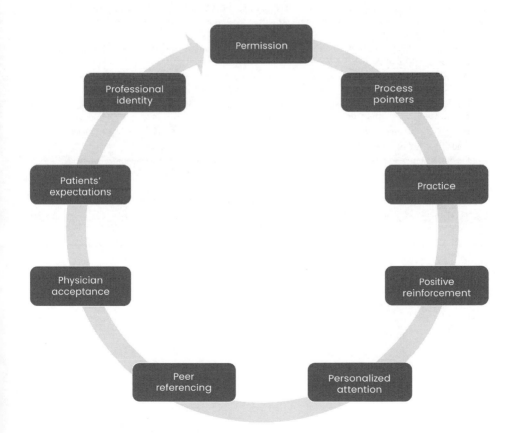

Summary

It is often said that the only constant is change, and this is particularly applicable to the profession of pharmacy. Change leadership is a critical element of any leader's role and will be a constant part of leadership. Leading change requires a sophisticated understanding of psychology, patience, energy, and dedicated time. One-size-fits-all generic change leadership models can provide some insights into the process, but more individualised, pharmacist-specific perspectives on change are more likely to lead to successful implementation.

References

1. Milella F *et al*. Change and innovation in healthcare: findings from the literature. *Clinicoecon Outcomes Res* 2021; 13: 395–408. https://doi.org/10.2147/CEOR.S301169

2. Nilsen P *et al*. Characteristics of successful changes in healthcare organizations. *BMC Health Services Research* 2020; 20: 147. https://doi.org/10.1186/s12913-020-4999-8

3. Igoe K (2021). *Change Management: Why it's so important and so challenging in health care environments*. Boston: Harvard TH Chan School of Public Health. https://www.hsph.harvard.edu/ecpe/change-management-why-its-so-important-and-so-challenging-in-health-care-environments/

4. Bamford D, Daniel S. A case study of change management effectiveness within the NHS. *J Change Management* 2005; 5(4): 391–406. https://doi.org/10.1080/14697010500287360

5. Dopson S *et al*. Understanding change and innovation in healthcare settings: reconceptualizing the active role of context. *J Change Management* 2008; 8(3-4): 213–231. https://doi.org/10.1080/14697010802133577

6. Varkey P, Antonio K. Change management for effective quality improvement: a primer. *Am J Medical Quality* 2010; 25(4): 268–273. https://doi.org/10.1177/1062860610361625

7. Bloom P, White P. The moral work of subversion. *Human Relations* 2015; 69(1): 5–31. https://doi.org/10.1177/0018726715576041

8. Ramasamy R, Ramaswamy G. A critical analysis of John P. Kotter's change management framework. *Asian J Res Business Economics and Management* 2017; 7(7): 181–203. https://doi.org/10.5958/2249-7307.2017.00106.2

9. Gregory P *et al*. What does it take to change practice? Perspectives of pharmacists in Ontario. *Can Pharm J* 2018; 151(1): 43–50. https://doi.org/10.1177/1715163517742677

CHAPTER 23

Addressing misinformation, conspiracies and lies

Upon completion of this chapter you should be able to:

- define the term misinformation
- list the criteria individuals use to determine if information is true
- outline the influence of the internet on misinformation
- explain the role of leaders in handling misinformation.

The COVID-19 pandemic fundamentally changed our world. Not only were civilian populations subject to a global lockdown, the introduction of public health measures such as mask mandates, and the introduction of the largest and fastest mass vaccination campaign in history, but humans became aware of and had to manage an uncomfortable reality regarding the spread of misinformation, conspiracies, and lies. While these realities are part of the human condition, the ferocity and intensity of their spread during COVID-19 has arguably become the greatest political, social, and leadership challenge of the 21st century.[1]

The challenges associated with misinformation, conspiracies, and lies are significant. Some of the most impactful political events of the last decade have in part been successful due to the spreading of false claims, clashes between a science-accepting 'elite' and an expertise-sceptical 'public', and the ongoing polarisation in society in general. Psychologists distinguish between 'misinformation' (sometimes called 'fake news') and 'disinformation'.[2] Misinformation refers to claims that are factually incorrect and based on erroneous but genuinely believed perceptions, while disinformation is deliberate deception intended to mislead. The fundamental problem with both misinformation and disinformation, of course, is that once it is accepted as truth, it can be very difficult for individuals to change their views and correct their perceptions. Layered upon these are the problems of conspiracies and lies: conspiracies refer to systematic and false conceptions of reality and motivations of others, while lies are deliberate falsehoods disseminated to mislead.

For 21st century leaders, the challenges posed by misinformation, conspiracies, and lies are amongst the most difficult ones to manage, and amongst the leading reasons why so many individuals choose not to become leaders in the first place.[3] The tenacity of misinformation, and the ferocity of those defending disinformation, is particularly troubling: research highlights how leaders who are women, visible minorities, and members of the LGBTQ2S+ communities are particularly vulnerable to hostility and violence for simply daring to tell the truth.[4] Today, one of the most important jobs of leaders is to defend the truth, advocate for science, protect those who are vulnerable from abuse and assault, and find ways of decreasing polarisation that characterises modern workplaces and societies. Even in the best of all possible worlds – which is not the one we currently inhabit – this is not an easy task.

Understanding misinformation

For over 50 years, psychologists have studied misinformation and its effects on thinking, feeling, and behaviour. These studies have highlighted the complexity and interdependence of logic, emotion, and action, and helps to explain the tenacity of misinformation once it has been accepted, and the challenges leaders (including teachers, health care professionals, and politicians) face in trying to reverse it. Psychologists have highlighted five criteria that most individuals use when deciding whether 'facts' or information presented to them is true and should be believed (rather than ignored). These criteria are:[5]

- *Compatibility with other known or accepted information:* When new information is consistent and aligned with other beliefs, it is more likely that this new information will be incorporated into an individual's belief system. This so called 'doubling-down' phenomenon means that individuals tend to prioritise information that actually reinforces existing beliefs, instead of information that may challenge or threaten existing opinions. This 'confirmation bias' means that individuals will literally see things more clearly, hear things more precisely and pay greater attention to information in their environment that provides them with psychological reassurance, or comfort, that what they have known and believed all along is actually true. This is one reason why it can be so difficult to address long-standing prejudices and beliefs with data, facts, and science. Where this data conflicts with existing beliefs, less attention and cognitive energy will be dedicated to examining it, and this dilutes its importance and value in helping to change minds and hearts.
- *Credibility of the source of information:* Human history has been the story of clans, families, and small groups battling one another. To this day, the notion that those closest to us are the most trustworthy (as opposed to those with advanced degrees, professional qualifications, or other forms of expertise) continues. Misinformation spreads and is tenacious because most individuals place outsized importance on believing what they are told by close friends and family members, rather than on distant, impersonal, leaders and experts. Further, individuals from 'other' groups (e.g. experts who may be women, members of the BIPOC/BAME communities, or LGBTQ2S+ people) may be marginalised and dismissed because 'they aren't like us'. Where an individual trusts, believes, and has faith in the source of information, the likelihood of it being believed and internalised rises significantly – and where there is a credibility, trust or belief gap between the 'expert' and the individual, misinformation can be difficult to counter.
- *Who else believes this?:* Psychologists describe how beliefs are socially constructed and reinforced. All human beings are part of different social networks, and there is a strong need to align with and support one's networks. Beliefs that are part of a social network's norms are more readily accepted than those that are outside those norms. One of the most widely described examples of this is with respect to Republicans and Democrats in the United States. While in most countries, voting patterns may vary depending on electoral issues and

circumstances, in the United States the connection between self-identification and voting is very strong. If a person self-identifies as a Republican or Democrat, they tend to be more open to believing everything of that 'tribe' espouse without necessarily questioning it.

- *Internal consistency – as opposed to external validation:* In our increasingly complex societies and relationships, beliefs are reinforced through focus on internal consistency, not necessarily through examination of evidence for external validation. So long as the new information continues a tradition of beliefs and behaviours from the past, that information will be privileged and prioritised. For example, no reputable psychological association or group has described homosexuality as a 'mental illness' for the last 40 years, and the vast majority of the psychological professions recognise it to be nothing more than simple human variation akin to left-handedness or being a ginger-haired individual. Despite this belief rooted in scientific consensus, evidence, and understanding, a significant number of individuals still cling to outdated – but internally consistent – views of homosexuality rooted in 'threats to the family' or 'undermining society'. Wilful disregard of actual scientific thought and evidence is required to maintain an internally coherent – but fundamentally flawed – belief system.
- *Searching for the 'right' evidence:* The final criteria for deciding whether news is true and ought to be believed involves a kind of intellectual gymnastics: contorting one's thinking to find the 'right' evidence to confirm beliefs and selectively ignoring all other forms of data and information, thereby providing a scientific veneer to one's beliefs. Selective searching for the 'right' evidence and ignoring all other information and facts is an active process requiring cognitive investment – and this in turn increases the stakes for individuals to actually find this 'right' evidence. Typically, this search for the 'right' evidence involves the weakest forms of evidence or science imaginable – anecdotes as opposed to data, or opinions as opposed to facts. Using a single case to generalise and thereby defend one's misinformed belief is common. For example, those who were opposed to COVID-19 vaccinations may point to relatively mild but frequently occurring vaccine induced side effects as 'proof' that all vaccines are unsafe and therefore should be avoided. Selective viewing and inappropriate prioritising/weighting of anecdotal evidence can give individuals false reassurance that their beliefs are correct.

Understanding how beliefs form and why misinformation is so tenacious is essential for leaders attempting to deal with this problem. As can be seen, the way human beings actually form their beliefs is part of the issue: the emphasis on anecdotes, local experience, and the need to confirm existing biases rather than challenge incorrect thinking, all make dealing with misinformation difficult, especially when leaders are not psychologically connected with individuals and do not have the benefit of the close relationship that can shape opinion.

Misinformation in the internet age

While psychologists have studied the spread and tenacity of misinformation for more than half a century, technological advances of the last 20 years have vastly expanded and accelerated the speed and extent of this problem in modern society. Since the 2016 Brexit vote in the UK and the American presidential election – when misinformation spread widely on social media platforms such as Facebook –

researchers have highlighted the new and unprecedented threats to truth and reality that have been unleashed in the internet age.[6]

At the core of the spread of misinformation are the various algorithms used by social media platforms – including Facebook, Twitter, TikTok, Google, etc. – designed to capture attention, lengthen the time individuals are engaged with the platform, and create a sense of virtual community online. These algorithms are designed to identify pre-existing preferences and interests, and direct users' attention to sites and topics that are aligned with and expand on that foundation of interest. Any internet user immediately recognises this process: one searches for something on Google, e.g. 'mango daiquiri recipes', then on Facebook an ad for the clothing store 'Mango' suddenly appears. The interconnectedness, seamlessness, and subtlety of these intersections are easily (and frequently) overlooked by users.

Whether this is a deliberate, calculated, and malicious use of computer algorithms by ubiquitous social media giants, continues to be a controversy and source of litigation around the world. Its impact on society, individuals, politics, and beliefs is, however, significant. This use of algorithms represents almost a perfect alignment with the criteria of how misinformation spreads and is consolidated. It creates an 'echo chamber' in which individual, isolated users of social media feel they have found a like-minded community online and therefore are more susceptible to believing what this (false) community believes. There is a selective presentation of confirming evidence rather than balanced representation of all sides of an issue with a focus on scientifically credible information. This echo chamber creates an internally consistent and coherent universe of belief which is at odds with the reality of a diverse, multicultural, and ever-evolving society. The isolating nature of social media means that those who are most lonely and vulnerable may be those who are most likely to succumb to misinformation since they do not have the benefit of a diverse 'live' community to challenge their thoughts and offer alternative perspectives.[7]

The Cambridge social decision-making lab in the UK has studied this phenomenon in detail and has described 'six degrees of manipulation' within social media that accelerate the spread of misinformation but also contribute to the growth of conspiracies and the propagation of lies and disinformation. These include:[8]

- *Impersonation:* From its earliest days, the internet has permitted anonymity for users, or at least made it very easy to hide one's real identity from the rest of the world. Initially this was heralded as a positive aspect – for example, communities of gay and lesbian individuals could 'meet' online in countries where homosexuality was illegal, without fear of being arrested and imprisoned. Today, impersonation means that no one can ever be certain of the actual person on the other end of our communication. Posing as 'experts', faking credentials, and even pretending to be family and friends, are all well-known tools of deception that are difficult to monitor and manage on social media.
- *Emotion:* Social media can allow for the expression of strong, negative, sometimes violent emotions in a way that would never be tolerated in the real world. Some of the most appalling thoughts, words, and beliefs can be shared online – because 'it's not real'. Some may argue that the amplification of emotion that occurs in social media is a necessary form of venting: rather than project it into the real world, it is safer in a virtual world. Most psychologists, however, believe the opposite: that emotional escalation, that has been prevalent on social media for a decade, means that what is acceptable in the real world has also changed – for the negative.[8] The

strong emotions expressed on social media paradoxically help build a certain kind of community and can produce connections between vulnerable or damaged individuals in unhelpful ways.

- *Discrediting:* One of the most significant challenges posed by social media is the ease with which discrediting or maligning the good reputation of another person can occur. A simple tweet, a random TikTok video or an email can trigger major reputational harm and perpetuate the spread of misinformation. For example, the mockery and vilification of Dr. Anthony Fauci (head of the American National Institute of Allergy and Infectious Disease during the COVID-19 pandemic) by tweet, Facebook, and other social media undermined his claims to expertise and caused significant harm in reducing public faith and understanding in science.

- *Trolling:* Unlike discrediting – which is focused on reputational harm – trolling is a malign action on social media aimed at triggering fear in individuals. Trolling behaviours include – for example – issuing anonymous threats of harm or physical violence online or publishing an individuals home address to incite protestors. The anonymity of the internet makes trolling a consequence free behaviour – for the troll – but an emotionally devastating experience for the victim. Fear of trolling will frequently lead experts and leaders to avoid statements or behaviours that are controversial, thereby lessening the impact of their expertise and leadership.

- *Polarisation:* The use of algorithms in social media has accelerated the trend towards polarisation – 'us' versus 'them' – in society, and created both a virtual and real world based on exclusion and demonising of those who are different or have different opinions. The ease with which individuals can 'find' others online who share their beliefs (no matter how extreme) provides a kind of social reinforcement and acceptability that did not exist in the past – which further amplifies these repugnant beliefs. Today, words like 'moderation', 'centrism', and 'compromise' are viewed by many as negative: a winner-takes-all attitude is emerging in which attempts to find middle-ground are dismissed as weak.

- *Conspiracies:* The rise of social media and its centrality in daily life today means that internally consistent and coherent worldviews are easier than ever to manufacture online – even if these worldviews are completely untethered from reality and ungrounded in fact. The Capitol Insurrection of January 6 2020 in Washington DC, following the legitimate election of Joe Biden as President, highlights the way in which social media can produce a (virtual) world of incredible power and unquestioned belief, leading average people to engage in the most abominable actions. While these individuals must, of course, take personal responsibility for their actions, the genesis of the thoughts that lead to these actions highlights the power and danger of social media. Conspiracies represent a packaged, internally coherent series of beliefs that attempt to explain a reality but are rooted in misinformation, disinformation, and lies. All of these are accelerated through social media in ways that can fundamentally threaten democracy and society as we have historically known it.

Despite growing awareness and discomfort with the ways in which social media perpetuates and accelerates the spread of misinformation, and some political action to control or at least provide some oversight to the proprietary algorithms that are the foundation of the social media business model, there has been very limited change in this area for the last decade. Arguably, the lockdowns of the COVID-19 era further isolated individuals and pushed them even deeper into social media, accelerating this trend.

Today, the internet continues to be one of the most important generators and perpetuators of misinformation – but also (perhaps) the best source of hope for addressing it. Attempts to educate young people on the dangers of the 'social media rabbit-hole' have expanded, as have certain safeguards around the application of algorithms. At the same time, however, dark-web materials have proliferated in ways never seen before. The ungovernable nature of the internet has historically been one of its most important features – if no one can govern it, no one can control it. However, this ungovernability also poses potential threats in terms of society's – and leaders' – inability to contain and control the threats and problems posed by it.

The infodemic – and how to deal with it

In September 2020, the World Health Organization, the United Nations, and a host of international organisations declared a global 'infodemic', arguing that misinformation and disinformation regarding COVID-19 was even more devastating than the virus itself.[9] During times of crisis and rapid change, individuals seek comfort from those they know and start sharing information to facilitate collective sense-making. While sometimes this can help us get through difficult times – in the case of COVID-19 it appears as though it had the opposite effect, perpetuating falsehoods, misinformation, and vilification of expertise. The consequences of the spread of misinformation, disinformation, and conspiracies was significant: witness the difference in COVID-19 related death rates between countries such as the United States and Canada, or between the United Kingdom and France.

The urgency of the pandemic and accompanying infodemic highlighted the importance of psychological research around countering misinformation. One of the more effective strategies that has been identified involves 'pre-bunking': inoculation against misinformation or fake news prior to actual exposure.[10] Like a vaccine, pre-bunking involves exposing individuals to small doses of misinformation as a way of helping them better understand how easy it can be to be mislead and end up in the world of disinformation, lies, and conspiracies.

Pre-bunking is best achieved by identifying and alerting individuals to specific pieces of misinformation that are false before they actually encounter it in the real world or online. Studies have highlighted the ways in which social media and online games can actually be powerful tools to support pre-bunking, teaching individuals how to differentiate real and fake news with respect to complex issues such as the European refugee crisis or climate change.

Another promising technique to address misinformation involves 'nudging'.[11] Regularly reminding individuals that they should not automatically believe everything they see and read online, can be enough of a small prod to help individuals engage in the kind of healthy scepticism and critical thinking necessary to provide some counterweight to misinformation. Importantly, the person delivering the nudge should not be an expert or anonymous leader, but instead someone who has credibility, personal connection with, and is part of the social network of the individual being nudged.

Media literacy has been proposed as an important technique for countering misinformation. Formal, systematic educational programs generally offered to teenagers in school have demonstrated some success in helping to prevent misinformation from succeeding; as a curricular intervention, it is complex and time-consuming and as a result may have limited applicability in other contexts – but it is an important tool to consider in battling the infodemic.

As scrutiny has increased on social media platforms and providers, they too have attempted to respond – albeit slowly. During the 2020 American presidential election, Twitter began flagging tweets that contained misinformation – a form of pre-bunking, and in December 2020, Facebook began removing posts with false claims regarding the COVID-19 vaccine. In one of the most breathtaking developments in corporate–social responsibility, multiple social media platforms suspended or banned former President Donald Trump for his role in inciting violence during the Capitol Insurrection. Arguably, social media platforms themselves have the greatest opportunity – and responsibility – to address the infodemic through more extensive moderation, controls over anonymity, swift punishment for trolling and discrediting, and more nuanced approaches to algorithm use. The simple fact that the former President of the United States was – and indeed had to be – banned from social media highlights the dimensions of this issue.

Leadership in an infodemic

Leaders have important responsibilities and opportunities surrounding misinformation and the infodemic, but it is within a context of the reality of the discrediting, trolling, and anonymity that is at the heart of social media and the internet age. Leaders need both authenticity and conviction to address misinformation and tackle the worst of disinformation and conspiracies. They also need to consider how best to apply the psychological research in this area to produce positive outcomes. Key considerations for leaders include:

- *The power of communication:* As described throughout this chapter, effective, empathic communication is the cornerstone of successful leadership. In the context of misinformation and lies, communication matters more than ever. It may be tempting to believe empathy should not be accorded to individuals with racist, homophobic, Islamaphobic, or sexist attitudes and behaviours, and that 'firmness' and 'strength' is the kind of leadership that should be communicated. While this is reasonable, the question of tone needs to also be considered. Effective leaders can use communication – and empathy – while still being clear, firm, and strong. Communication that belittles or denigrates those with opposing views simply adds fuel to fire and risks escalation. Worse, it may drive individuals further away from reality and towards their own echo chambers. While passive agreement to misinformation, or even tacit acceptance of lies should never be considered, respectful but firm disagreement is often appropriate. Leaders should seek to use communication that helps establish common ground: a foundation of some mutual acceptance and understanding rather than focus entirely on differences. Concepts such as pre-bunking (previously discussed in this chapter) can be particularly useful as a communication method for leaders. Clarity in messaging is essential: overly convoluted, jingoistic, and ever-changing messages frequently build mistrust in leaders (and likely contributed to the growing distrust of public health during the pandemic). Very careful consideration of clear, simple, powerful messages as a way to counter the clear, simple, and powerful lies of others, need to be crafted. One communication technique that can be helpful in this regard is curation: selective prioritisation of what messages are most important to convey in what sequence so as to minimise the risk of overburdening individuals. Curation requires leaders to work collaboratively with diverse teams to bring forth expertise, opinions, and consensus, but has the benefit of reducing cognitive and emotional burden on members of the public for whom curation can help reduce stress – and reduce the risk of succumbing to falsely simplistic misinformation or lies.

- *Tone:* One of the most important elements of communication for leaders to consider is the question of tone. Tone is difficult to precisely define, and involves a complex amalgam of word choice, vocal inflection, gestures and other non-verbal cues, and environmental context. Individuals most often react subconsciously – and disproportionately strongly – to tone rather than content, and in addressing misinformation and lies, tone is essential. Part of the success of misinformation spreaders is their breathless self-confidence in their own righteousness – a confidence that inspired confidence and belief in listeners. Their polarising tone is strangely effective for some in society, while powerfully off putting for others – and these individuals don't particularly care because they are not interested in social consensus in the first place. Countering this kind of hubristic tone is difficult: fighting fire with fire and reproducing that same hubristic tone makes leaders feel inauthentic and can sully their reputations, but 'playing by the rules' and maintaining respectful decorum, also runs the risk of looking weak and potentially being shouted down. Finding a balance that is unique and authentic to the individual leader is essential. Equally important is the necessity to avoid vapid, inspirational – but substance-free – messaging. A reassuring tone can be important in some leadership contexts but if it fails to recognise legitimate grievances and concerns of those susceptible to misinformation, it will be dismissed as 'elitist'.
- *The power of the network:* Relationships are integral to success at debunking misinformation: without a consistent foundation of empathy, respect, and trust, individuals will be less likely to believe a leader than someone else they know spreading misinformation. This introduces a major challenge for leaders: it may be mathematically impossible to create meaningful relationships with the numbers of individuals or groups needed to debunk misinformation, while those spreading misinformation need only establish relationships with a far fewer number of individuals. One of the ways in which misinformation amplifies is through network effects: friends of friends of friends who post on Facebook or tweet take on the mantle of believability and so super-spreading of misinformation is facilitated through a network. Those trying to counter the spread of misinformation have not yet identified ways of using networks in this way to pre-bunk or debunk misinformation, but it remains an important potential tool for leaders to consider. Finding ways of engaging a broader network to support truth and reality in the face of misinformation requires new models of communication and leadership, and willingness to cede control to others, but can be a powerful antidote to lies.
- *Clearly define lines in the sand – and stick with them:* Amongst the most important decisions leaders must make in the face of misinformation is to determine what can be ignored, what can be safely overlooked, and what must be addressed. Does the occasional sexist 'joke' merit intervention? Should a single employee refusing vaccination be terminated? Leaders need to carefully consider, deliberate, and build consensus across their teams and organisations to understand where the 'lines in the sand' exist – what are the specific actions and behaviours that will warrant clear, swift and consistent responses. Where leaders have not pre-defined these lines in the sand, they will likely be inconsistent and reactive, which produces its own problems

and diminishes trust amongst others. Where lines in the sand are too rigid and inflexible, this can produce fear which encourages subversion. Anticipating and defining these lines in the sand, both in advance and in a way that encourages by-in across a team and organisation, is critical – the support of others can help leaders endure the blowback when enforcement is required. One important element to consider is the role of 'super-spreaders' of misinformation, particularly in larger organisations. Research suggests that in social and occupational settings, a surprisingly few number of identifiable individuals are responsible for disproportionately large numbers of lies and spreading of misinformation. These 'super-spreaders' represent an interesting opportunity for leadership: finding ways of identifying and stopping super-spreaders can have positive effects across a workplace or a community. Swiftly addressing rumours and innuendo can help reduce the power super-spreaders have within their networks and can help isolate and reduce their influence over others.

- *Empower others:* While this chapter is written in the context of leadership to prevent the spread of misinformation, it is abundantly clear that leaders – no matter how powerful they may be – have surprisingly limited scope to address this complex issue. Successful leaders must mobilise, empower, and motivate others at all levels of an organisation or community, to work with them to address misinformation and lies. In part, this reflects the idea of the power of the network, but it goes beyond that: empowerment means engaging as many people as possible to think of themselves as leaders in the campaign to debunk misinformation. Such empowerment requires leaders to be inspirational, motivational, adopt a coaching mindset, and find ways of engaging the broadest group of individuals in co-equal ways to tackle these issues.

- *Use social media more effectively:* The acceleration of misinformation in the past decade has been connected to the proliferation of social media across the globe, and while platforms have been making small steps towards trying to control the worst abuses online, the reality is that super-spreaders and others will continue to find ways of manipulating web-based communication in new ways. Savvy leaders need to recognise that traditional methods of communication – lectures, newspaper articles, TV broadcasts, etc. – cannot compete with social media, and need to learn to use social media more effectively as a tool to counteract malign influences of misinformation. Many of the techniques that allow for the spread of online misinformation and lies could potentially be used to pre-bunk or inoculate individuals from the worst effects of super-spreaders. Many leaders may not have great personal experience or comfort with the effective use of social media platforms, but will need to rely on communications experts and others to support this effort. Finding and engaging in the very echo-chambers that perpetuate misinformation brings risks but is essential. Fighting the misinformation battle on the field of social media is an essential tactic for reducing its influence on others.

- *Lead with values:* Ultimately, leadership to address misinformation, conspiracy, and lies is rooted in genuine and deeply held convictions regarding the foundational principles of our society related to fairness, equity, respect for science and expertise and democratic values. In chaotic times such as these, where many individuals feel threatened, vulnerable, and confused, these foundational principles can sometimes be forgotten. Leaders need to be authentic in their expression of values, and consistent in their behaviours and actions. Genuine belief that – in the end – these enduring values will triumph needs to be the foundation of action.

It is tempting to wish that a list, such as the one just presented, can be a roadmap or checklist to address and prevent the spread of misinformation and lies. Of course, it is far more nuanced and complex than any list can encapsulate. The considerations presented above are merely a starting point, not an action plan. Each leader, each context, and each situation is different and will require different approaches. Importantly, spreaders of misinformation and lies are clever and will adapt rapidly to approaches taken by leaders to call them out: this is an ever-shifting target and leaders must be ready to invest the cognitive and emotional energy necessary to constantly address these issues, recognising it may literally never end. Still, the responsibilities – and opportunities – of a leader means that they must address some of the most divisive and pernicious aspects of modern life (including sexism, homophobia, racism, anti-vaxx sentiment, anti-science beliefs, etc.); this is empowering in its own way and can provide the psychological fuel leaders need to sustain this most important of good and noble battles.

Summary

Perhaps the most significant threat facing communities, workplaces, organisations, and societies today is the spread of misinformation, lies, and conspiracies. In many places, these fundamentally threaten the foundations of the world as we have known it to be. Leadership is absolutely necessary to counteract and debunk the kinds of pernicious, malicious, and devastating lies that can spread quickly, especially by social media. Wilful ignorance, wishful thinking, and studious avoidance are not options that should be considered. Though difficult and draining, the importance of leadership to address these issues cannot be overstated.

References

1. Stoller J. Reflections on leadership in the time of COVID-19. *BMJ Leader* 2020; 4(2): 77–79. https://doi.org/10.1136/leader-2020-000244

2. Petratos P. Misinformation, disinformation and fake news: cyber risks to business. *Business Horizons* 2021; 64(6): 763–774. https://doi.org/10.1016/j.bushor.2021.07.012

3. Shikaze D *et al.* Community pharmacists' attitudes, opinions, and beliefs about leadership in the profession: an exploratory study. *Can Pharm J* 2018; 151(5): 315–321. https://doi.org/10.1177/1715163518790984

4. Cheng J *et al.* Anyone can become a troll: causes of trolling behaviour in online discussions. *CSCW Conf Comput Support Coop Work* 2017; 2-3: 1217-1230. https://doi.org/10.1145/2998181.2998213

5. Adjin-Tettey T. Combatting fake news, disinformation, and misinformation: experimental evidence for media literacy education. *Cogent Arts Humanities* [online] 2022; 9(1): 2037229. https://doi.org/10.108023311983.2022.2037229

6. Marshall H, Drieschova A. Post-truth politics in the UK's Brexit referendum. *New Perspectives* 2018; 26(3): 89–106.

7. Allen J *et al.* Evaluating the fake news problem at the scale of the information ecosystem. *Science Advances* [online] 2020; 6(14): eaay339. https://doi.org/10.1126/sciadv.aay3539

8. van der Linden S. *Foolproof: Why misinformation infects our minds and how to build immunity.* New York: WW Norton, 2023.

9. Editorial. The COVID-19 infodemic. *The Lancet Infectious Diseases* 2020; 20(8): 875. https://doi.org/10.1016/S1473-3099(20)30565-X

10. Roozenbeek J *et al.* Prebunking interventions based on inoculation theory can reduce susceptibility to misinformation across cultures. *Harvard Kennedy School Misinformation Review* 2020; 1(2): 1–23. https://doi.org/10.37016/mr-2020-008.

11. Vlaev I *et al.* The theory and practice of nudging: changing health behaviors. *Public Administration Review* 2016; 76(4): 550–561. https://doi.org/10.1111/puar.12564

CHAPTER 24

Wicked problems – sustainability

Upon completion of this chapter you should be able to:

- understand the importance of leaders in pharmacy addressing climate breakdown
- outline the significance of the global climate and ecological emergency
- recognise the role of health care professions in climate breakdown
- explain how sustainability in pharmacy can be improved
- detail how leaders should approach wicked and super-wicked problems.

In a complex, sometimes frightening, world filled with potential problems and threats, it can be easy for leaders (and individuals) to feel overwhelmed by the magnitude and scale of issues. Beyond political instability, societal unrest, and economic precarity, one concern in particular has emerged as a dominant issue for leaders across all sectors: climate breakdown and environmental sustainability. Regardless of one's leadership title or role, understanding the dimensions of climate breakdown and identifying strategies to lead change across organisations to support sustainability related initiatives, is essential. Leadership in mobilising individuals, organisations, and resources to support sustainability is not simply a general case study of change management or misinformation, it is an existential threat that requires strategic thinking, bold commitments, and a type of leadership that is unique.

Why is leadership to address climate breakdown through pharmacy and health care so important? In part, it is because there are so many problems, so many options, so many possibilities, and no discernible way to identify shared priorities, find common ground, and actually start somewhere. In some ways, climate breakdown represents the perfect leadership problem that defies action or solution: too big, too impersonal, too beyond anyone's control – yet absolutely essential to address for all of us. The term 'wicked problem' is sometimes used to describe a leadership challenge that is difficult or impossible to actually solve because requirements are constantly changing, allegiances are frequently shifting, and information is constantly evolving.[1] It is 'wicked' because it defies a solution, not because it is evil. An alternative definition of a wicked problem is '...a problem whose social complexity means it has no determinable stopping point'; due to the complexity and interdependency of the problem (colloquially, 'too many moving parts'), solving one aspect of a wicked problem often creates other, unanticipated problems.[2] Other key elements of a wicked problem that makes them difficult for leaders includes:[1,2]

- *It is challenging to actually define the problem clearly:* 'Climate breakdown' is such a broad and all encompassing term, that it is almost difficult to explain what the problem that can be solved actually is.
- *There are rarely 'right answers' only 'least worst alternatives':* Even if carbon emissions dropped to zero today, the legacy of the 20th century means that aspects of climate breakdown are likely inevitable. Mobilising interest to change current behaviour when there is a certain element of futility involved, makes 'right answers' impossible.
- *The wicked problem itself is a symptom of other wicked problems:* Climate breakdown may accelerate future pandemics, trigger global hunger, and wreak havoc on political and social systems…. all of which are their own wicked problems. The connections and interdependencies are so complex and defy explanation, comprehension, and sometimes even imagination.
- *There is no endpoint:* Where simple problems have solutions, there is a way of knowing when we are finished. How can we know when we have solved climate breakdown? The reality is – never. There is no endpoint, no metric, and no clear way of defining when it is appropriate to stop.

Traditional change leadership models may struggle to support those interested in moving forward but lessons from these models are clearly applicable in this context. Roberts has identified three major approaches leaders can take to tackling wicked problems:[3]

- *Authoritative:* Taming wicked problems by allocating responsibility (and authority) to a few people or a single person is thought to help reduce complexity, eliminate competing views, and allow for swift action. The idea of a 'climate czar', with the tools and power necessary to make and swiftly enact bold decisions, is tempting as a way of circumventing inevitable discussion and debate. Of course, this approach is open to abuse and misuse and is fundamentally unrepresentative and undemocratic. Arguably, the wickedness of so many current problems (including climate breakdown) has primed citizens in many democracies to actually vote away their democratic privileges by selecting strong men who are dismissive of consultation and consensus. The illusion that authoritative leadership can 'solve' problems is a timeless issue and one that risks significant social consequences.
- *Competitive:* Solving wicked problems by pitting opposing perspectives and determining who the winner is, can be one approach. This approach forces each side to justify, defend, and promote their perspectives, and when fairly implemented, competition can actually produce better outcomes. It is inherently confrontational, can make compromise difficult, and the winner-take-all nature of it can be problematic. Competitive strategies to wicked problems may ultimately end up becoming authoritative after the winner is announced.
- *Collaborative:* This approach attempts to authentically engage as many stakeholders as possible to find consensus and compromise. It is strongly rooted in democratic ideals and emphasises the creation of transparent and open communication systems designed to build relationships and empathy, which support trustful resolution. Of course, collaborative approaches can easily become paralysed, the time required can be intolerable, and individual patience for hearing so many different viewpoints can lead people to lose interest. Current systems for managing climate breakdown include strong collaborative elements but the time required for this approach to produce positive outcomes means it may be too late to stop the worst effects from occurring.

While climate breakdown may be amongst the most significant and globally impactful wicked problems that leaders must address, it is by no means the only one. Other wicked problems of our time include income and wealth inequalities, racial justice, and pandemic/disaster preparedness. For this chapter, climate breakdown is presented as a sample wicked problem to consider ways leaders can approach it, and as a way of priming leaders for the many other wicked problems they will likely encounter.

What's the problem?

In September 2021, the Royal Pharmaceutical Society (RPS) formally recognised the scale and significance of the climate and ecological emergency facing the globe by publishing a climate declaration.[4] 'Pharmacy's role in climate action and sustainable healthcare' highlighted not only the dimensions of the issue but the central role health care (including pharmacy) has played in contributing to the problem. As noted in the report, '…climate change is the most significant health threat modern society has ever faced'.[4] The magnitude of this issue is truly alarming: modelling suggests that the last 50 years of health-related improvements in mortality, morbidity, longevity, and quality of life will be erased and reversed unless immediate action is taken to address the consequences of climate breakdown on clean air, safe drinking water, access to quality food, and secure shelter. There is risk of a vicious downward spiral: as climate breakdown accelerates in the years ahead, demands on health care services will increase.[4]

The Intergovernmental Panel of Climate Change (IPCC) has calculated that there must be a global limit of temperature rise to no more than 1.5°C in order to prevent catastrophic health-related deaths globally.[5] The nature of climate breakdown means that our historic patterns of the 20th century will only begin to exert their full effects in the 21st century, so even with controls to prevent any further pollution, climate breakdown will be inevitable. Still, it is essential we mitigate future risk by changing current patterns and reducing emissions to best manage future events.

Climate sensitive health risks are significant and include:

1. Direct injuries associated with extreme weather events (such as an increasing intensity and frequency of hurricanes and floods).
2. Heat related illness due to shifting climate patterns, especially in regions without infrastructure to manage this appropriately.
3. Respiratory illnesses such as asthma and chronic obstructive pulmonary disease, triggered by ever increasing particulate pollution.
4. Water-borne diseases and related health impacts, as access to safe potable water sources decrease.
5. Animal-borne illnesses or zoonoses, such as swine and bird flu – and the risk of future pandemics brought about by propagation of new and unknown pathogens.
6. Vector-borne illnesses transmitted by mosquitos and other insects, such as the spread of lyme disease to the reaches of North America.
7. Changes in the pattern of agriculture leading to food shortages and starvation as formerly arable land becomes untillable.

These, and other risks, in turn feed into social problems such as political polarisation, significant increases in mental health issues, and psycho-social problems across society. Despite overwhelming evidence to the contrary, some politicians and others continue to reject scientific consensus, so it is important for leaders and health care professionals to unequivocally and clearly affirm that climate breakdown negatively affects human health in myriad ways. The brunt of climate breakdown is being disproportionately experienced in those most vulnerable. The elderly, those living in low-lying areas prone to flooding or wild temperature swings, and those with socio-economic and educational disadvantages are more likely to directly experience the effects of climate sensitive health risks. Recently there has been interest in building health system and societal capacity and resilience to deal with climate breakdown – a subtle but important shift that suggests the time for actually preventing climate breakdown through carbon emission control may be passing.

As individual citizens, this data can be overwhelming and paralysing: the thought that something as big, global, and pervasive as the 'climate' can be breaking down, can sadly leave many individuals feeling nothing can be done, and the best approach is to simply look out for oneself and one's family and let everyone else fend for themselves. While understandable, this head-in-the-sand approach is actually unworkable: climate breakdown cannot be avoided by anyone (so long as they remain on the planet) and the interdependence of modern life means that collective action – and strong leadership – is needed.

Health care and climate breakdown

It has been noted that, if health care were a country, it would be the 4th biggest polluter in the world.[6] Health care provision itself is a significant cause of carbon production and pollution in ways that individual health care providers may not fully grasp. From a pharmacy perspective, medicines are amongst the most relied upon interventions in health care – yet pharmaceutical products have significant, often hidden impacts on climate breakdown. Three major sources of concern include the actual chemical and biological effects of active pharmaceutical agents, the extraordinary carbon footprint and risks of pollution associated with pharmaceutical manufacturing, storage and distribution, and the issue of safe disposal of pharmaceutical wastes. The need for a safe and sterile supply and distribution chain in pharmacy has historically led to measures that have significantly increased carbon footprint; for example, the safety and efficiency of a unit-dose (or unit-of-use medication distribution system) produces astonishing volumes of packaging that must be manufactured, transported, and disposed of...all of which contribute to carbon footprint and ecological waste. It is estimated that medicines alone account for approximately 25% of carbon emissions in most health care systems. This provides pharmacy leaders with unique responsibilities and opportunities to consider how best to mitigate, minimise, and manage these impacts on global climate.[4,6]

The RPS has identified four primary pathways by which pharmacy (as a profession) can support sustainability and positively contribute to mitigation of the worst impacts of climate breakdown: a) improving prescribing and medicines use; b) tackling medicines waste; c) preventing ill health; d) improving infrastructure and ways of working.[4] As they have noted, some of these pathways can be influenced directly and relatively quickly by individuals who work in mindful and informed ways, while others require organisations to enact new systems. At the macro level, some of these pathways require pharmacists to advocate vigorously in new ways and engage politically at the national and international levels to influence change. The RPS has also noted the pivotal role of leadership in advancing a sustainability agenda within pharmacy.[4] In this context, 'leadership' is not simply limited to those with specific titles or job descriptions: every single member of the pharmacy profession (including 'average' pharmacists and technicians) can and should imagine themselves as sustainability leaders. There is, however, also an important role for titled leaders to educate themselves, advocate relentlessly, plan and think strategically about how sustainability must be incorporated in all aspects of their work, and marshal resources that are necessary.

Sustainability in pharmacy

Improving prescribing and medicines use

Researchers have noted that the environmental impacts of research, development, manufacturing, storage and distribution of medicines have historically been overlooked or downplayed, with the veneer of 'life-saving drugs' used to justify unsustainable practices.[7] Most pharmacists are simply not aware that the medicines they dispense, on a routine basis, have an enormous carbon footprint that began decades before the medicine was ever even marketed. An important policy priority for the RPS is one that is entirely aligned with the profession of pharmacy's remit: to improve prescribing and medicines use but highlight the importance of significant data and awareness gaps that currently exist.

Environmental risks, costs, and consequences of medicines is not transparent or readily available to prescribers, dispensers, or patients. For example, the simple and common act of using certain kinds of inhalers for asthma contributes meaningfully to particulate pollution globally – and when used by millions of people in the world, this is part of the climate breakdown issue. Further, disposal of canisters containing certain kinds of propellants or plastic sheaths, contribute to climate breakdown in years to come. While individuals undoubtedly benefit immensely from access to high quality medicines, there are costs and consequences of this access that need to be more transparent to all – including patients – so environmentally informed choices can be made. Just as patients need to provide informed consent for the use of medicines, informed environmental awareness needs to be considered as part of 'appropriate' medicine use. Currently, this may be a challenge: there is insufficient and disaggregated data from pharmaceutical researchers, manufacturers, and wholesalers and so the actual environmental impacts of medicines are difficult to confidently quantify. Further research and the development of robust and trustworthy systems to monitor and report are necessary to allow prescribers, dispensers, and patients to make environmentally informed choices.

A key consideration is also the effective use of existing supports to ensure optimal medication use for all. While this has been a health consideration for many years, it is increasingly clear that many patients continue to be on medications that are only marginally beneficial, if at all. While the environmental consequence of this at the individual level may appear trivial, when it is replicated millions (or billions) of times globally, it is part of the reason why health care is such an important contributor to global pollution. Use of pharmacogenomic screening or other tools, in conjunction with active de-prescribing programs focused on ensuring patients receive only the exact amount of the correct and necessary medications required to manage their health care, is essential. A final area of importance relates to the use of medicines in veterinary and agricultural contexts. Many pharmacists may not recognise that most pharmaceutically active agents (such as antibiotics) are actually used in farming and livestock, not in human beings. The carbon footprint of this part of the medication chain needs to be further researched and more data available to permit environmentally responsible use in these contexts.

Pharmacy leaders (titled and untitled) can support sustainability action in this area by re-doubling efforts around person-centred care provision. Expanding the concept of 'informed consent' and education to include environmental awareness is important. A strong focus on de-prescribing practices, with an eye to switching from high-carbon to low-carbon products, fits within the pharmacist's role and scope of practice but requires leadership and dedication to implement widely. Hospital pharmacists and pharmacy leaders, in particular, have important roles to play in the context of inhalers and medical/anaesthetic gases. In the same way that pharmacists support effective resource utilisation by considering cost-effectiveness outcomes, incorporating environmental sustainability indices into formulary and prescribing considerations is essential.

Medical waste

One of the hallmarks of the pharmacy profession has historically been safety and integrity of the pharmaceutical supply chain – with particular emphasis on purity and sterility to prevent transmission of infection. This mandate has traditionally been interpreted as a rationale for introducing layers upon layers of protection (for example, the use of gloves and masks while preparing intravenous solutions, or the use of packaging so that human hands do not touch and contaminate pills being dispensed). The use of single-use products such as these in pharmacy has created an enormous industry in disposal of medical waste – and contributed significantly to the environmental sustainability problem of today.

This is an area of considerable debate and interest, and an opportunity for pharmacy leadership: how can the principles of stability, safety, integrity, and sterility be maintained without over-reliance on single-use (frequently plastic) products? While recycling initiatives have become more common in pharmacy, it is important to note that 'recycling' is the last and arguably least effective of the three R's: 'reducing' and 'reusing' have far more impact on the environment, yet pharmacy has not demonstrated sufficient leadership in identifying ways of reducing volumes of single-use plastics or identifying safe, effective and consumer-acceptable alternatives for re-use.

One area of particular importance in pharmacy is the paper-intensivity of current practices, related to record keeping and patient information. While considerable shifts towards electronic formats has occurred, there are certain legislative and consumer preferences that means pharmacy is not as 'paperless' as it could be – and as many other industries already are. In particular, the use of technologies such as QR codes on medicines packaging could be expanded further. Further work in confirming the source of electricity ('the grid') used to power electronic offices is essential: in some cases, polluting electricity generation (e.g. through coal or other fossil fuels) may actually be less environmentally friendly than using paper which can be recycled.

Another important area of focus relates to the safe disposal of medicines both by patients and pharmacies. There is only limited information regarding how frequently patients dispose of expired or unused medicines by flushing them down the toilet or tossing down a sink. Inconvenient medication returns systems sometimes drive patients to these behaviours, which have significant risks in terms of contamination of waterways and soil. Pharmacy leadership in this area needs to expand, as does concerted public education and awareness: rather than simply saying 'don't do this', actually explaining environmental consequences of improper disposal as part of patient education, can be useful to change behaviours. Another area for pharmacy leadership focuses on advocacy to mandate that pharmaceutical and medical product manufacturers make publicly available information regarding carbon footprints and environmental impacts of the research, development, manufacturing, distribution, storage, and procurement processes involved prior to dispensing to patients. Like labelling on food products outlining calorie counts, fat content, etc. of grocery store items, this kind of information can support more informed decision making to reduce environmental impacts.

There are many opportunities for pharmacy and pharmacists to improve management of medical and pharmaceutical waste. While everything is a priority, leadership in actually getting started with something is necessary to overcome paralysis that prevents action.

Preventing ill health

Given the issues of medical waste and inappropriate use of medicines, an important environmental stewardship activity for all health care professionals (including pharmacists) is to consider ways to actually reduce the need for medical interventions (including pharmaceuticals) in the first place, to keep citizens healthy and active. Preventing illness is both more sustainable and cost effective than treating it, yet the health care system has evolved in ways that make this difficult. Fortunately, there are ongoing developments – ranging from 'social prescribing' to public health awareness campaigns – designed to prevent small health problems escalating to larger ones which require more extensive (and unsustainable) kinds of interventions.

Exploring the social prescribing roles of pharmacists and technicians to keep populations healthy is relatively new. Particular emphasis on social care in conjunction with traditional medical interventions (e.g. vaccination and infection prevention) is especially showing promise. Leaders have unique opportunities to implement pilot projects, share findings, and mobilise resources to shift the pharmacy profession's remit away from a highly medically oriented form of problem-solving, to a more holistic philosophy of problem prevention.

In the for-profit community pharmacy sector, this will require a particular kind of bold leadership: existing policies clearly reward pharmacies for dispensing more medicines and performing more clinical interventions that are paid. New models for incentivising and rewarding practices that emphasise public health, social prescribing and disease prevention are relatively rare and not widely disseminated across the profession. Change leadership will be required to advance these kinds of initiatives in ways that will actually lead to broader uptake across the pharmacy profession.

Improving infrastructure

The final priority area in the RPS policy statement focuses on infrastructure, teamwork and systems. These are amongst the most impactful – but most logistically complex – areas in which to positively influence and drive sustainability practices. In part, the complexity relates to the scale of infrastructure changes that can be considered: this includes a greater reliance on virtual consultations, enhanced electronic medical/health record use, expansion of electronic prescription systems, and significant changes to purchasing and procurement decision making to emphasise sustainability in manufacturing and reward it in action. Other infrastructural elements include changing educational and continuing professional development processes to embed sustainability in both curriculum and program delivery.

At the heart of this is the recognition that there are significant unmet opportunities to enact climate favourable changes in health care delivery and systems through the use of digital/virtual/electronic tools. For example, expanded use of work-from-home options, virtual patient/caregiver consultations, and other existing practices refined during the COVID-19 pandemic, can be more broadly embraced in day to day practice. A system of building a culture of 'carbon literacy' in pharmacy personnel, other health care professionals, and patients is necessary so that climate consciousness in decision making becomes more commonplace.

Where to start with a wicked problem?

The RPS is one of several organisations in pharmacy that are raising awareness and initiating practices and policies aimed at sustainability. Within both the private and public sector, there is increasing awareness of the issue and resources are being mobilised to support climate conscious practice evolution. This will likely accelerate over time – as will climate breakdown and the consequences of decades of neglect of this issue.

The term 'super-wicked problem' was coined in 2007 and characterises the issues facing leaders interested in climate breakdown.[8] These super-wicked problems are ones that:

- have a significant time-pressure to finding and implementing a solution
- have no central authority with the job of actually finding and implementing solutions
- involve individuals and groups who simultaneously seek to solve the problem but are also the cause of it.

All of this may suggest that leaders interested in staying leaders should simply avoid climate breakdown and concentrate on things they can actually get done...and sadly, this is what some pharmacy leaders have elected to do, unaware of the reality that simply ignoring the problem won't solve it or leave individual leaders alone and unaffected by it. Understanding the nature of wicked and super-wicked problems, and the specific issues, dimensions, and opportunities of pharmacy practice to meaningfully lead improvement, leaders can consider certain approaches:

- *Staking a position as an environmental leader:* Boldly and authentically stating one's commitments to the environment and sustainability are essential. Not only is this inspirational, it introduces a level of accountability, and provides clarity that leaders accept not only the facts of the problem but personal responsibility to do something to address it. Leaders who ignore, avoid, trivialise, or minimise wicked problems risk being ignored themselves or disrespected by others. Worse, leaders who actually deny that wicked problems are even problems at all (for example, as certain climate breakdown denying politicians attempt to do), demonstrate lack of accountability and a mendacity that will ultimately undermine any claims to authority. The reality is that leaders cannot avoid or ignore a problem as large and impactful as climate breakdown – and denying its existence is even more counterproductive. It is actually in leaders' best interests to get ahead of the issue, stake a position, and be bold about it. Most people recognise that a wicked problem such as this defies simplistic solutions and will respect leaders' genuine attempts and authentic interest in the issue, even if 'perfect' solutions are not realistic.

- *Personal journey from the global to the local:* A key consideration for a wicked problem of the magnitude of climate breakdown is, of course, that the issue does not respect borders. In some circles, this leads some leaders to try to avoid responsibility by saying 'our country only produces 2% of global emissions so nothing we do, or sacrifice will matter anyway... so let's do nothing'. Wicked problems require both a macro-level understanding and micro-level actions: leaders themselves have to be able to recognise and accept that small changes under their direct sphere of influence may indeed be painful and may indeed be just a 'drop in the bucket' but for practical and inspirational reasons...every small step matters. Personal sacrifices and being part of the same journey as everyone else in abiding by changes is essential.

- *Environmental leadership is for everyone:* The scale and daunting complexity of climate breakdown means that titled leaders alone will have only limited impact and influence on outcomes, even if everyone around them follows their guidance and direction. A key insight for leaders is that wicked problems will only be addressed if titled leaders find ways of inspiring everyone and every level to think of themselves as leaders, and apply their own creativity, problem-solving, insights, experience, and commitments to the cause. Distributed rather than centralised leadership is essential for wicked problems, and creating space for everyone to think, act, and be recognised as a leader in some way, shape or form is essential.

- *Understand and commit:* Leaders have an essential responsibility to actually do their homework and truly comprehend the causes, consequences and dynamics of the wicked problem they are trying to address. In some cases, leaders can rely on others to digest and synthesise complex information, or to simply trust the guidance of advisors and follow it (as a leader) without question. The complexity of a wicked problem such as climate breakdown inverts this dynamic: leaders themselves need to invest the time necessary to understand the issues fully and then commit to sharing this understanding with others. Attempting to manage wicked problems by relying on second hand synthesis will often mean key issues are overlooked or underappreciated and this may reduce the leader's effectiveness in attempting to move forward in a positive way.

- *Recruit and network:* Wicked problems cannot be solved by sheer force of will, charisma, or by issuing orders to others. Social networks that mobilise mass populations are essential to moving forward with a problem such as climate breakdown. The leader's role is not to issue binding orders on others or to develop elaborate rewards and punishments to inflict on those who comply or do not comply. Instead, the leader needs to persuade large numbers of individuals, recruit them to the cause and help build and nurture networks that in turn can generate ideas, produce new leaders, and sustain the change effort effectively and authentically. It is a mistake for leaders to believe that centralised, top-down leadership can work with wicked problems: such problems are intractable, enduring, chronic, and ever-changing and no single individual (no matter how powerful they may think they are) can ever hope to address climate breakdown in isolation.

- *Measure:* Leaders need to be realistic in recognising that a wicked problem like climate breakdown is not going to be 'solved', or perhaps even 'managed'. Having staked one's name and integrity on an issue such as this may be important for accountability and inspiration, but for some leaders there may be nervousness regarding failure. If indeed a wicked problem is so intractable as to defy solution – why commit to it wholeheartedly and why engage with it knowing that ultimately failure will be the result? Some leaders attempt to reconcile this issue by making vague, generalised pronouncements of support then quickly moving forward without following up. Paradoxically, such leadership attempts to save face may have exactly the opposite outcome and reduce trust and belief in leadership. Instead, active, impartial, and transparent measurements of success with respect to goals and objectives is important. In the climate breakdown context, this is one reason why Conference of the Parties 2021 (or COP-21, in reference to the Paris Climate Change Conference to discuss the United Nations Framework Convention on Climate Change (UNFCCC)) has so many highly specific quantitative measurement goals. For example, the need to reduce global warming to between 1.5–2°C is a very specific, quantitative and (arguably) unrealistic goal...yet leaders need to promote it, measure it, and report on it to be taken seriously and to engage everyone in the process of trying to achieve it. Failure to set quantitative goals, measure them, and report them diminishes the likelihood of any improvement – and also diminishes the leader's credibility and trustworthiness as an authentic advocate of the cause.
- *Promote and make your own work sustainable after you:* Leaders recognise that wicked problems have no clear solution and that even improvement is a generations long activity that will outlive leaders themselves. As a result, leadership in the area of climate breakdown needs to recognise the importance of promoting others to assume leadership roles to make the effort itself multi-generational and sustainable beyond any individual leader.

Summary

Wicked and super-wicked problems – like climate breakdown – are defining moments and events for leaders and for society. The kinds of leadership that may be effective for other, short-term, or acute issues cannot work for the complex, multi-dimensional and frustrating insoluble problems of the world like climate breakdown, economic inequalities, and racial justice. The kind of leadership needed in situations such as these are rooted in understanding, relationship-building, persuasion, and distributed responsibility rather than centralised power and authority. Leaders themselves need to actively manage the reality that they will be leading – and therefore will be the 'face' of the problem to others – in an arena where failure to actually solve a problem is likely. Rather than avoid or ignore it, leaders need to find ways of authentically engaging with these big issues that plague our world and build trust, respect, and understanding with others as a way of making incremental improvements in meaningful and sustainable ways.

References

1. Ritchey T. Wicked problems: modelling social messes with morphological analysis. *Acta Morphologica Generalis* 2013; 2(1): 1–8.

2. Termeer C *et al*. A critical assessment of the wicked problem concept: relevance and usefulness for policy, science and practice. *Policy and Society* 2019; 38(2): 167–179. https://doi.org/10.1080/14494035.2019.1617971

3. Roberts N. Wicked problems and network approaches to resolution. *Int Public Management Review* 2000; 1(1): 1–20.

4. Royal Pharmaceutical Society (2022). *RPS Declaration of Climate and Ecological Emergency*. London: Royal Pharmaceutical Society. https://www.rpharms.com/about-us/sustainability/declaration

5. Watts N *et al*. The 2020 report of The Lancet Countdown on health and climate change: responding to converging crises. *Lancet* 2021; 397(10269): 129–170. https://doi.org/10.1016/S0140-6736(20)32290-X

6. Eckelman M *et al*. Health care pollution and public health damage in the United States: an update. *Health Affairs* 2020; 39(12): 2071–2079. https://doi.org/10.1377/hlthaff.2020.01247

7. Crespo-Gonzalez C *et al*. Sustainability of innovations in healthcare: a systematic review and conceptual framework for professional pharmacy services. *Res Social Admin Pharm* 2020; 16(10): 1331–1343. https://doi.org/10.1016/j.sapharm.2020.01.015

8. Lazarus R. Super wicked problems and climate change: restraining the present to liberate the future. *Cornell L Rev* 2009; 94: 1153–1234.

CHAPTER 25

Advocacy

Upon completion of this chapter you should be able to:

- define the term advocacy
- understand the impact of political advocacy in pharmacy and health care
- explain the terms legislation, regulation and policy and how they create change
- outline the key areas leaders should consider in political advocacy.

One of the more important activities leaders do involves advocacy to diverse constituencies and in different contexts. A common definition of advocacy involves generating public support for particular causes, recommendations or policies.[1] One example of advocacy involves politics and government: leaders may be required to convince politicians and bureaucrats of a specific idea or recommendation and work effectively to translate 'agreement' into political action – including changes to legislation or regulations. Another example of advocacy involves building public understanding or awareness: at the outset of the mass public vaccination campaign associated with COVID-19, pharmacists and other health care professionals had to advocate vigorously with different segments of the public to build consensus regarding safety and efficacy of vaccines – then translate that consensus into actual action involving individuals receiving the vaccine.

Advocacy is both a concrete action and a philosophy; it is equally a communication technique and a political tactic.[2] Effective advocates learn to balance evidence and story-telling, appealing to emotion and clear-eyed facts and figures.[3] The art of advocacy can be difficult to master, but the outcomes of successful advocacy can transform professions and societies. Importantly, advocacy is a skill that can be learned, and one that builds upon a foundation of each individual leader's own interests and strengths. It is usually least effective when approached in a cookie-cutter way as a checklist of tasks to be accomplished. It is often most successful when leaders find ways of infusing their own dedication and passion into an issue to present compelling cases for change.

Ultimately, advocacy requires leaders to be heard, capture the attention of busy and distracted stakeholders, generate interest in issues that may not be inherently interesting to others, and cut through the noise of other advocates trying to do exactly the same thing. Effective leaders find ways of leveraging their personal strengths, talents, and emotional intelligence in the service of advocacy for causes that are authentically relevant to themselves.

Understanding political advocacy

In the past decade, some of the most impactful changes in pharmacy and health care have been a direct result of successful advocacy work undertaken by dedicated leaders in these fields.[4]

The evolution of the scope of practice of pharmacists, the growth in the role of the regulated pharmacy technician, changes in pharmacy education to emphasise clinical skills development, and expansion of remuneration to pharmacists for clinical (rather than dispensing) work, all have occurred because of advocacy at various political levels.

At the root of understanding political advocacy is an understanding of how government works and how laws, regulations, and policies are made, enacted, and enforced. Importantly, political advocacy rarely works if it is solely based on shouting, emotions, or insistent demands. Equally, political advocacy is usually unsuccessful if it only deals in hard quantitative evidence with limited opportunity to tell real world stories.

Political advocacy recognises three distinct groups: the state, the bureaucracy, and the government. States are served by a continuous succession of governments, often (in a functioning democracy at least) representing different political parties and political perspectives (e.g. Conservatives versus Labour). In contrast, the bureaucracy is the group of civil servants that simultaneously serve the government of the day while controlling the mechanics of the state at a given time. The interests of the state are usually long-term and enduring: peace, order, efficiency and effectiveness are the general objectives that define a successful and functioning state. Today, in most democracies the State's interests are represented by enduring documents such as a constitution, and institutions such as courts which interpret the state's longer-term interests through the filter of constitutional principles. In contrast, governments may change relatively quickly, and may be more interested in short-term 'wins' even if this may, in the longer term, undermine the interests and objectives of the state. Governments – and the politicians that populate them – must face regular periodic election, the opprobrium of their constituents, and the intense scrutiny of the media; as a result, they tend to react and respond to short-term opportunities with a crisis-avoidant emphasis. The bureaucracy consists of long-term employees: civil servants who are required to abide by the wishes of the government of the day whilst still trying to safeguard the state's longer-term objectives and needs. The bureaucracy serves at the pleasure of the government, not the state, yet the bureaucracy gains its power due to the longevity of the state. There are many different political configurations in the democratic world today. For example, constitutional monarchies such as the United Kingdom invest the 'state' function in the monarch (i.e. King Charles III who serves as a figurehead representing continuity, tradition, and an appeal to loftier ideals of peace and order), the 'government' function is the political party that wins the most seats at election time (e.g. Conservatives, Labour, Liberal Democrat, etc.), and the 'bureaucracy' function with the civil service centred in Whitehall but distributed throughout the four nations. Constitutional monarchies in countries like Canada and Australia follow similar structures involving elected parliaments, hired and qualified civil servants, and appointment of a Governor–General to act as the King's representative of State. In contrast, republics (such as India or the United States) have elected Presidents and different structures of government involving, for example, in the United States, a Senate and a separate House of Representatives at both the national and state level. The republic system uses an elected head-of-state (as opposed to a monarch or appointed individual) and is therefore typically aligned with partisan politics. Arguably this produces a more political state and politicised bureaucracy.

This confusing picture of politics accounts, in part, for why it can be so frustrating and challenging for those trying to advocate for change requiring political input. While the distinction between state, bureaucracy and government may seem like a recipe for gridlock, indecision, and acrimony, these distinctions are essential to ensure that political change is measured, incremental, and manageable. It is essential for leaders to understand the specific characteristics of their own state, bureaucracy, and government. In order to advocate effectively, leaders need to understand and appreciate how these three different arms or branches of the political interact, intersect, reinforce one another, and are at odds with one another.

Understanding legislation, regulation, and policy

Many of the things that leaders advocate for at the political level involve development of new, or changes to existing, legislation, regulation, and policy. Over the past decade, some of the most important developments in the profession of pharmacy have included legislative initiatives to create new professions (such as the regulated pharmacy technician), regulatory changes that have enabled scope of practice evolution, and policy development to support different kinds of clinical services payments by the National Health Service (NHS). Each of these changes – which have directly influenced patient care and the day to day work of pharmacists – have only been possible due to tireless and successful advocacy efforts of pharmacy leaders.

Legislation describes the laws of a country or jurisdiction (like a state or province) that apply to and govern everyone equally. Legislation provides a description of legal expectations and requirements as well as punishments associated with violations. Legislation is the most overarching and therefore the most challenging kind of advocacy to engage with because it is so far reaching, so politicised, and so scrutinised by the public, the media, political parties and the general public. High-profile examples of legislation include recent laws in the United States that have criminalised the provision of abortion in some American states. What (in most democratic countries) had historically been considered a private matter between a woman and her physician was vaulted into the legislative arena in some states, and laws were passed prohibiting and criminalising this procedure. Prior to this change, decades long, highly polarised, and highly publicised media battles consumed much of the country's attention. In contrast, regulations are specified legally binding actions focused on specific administrative agencies (such as a health professions regulatory body like the General Pharmaceutical Council or the State Board of Pharmacy) that generally affect only those who deal directly with the agency enforcing the regulation (in this case, a pharmacist or pharmacy technician). Regulations are typically less sweeping and public, and therefore less politicised, than legislation, but can have significant impact. For example, in jurisdictions where pharmacists are allowed to prescribe medications independently, legislative change has usually been required first to permit a new scope of practice. Once legislation has been changed to allow for prescribing, then detailed regulations may be developed that focus on specific medication-related issues (i.e. are pharmacists allowed to prescribe all categories of medications or just certain limited ones, or if a new type of medication is introduced on the market, regulation can be amended without re-opening the original enabling legislation itself). Finally, policies describe the specifics of how legislation and regulation are to be implemented and are designed to support effective and efficient enactment.

The intersection of legislation, regulation, and policy with state, government and bureaucracy produces significant issues for advocacy, and requires leaders to have a sophisticated knowledge of both the processes involved and the personalities of different individuals involved. Purists would argue that government is interested in and controls legislation, bureaucrats control policy, and both negotiate around regulation, all under the watchful benevolent gaze of the state. In reality, of course, it is far more complicated, with elected politicians intervening at the policy level to make their point, bureaucrats tacitly and inappropriately exerting force or influencing naïve politicians at the legislative level and the state's role becoming progressively less and less clear, yet more and more legalistic and court-focused. In many countries, the democratic dysfunction that has become all too apparent in the early part of the 21st century, reflects this confusing, contradictory, and at times, self-defeating structure and intersections that can make advocacy for change difficult. Still, and despite these obstacles, leaders must find ways to effectively work through this chaos and find opportunities to address changes the profession and patients need.

How do policy, regulation, and legislation actually change?

The complex interplay between state, government, and bureaucracy means there is no simple and reliable roadmap that advocates can use to navigate and negotiate change. Democratic safeguards in most jurisdictions exist to prevent single individuals from having outsized influence on change processes, though in recent times these have been tested as never before. For example, in many cities there is a shift towards centralising power and authority in 'strong mayors' to deal with what is described as municipal gridlock or paralysis. In parliamentary systems such as Britain and Canada, power and decision making authority has been increasingly concentrated in the hands of Prime Ministers and a select number of high-level cabinet officials. In republics such as the United States or India, the role of the President has become amplified to (ironically) the point where some believe they have powers akin to royalty to enact change. Centralisation of decision making power in single individuals is, of course, the hallmark of dictatorships, not democracies, and while this trend towards centralisation has been accelerating in many jurisdictions, it is a mistake to believe it has actually fully succeeded (yet).

Traditionally, governments of the day have initiated changes using legislation and often in response to political advocacy, voter demands, or results of referenda. The legislative change initiated by government would then be handed over to bureaucrats who would develop regulatory and policy changes necessary to support uptake and implementation of new legislation. Legislation, regulation, and policy would then be overseen by the state, often through courts, administrative agencies (including regulatory bodies) or other similar bodies. More recently, this process has become less clear-cut. For example, bureaucrats are often involved in assessing the impacts of proposed legislative change prior to governments enacting them; in some cases, it is actually bureaucrats who push forward legislative change in response to identified needs. The role of the state and its agencies, such as courts and regulatory bodies, has also shifted; in the context of a profession such as pharmacy, it has often been regulatory bodies that have actually advocated politically to drive legislative change which ultimately, they would enact through regulation and policy developed by bureaucrats.

This blurry reality means that those advocating for change must consider the needs and interests of the state, the government, and the bureaucracy, and often this means tailoring or customising advocacy approaches to three distinct groups whilst maintaining clarity and consistency since these groups interact with one another. Political advocacy involving an elected government can only go so far if the bureaucracy and the state are uninvolved or opposed; similarly, attempting to enact change through the state (for example, a court battle involving litigation) may provide some measure of immediate victory but if it triggers resistance from government and the bureaucracy, sustainable and meaningful change may be difficult. This reality means there are many different approaches advocacy can take, and different priority audiences depending upon the specific issue at the heart of the advocacy effort. Thinking in terms of multiple intersecting audiences with different needs and interests, and finding ways of capturing interest, delivering focused messages, and advancing an agenda, is the real work of advocates for change.

Lessons for leaders in political advocacy

While there are many different fora and audiences for advocacy, political advocacy is arguably the most impactful given the control it has over legislation, regulation, and policy. Understanding the nuances and complexities of how government, bureaucracy, and the state intersect with one another, leaders need to approach advocacy work with both precision and flexibility. Key lessons to consider are detailed below.[5,6]

Be strategic

Advocacy is not an ad-hoc, on-the-fly activity involving glib talk and glad-handing. Recognising that the pharmacist advocate is a very small player in a large and complex ecosystem of moving parts, means that leaders need to be strategic in prioritising the topics for their advocacy and the way these will be presented. In the context of advocacy, being strategic means having a clear mission, vision, and goals that can be easily and clearly articulated to diverse audiences. These missions, visions, and goals need to be developed carefully, using a strategic planning process to ensure they are representative of the aspirations of the group/profession, and that they are framed in ways that resonate with different constituencies. Leaders who advocate for topics that are irrelevant to those they lead, or use language, concepts or framing that is not resonant will find it difficult to advance their cause. Before ever speaking to an elected official, a regulator, or a bureaucrat, systematic strategic planning is required that involves diverse constituencies within the profession, resulting in clearly articulated and prioritised missions, values, and goals aligned with professional and personal values.

Know your audience

As discussed previously, the diverse audiences of government, state, and the bureaucracy will want different things, have different questions, and respond to different triggers. Anticipating these differences means a one-size-fits-all approach to advocacy is seldom successful. Bureaucrats may be most interested in details, implementation, operational issues, costs, and potential risks to existing systems. In contrast, governments are often most sensitive to public opinion, voter impressions, and addressing the needs of their specific constituents (not necessarily the 'majority' of voters, but only that slice of the electorate that actually voted for them in the last election). The state is interested in precedent, procedural fairness, and the upholding of legal principles. When advocating for change, it is essential to understand how to explain the rationale, potential value, and impact of a proposed change to each of these different stakeholders in ways that resonate with them using language that is appropriate for their contexts. Simply presenting a great idea that makes good sense is rarely sufficient to move all three of these audiences. Attempting to use the same advocacy 'pitch' is equally unlikely to be successful since each audience has a different set of pressures they face. Perhaps most importantly, it is essential to prioritise and sequence audiences for advocacy: in some cases, it may be appropriate and most effective to begin advocacy work with the bureaucracy, to start to work through cumbersome logistics or implementation issues that politicians may cite as a reason to disagree with a proposed change. In other specific situations, it may be prudent to begin advocacy efforts directly with politicians, leveraging the interests and opinions of their voters to build their interest and attention: when politicians prioritise certain issues, they may be able to pull reluctant bureaucrats along with them, rather than the other way around. In some cases, advocates have found greater success appealing directly to the state, in order to overcome reluctant politicians and resistant bureaucrats. Compelling court cases can sometimes shift legal understanding of issues in ways that compel politicians and bureaucrats to act, even if they actually are opposed to a change.

Understand and leverage your powers

Advocacy is an art and a skill, and each individual person who acts as an advocate needs to understand themselves and the powers they leverage. Some advocates may enjoy certain privileges due to their professional designation, academic qualification, or status in the scientific community: those who rely on expertise as a tool for advocacy can convince others to move forward with change because of their authority in the field. In contrast, some advocates are effective because of their personal experiences and life history; for example, advocates for change who represent different patient groups are often extraordinarily sympathetic public figures who move voters – and this in turn can move politicians to act. One of the most challenging aspects of advocacy is when individuals represent personal or professional self-interests. For example, a pharmacist advocate who is trying to persuade others that pharmacists should be allowed to independently prescribe could easily be accused of simply wanting more money or status – unless that advocate can clearly make the case for why independent prescribing is in society's, patients' and even physicians' best interests. As part of a plan for advocacy, individual advocates need to carefully reflect upon their own powers and how these may be perceived by others. Where advocacy power is seen as being motivated by naked ambition or shameless self-interest, it will not be successful and alternative approaches should be considered – including considering changing the messenger and identifying alternative advocates for change without the same self-interest issues.

Be focused/targeted messaging/know what you want

Messaging is central to advocacy efforts. Complex, polarising, and uncomfortable issues are exactly the topics that governments, bureaucrats, and the state prefer to avoid, for fear of triggering dissension or hostility. Where advocacy work is focused on change, there is an implicit criticism that current practices are inadequate – and this in turn can feel like a criticism of those in power who oversee the current practices. Careful messaging that highlights the benefits of change without being insulting or denigrating to those with an investment in the status quo, is an essential element of targeted messaging. Coupled with this, is the need to ensure complex, multi-factor problems are explained clearly and concisely in ways that do not overwhelm or confuse diverse audiences. In essence, this means identifying and prioritising 'asks' carefully and pragmatically: incremental, step-by-step change is usually more palatable to politicians, bureaucrats, and courts than sweeping, radical, all-encompassing changes. Care must be taken by advocates to not descend into crass advertising or sloganeering – but the value of a clear, pithy, and memorable slogan to identify one's cause and one's ask is essential. In many cases, advocates work closely with marketing and advertising firms to help refine messages, tailor messages to specific audiences, and find ways of prioritising 'asks' in ways that are palatable to all parties.

Every word counts

Advocacy means paying very close attention to the choice and use of words, in all interpersonal and written communication. Improper word use can scupper attempts to persuade politicians, bureaucrats, and the public. A single misplaced word or poorly phrased sentence can undo months or years of careful relationship and trust building. One of the most significant challenges for advocates is recognising how every word –whether intended or accidental – shapes perceptions of not only the individual but the issue for which advocacy is being deployed. Use of strong or profane language, being overly dismissive of others, or peculiar word choices, raise questions as to the credibility of the individual – and by extension the value of the cause itself. This is particularly important in written communication including emails, media releases, letters to the editor, etc. Importantly, the words advocates choose and use need to be consistent across different formats and fora; the targeted focused messaging described above needs to be highly crafted and used in a disciplined and consistent manner. In the event of an issue – a misplaced word or unfortunate turn of phrase – immediate attention to 'damage control' is essential. Individuals who have difficulties maintaining self-discipline around word use and choice, who resist attempts to stay on point and use targeted messaging, and who have a tendency to speak off-the-cuff may not be the most effective advocates, or will need to be paired with other advocates who can smooth some of these rougher edges that could cause problems.

Reinforcement of messaging

It is important to recognise that decision and policy makers – including politicians, bureaucrats and even judges – have multiple issues jockeying for their time and attention. It is a mistake to assume that simply because an issue has been presented or discussed once, twice, or even three times, that it will be remembered and recalled. Advocates need to prepare themselves for the reality that gentle, respectful repetition of messaging is important and identify methods to engage in repetition without coming across as tedious. The key to successful reinforcement messaging is to ensure the content is consistent but the manner of delivery is subtly varied, in order to engage listeners when hearing the same message repeated. Clever use of non-verbal messaging (e.g. pictures or photographs) can also be a useful tool to consider to help reinforce verbal messaging. It is easy for advocates to become frustrated by the amount of repetition that is necessary to allow messages to eventually be heard and internalised, but if this frustration comes across in verbal or non-verbal ways, it can undermine attempts at building trust and relationships with decision makers. Pleasant, polite, but clear reinforcement of key messages, using different approaches while still maintaining consistency in the core content, is essential.

Mobilise others including media

The role of the media – including mass media (television, movies, radio), social media (Facebook, Twitter, LinkedIn) and targeted media (mail-outs, direct-to-voter solicitations) all have an important role in advocacy. In many cases, media relations will be an expertise that most pharmacist advocates will lack: fortunately, media training programs and expertise are available, and depending on the nature of the advocacy work, should be considered. Similarly, social influencers are adept at leveraging social and targeted media channels as a way of mobilising public and voter support for the advocate's cause. It is important for advocates to recognise that media mobilisation is a unique and professional expertise: simply being a Facebook user in one's personal life does not mean an individual is adept or qualified to mobilise media for advocacy purposes. Recognising that professional assistance in media mobilisation is necessary to build awareness around causes, most advocates will hire or partner with professional services firms with expertise and experience in this area. Learning how to speak with media is equally important – a television interview is different from a radio interview, and a 'hosted' interview (i.e. on a talk show) is different than an on-the-street interaction with a reporter. Media training requires advocates to constantly and mindfully self reflect on their verbal and non-verbal communication, particularly knowing that video clips will last forever and be played repeatedly online, and that filmed interviews focusing on an individuals head means that even the slightest non-verbal 'tell' will be projected immediately to an audience. The potential role of advocacy in media is enormous: arguably, sophisticated and principled use of media is one of the most powerful tools advocates have to persuade politicians, bureaucrats and perhaps even judges. The need to manage this power professionally, be professionally trained and ready, and leverage its potential fully is important and should not be undertaken in an amateurish manner.

Stories versus evidence

One of the most challenging issues for pharmacist advocates to reconcile is the differential weighting of stories versus evidence in political decision making. As scientifically trained health care professionals, pharmacists place a high premium on good quality evidence and rigorous data to drive decision making: this is the foundation for pharmacotherapy decision making at the root of the profession. Advocates are frequently startled by the way in which 'evidence' is perceived and treated by politicians, bureaucrats and even judges. For example, for a generation there has been strong evidence to support the impact pharmacists could have by being directly involved in prescribing decisions at the patient interface (rather than in the pharmacy once a prescription is already written). High quality studies have consistently demonstrated that pharmacist involvement in prescribing reduces errors, improves health outcomes, and saves money.... yet for decades, politicians and bureaucrats seemed indifferent to this evidence and were slow to respond to calls to increase pharmacists' scope of practice in line with the evidence. What finally motivated politicians and bureaucrats to pay attention to the evidence were stories from patients involving problems accessing primary care providers, delays in starting treatment, and frustration with government and bureaucrats for being indifferent to their plight. It is sometimes said that stories provide the spark that lights the fire for change: without stories of real people and the problems and suffering they endure, there can often be too many other priorities for politicians and policy makers to pay any attention to 'studies'. Once that fire is lit, however, high quality evidence can provide the fuel necessary to make change happen quickly. Once political and bureaucratic interest in solving primary care problems faced by an angry electorate was established, it was fortunate that pharmacist advocates had high quality evidence to help solve this problem by expanding pharmacists' scope of practice. Advocates who believe evidence alone should be sufficient to drive change will rarely be successful: similarly, those who rely only on stories will often find politicians agreeing with them but bureaucrats resisting change (for good reason). Learning how to manage both stories and evidence in a nuanced way that meets the needs of diverse audiences, is an essential skill for advocates.

Build relationships not transactions

At the core of advocacy work are advocates themselves: those who speak on behalf of a cause or initiative reflect the issue itself. As such, advocates invest considerable time in building relationships with key stakeholders in government, the bureaucracy and the state in order to understand their needs, interests, and concerns. Relationship building takes time, focused attention, and dedicated communication. It is not established after a single meeting or a few interactions. Relationships, however, build trust between individuals and trust is ultimately necessary for decision makers to believe in the same causes and ideas that advocates do. Advocacy work that is transactional in orientation and focused on getting something done immediately is rarely successful. No matter how compelling evidence or stories are, advocates themselves need to establish their trustworthiness and credibility as individuals who are speaking on behalf of others. Relationship building and nurturing is inherently interpersonal work, and some passionate advocates actually find this difficult and irritating to sustain over time. It is essential that someone on a team of advocates has the skills, propensities, time, and patience to dedicate to building relationships with diverse stakeholders in order to move change forward. In the context of government and politicians, it is essential to remember that governments come and go: voters elect and sometimes reject individual politicians and political parties, so over investing in specific political parties can backfire at election time. Building non-partisan relationships focused on issues and causes – not on personalities – is important to ensure that an election cycle does not disrupt an advocate's progress. Similarly, being overly focused on transactions or specific 'asks' does little to build trust or relationships and this can be problematic in the long run.

Solve other people's problems, not just yours

In most cases, advocates adopt this role because they have strong feelings and particular passions about a specific cause or issue. In most cases, they believe their idea will solve a problem. It is essential for advocates to reframe their thinking to ensure the problem being solved is not one of self-interest. For example, in the early days for advocacy around expanding the scope of practice for pharmacists, there was a tendency for advocates to say that pharmacists were 'underutilised', and not working to the fullest potential of their education to help patients. While this was (and is) undoubtedly true, that framing of the issue makes it sound like scope of practice expansion solves a problem for pharmacists feeling underappreciated. Frankly, government and bureaucrats don't care if pharmacists feel underappreciated – nor should they. This self-interested expression of a problem did little to gain interest in advancing ideas like pharmacists prescribing or administering vaccines. When the issue was reframed as one of solving the problem of access in primary care, then politicians and bureaucrats became interested: expanding scope of practice could help solve their problem instead. Careful attention to how problems are framed, and ensuring that advocates focus on other peoples' issues and not their own, is important for advancing causes and issues.

Be resilient

Advocacy work is not for those with thin skin or who fear rejection. Many advocates work for years, sometimes decades, before the fruits of their labour are realised. Advocates must endure disappointment, being dismissed, and sometimes being misled or lied to by others. All of this is part of the work of advocacy – maintaining positivity, optimism, and belief in one's cause despite the reality of what advocacy work involves. Resilience is essential. Most advocates cope by developing social networks and systems to help them absorb the many ups and downs of the process: a network of trusted friends and confidantes is essential to allow an advocate to blow-off steam, vent their frustration, and rehearse forbearance. Not everyone is well suited for this work, and resilience can be a reason why individuals hesitate to undertake advocacy work. Understanding oneself and establishing systems to help manage the inevitable disappointments associated with advocacy, is essential.

Compromise is not a dirty word

Political reality in the early 21st century has become quite dispiriting for many. A 'winner-takes-all' view of politics now prevails in which those who compromise on their objectives are seen as weak. Unfortunately, this current reality flies in the face of the experience of most advocates, who recognise that compromise is an essential part of advocacy work and that 'half a sandwich is still better than no sandwich'. Expecting that compromise will – eventually – be the outcome of advocacy work, helps advocates plan for and anticipate what compromises are acceptable and which ones are not. Compromise per se is often the best way forward, representing incremental improvement that allows broader reaches of society to get used to new practices or ideas. Of course in some situations, compromise may not be possible: 'compromise' in the context of racist, sexist, homophobic or discriminatory behaviour or policy is difficult to accept. In other cases, compromise, negotiation, and bargaining are all part of advocacy work and should be anticipated and expected.

Hold your coalition together

One of the realities of compromise, of course, is that it can make it difficult to continue to keep advocates and their supporters engaged and committed to a cause. One of the challenges for leaders in advocacy is recognising that compromise is a likely outcome, identifying least-worst options and acceptable alternatives, and finding ways of keeping a team or a group on-side and committed even though some will view compromise as failure. Holding a coalition together is usually facilitated by strong pre-existing relationships and trust amongst coalition members. Transparency and honesty in communication throughout a negotiation process can be helpful in preparing a coalition for the results of a compromise, though in some cases, such transparency can result in interference in the negotiation process itself. There are few easy or formulaic answers as to how one balances the reality of compromise with the necessity of holding a coalition together...but it is an essential part of the advocacy process itself.

Know yourself and actually believe what you are saying

Perhaps it is obvious...but in a surprisingly large number of situations, many advocates appear to be less committed to the cause they espouse than they would like others to believe. For example, there are questions as to whether some politicians who supported the Brexit movement in the UK did so simply to win votes and elections or because they actually truly and deeply believed in the cause itself. When advocates have selfish reasons for supporting a cause, that are unrelated to the cause itself, it is often transparent to others – including stakeholders. Knowing oneself and one's beliefs and advocating for those beliefs makes advocacy work not only more effective but ultimately more personally fulfilling. Inauthentic advocacy can be soul-crushing – and it is often unsuccessful. Ensuring you are not 'trapped' into advocating for causes you have no interest in – or worse, actually are opposed to – is essential.

Summary

Advocacy is one of the most important tools available to advance change, and leaders have unique responsibilities and opportunities in this area. Advocacy is not simply about a great idea or about high-quality evidence: it is a complex, interpersonal dynamic that relies upon a sophisticated understanding of government, the state, and bureaucracy, a wide variety of skills, and a dedicated team of committed individuals who understand it is a long game, not a short battle. When successful, advocacy has tremendous potential to transform and improve communities and societies. Mindful and intentional focus on the structure, function, and nature of effective advocacy can help support leaders in advancing change at the highest levels.

References

1. Boechler L *et al*. Advocacy in pharmacy: changing 'what is' into 'what should be'. *Can Pharm J* 2015; 148(3): 138–141. https://doi.org/10.1177/1715163515577693

2. McDonough R. Advocacy: an essential skill for all pharmacists. *Pharmacy Today* 2014; 20(3): 42. https://dx.doi.org/10.1016/S1042-0991(15)30953-1

3. Knoer S, Fox E. Advocacy as a professional obligation: practical applications. *Am J Health Syst Pharm* 2020; 77(5): 378–382. https://doi.org/10.1093/ajhp/zxz328

4. Apollonio D. Political advocacy in pharmacy: challenges and opportunities. *Integrated Pharmacy Research and Practice* 2014; 3: 89–95. https://doi.org/10.2147/IPRP.S47334

5. Murphy E *et al*. Three ways to advocate for the economic value of the pharmacist in health care. *J Am Pharm Assoc* [online] 2020; 60(6): e116–e124. https://doi.org/10.1016/j.japh.2020.08.006

6. Murphy E *et al*. Integration, perceptions, and implementation of legislative advocacy within US schools and colleges of pharmacy. *Am J Pharm Educ* 2022; 86(5): 8668. https://doi.org/10.5688/ajpe8668

CHAPTER 26

What kind of a leader are you – and do you want to be?

Upon completion of this chapter you should be able to:

- understand the challenges leadership in pharmacy is facing
- outline the challenges women face in becoming leaders
- recognise the challenges minority communities face in becoming leaders
- explain the model of leadership styles.

It is important to have self-awareness, self-reflection, and authenticity as a leader. Whether in the context of difficult conversations, understanding one's sources of power, or in work as an advocate, knowing oneself and behaving in ways that are consistent with that self realisation are essential to success as a leader.[1]

There is a strong emphasis on the interconnectedness of personality and leadership, as though the two are conjoined or the flip side of the same coin.[1,2] Attempts to reduce leadership training to a one-size-fits-all checklist of tasks and steps are usually unsuccessful and reflect an important reality that there is no formula for becoming and being successful as a leader. Most leadership training programs emphasise deep introspection, honest self-appraisal, and a psychological perspective on barriers and facilitators to leadership.[2]

Historically, this has not always been the case. As recently as the 1970s, there was a general belief that leadership was a function of one's characteristics, that only individuals with certain traits were 'born' to lead and everyone else was destined to follow. These characteristics frequently focused on demographic characteristics, so white, privileged, Christian, cis-gendered heterosexual men enjoyed certain advantages – but equally suffered from harsh expectations – regarding their preordained role as leaders. As massive social change evolved across many societies and awareness grew of systemic bias against the majority of the population, it became clear that old models of leadership built on a foundation of 'characteristics' were not workable. High-profile and impactful political, economic, and social leadership failures made many people question 'who should be a leader?', and this lead to an evaluation of the importance of character, rather than characteristics, in leadership.

Today, there is not only tolerance and acceptance of diversity in leadership but the recognition that it should be embraced by everyone. Awareness of multiple models and types of leaders, and that leadership is available and open to everyone regardless of their characteristics, has transformed modern society. It has also increased the complexity of leadership itself, triggered a psychological approach to leadership, and heightened the importance of honesty and authenticity as tools for successful leadership.[3] Today, there is a general belief that everyone should have the right, privilege and ability to lead, and that what is more important than characteristics or character is the context in which leadership is demonstrated.

'I'm not a leader'

One of the most important challenges facing the pharmacy profession today is a dispiritingly widespread belief (particularly amongst students) that they simply do not have the 'right stuff' to be a leader.[4] In some cases, this is phrased differently – 'I don't want the pressure', or 'I just want to have a simple and nice life'. In other cases, leadership is actually viewed suspiciously or negatively: 'all leaders are crooks', or 'what's the point anyway, they're just going to bring you down'. A central challenge for the profession – and for the pharmacists in this profession – is the recognition that a profession that cannot produce its own leaders is likely to fade from significance and not be around much longer.[5] This pervasive belief in the futility of leadership is not confined to pharmacy. Enoch Powell, a controversial 20th century British politician often remembered for incendiary rhetoric around immigration and multiculturalism in the United Kingdom, is credited with saying 'all political lives...end in failure', highlighting a growing sentiment that leadership is exhausting, soul-crushing, and ultimately pointless. Today, more than ever, many share this sentiment particularly in light of the abuse suffered by leaders across all fields.

At the core of this pessimism towards leadership, however, may actually be a lack of confidence and self-doubt. When individuals proclaim 'I'm not a leader', what are they actually saying? 'I don't want the pressure and stress', or 'I fear I am not going to be successful', or perhaps 'no one is ever successful so why bother?'. A central challenge then is to overcome internalised biases and misperceptions – including lack of self-confidence – that can self-handicap individuals, driving them to quit even before they start.

The pervasiveness of 'I'm not a leader' in pharmacy may be due, in part, to the diversity of the pharmacy profession itself. Amongst major health professions, pharmacy has a unique role in leading and embracing demographic change. Historically, in western democracies, pharmacy (like most professions) was the domain of straight white Christian men, those deemed to have suitable characteristics to be trusted by others in their communities to undertake important jobs. Uniquely, at a time when women and Jewish people were forbidden from becoming doctors, the pharmacy profession demonstrated openness to diversity. While pharmacy never officially lowered its barriers to entry for individuals with different characteristics, it nevertheless did not interfere in ways that were as obvious as the medical profession. In Canada, there is literature that highlights the unique, powerful, and impactful role that Roman Catholic nuns had on the profession of pharmacy and the health care system as a whole.[6] In the 1930s and 1940s, at a time when admission to professional education programs was still highly restricted for women, clever, dedicated, and hard-working women became pharmacists because this was deemed as 'acceptable' and 'tolerable' within their Catholic orders and society as a whole. These women worked in Catholic hospitals, built Catholic health care systems and values and – even though they didn't use the term – led the evolution of pharmacy in Canada away from dispensing and products and towards pharmaceutical care. By the 1960s and 1970s, some of the nuns became vice-presidents of Catholic hospitals, leading institutional reforms in a time that was more accepting of women in leadership roles.

Similarly, in the 1970s and 1980s, pharmacy was amongst the first professions to experience significant ethno-cultural diversification as large numbers of Asian and minority ethnic individuals enrolled in university programs and became part of the professional community. Pharmacy was amongst the first major professions to become 'majority minority' – where white, Christian males numerically were under-represented in the profession. Today, in many parts of the world, pharmacy as a profession leads the integration of LGBTQ2S+ individuals in health care work.[7]

The diversity of the pharmacy workforce is a significant asset – and is being accompanied by increasingly more diverse leadership within and across the profession. The lesson from this is the importance of representation in leadership: when young professionals see people like them in leadership roles, it helps them recognise that they too can be a leader. When young people see respected leaders with similar backgrounds, life stories, and experiences, it makes leadership seem more attainable.

This is not to say that the path towards leadership is straightforward or easy for anyone. Across diverse fields, studies suggest that women, Minority Ethnic, LGBTQ2S+ and other historically disadvantaged groups suffer greater criticism and hostility than white Christian men in similar roles[8] (though importantly, white Christian men must also endure significant criticism and hostility). Part of one's reflections around a future career involving leadership must consider personal and demographic realities and the way individuals will navigate them, rather than simply saying, 'I'm not a leader'.

Women in leadership

The story of Catholic nuns in Canada leading the evolution of the pharmacy profession reminds us of how important diversity in leadership actually can be. The caring ethos of these women infused their approach to their profession, anticipating broader changes in scope of practice in years to come. While it may appear oversimplistic to say 'men are like this and women are like that', there is some evidence to suggest that women in leadership roles may bring different perspectives, skills, and values than men...and in turn they must sometimes endure different kinds of resistance than men.

A key factor that is frequently highlighted is the different ways women may have of communicating, building teams, and interacting with others in leadership roles. Caution must be exercised to avoid the pitfalls of sweeping generalisations and stereotyped thinking that ALL men do X while ALL women do Y. However, there is sufficient data from different fields and contexts to suggest that female leaders do value conversation, interaction, cooperation and do leverage effective listening more frequently than similarly qualified men.[9] In contrast, many male leaders may have a view of leadership that is rooted in power and control, decisiveness, and competition.[9] While this may be more or less true for specific individuals, social expectations regarding male versus female styles of leadership do persist and do influence effectiveness of the leader, particularly in health care professions like pharmacy.[9]

A significant issue for women considering leadership continues to be systemic barriers related to family planning. Despite great strides in social understanding over the past decades, there is still significant asymmetry in individual households regarding male and female roles around child-rearing and other domestic responsibilities – the majority of which frequently falls to women. While some individual women may have support from a partner or family to pursue leadership aspirations without unduly sacrificing family dreams, others do not and must make hard choices regarding personal career ambitions. Further, systemic bias continues to exist in many jurisdictions. While some countries have broad and inclusive parental leave provisions that support either parent in taking time off (up to two years in some places) after the birth or adoption of a child, other jurisdictions have no legal protections and expect that mothers will return to work within 4–6 weeks after delivery. In some places, public subsidies for day care or universally accessible pre- or junior-kindergarten exist, allowing women to contemplate greater career leadership opportunities, while in other places, day care costs are prohibitive and force one parent (often the mother) to give up career growth for a period of time.

There is evidence across all professions – even health care – that a persistent pay and career potential gap exists between equally qualified men and women.[9] Exact causes are not known, but it is generally believed to be a combination of social factors, family issues, as well as the fact that women typically spend more time in caring interactions with individuals (like patients) which in many remuneration systems reduces income potential and career prospects, despite paradoxically improving patient outcomes. For these and other reasons, some women may decide, 'I'm not a leader', and forego exploration of their own leadership potential, viewing it as too difficult and not worth the effort. To address this issue, structured mentorship programs have demonstrated great effectiveness: women learning from other female leaders, sharing their self-doubts, learning from their experiences, and seeing how work-life balance can be reconciled, is a powerful way of showing younger women what might be possible. Structural changes to provide humane parental leave, support more accessible and affordable day care, and provide support for work-life balance to enable leadership aspirations, are evolving in large and small corporations and organisations.

In the past, there may have been a perception that for women to succeed as leaders, they had to think and behave like men – that is, shift away from relational to transactional ways of relating to others, focus on power and control, and favour competition over cooperation. While, of course, some women are naturally inclined to behave that way (and some men are naturally inclined to behave in the opposite way), the notion that 'women need to be more like men' to succeed needs to be challenged. Understanding one's strengths (as a man, woman, or non-binary identifying individual) is far more important than clinging to outdated behavioural stereotypes. Playing to strengths rather than focusing on deficiencies helps define successful leadership – and allows for honest self-appraisal of how to build a supportive team around a leader that mitigates issues that may arise.

Recently there has been significant public interest in the unique forms of resistance, hostility, and sometimes violence faced by women leaders in fields such as politics and journalism. Undeniably, there are certain forms of behaviours that target women specifically because they are leaders, and attempt to threaten or intimidate them through anonymous threats to themselves or family members. It takes extraordinary courage and a strong support network to endure such hostility – and it is a sad reality that this may occur. Women mentors can be extremely helpful in this regard as they have likely experienced and managed situations such as this. Structural supports (ranging from aggressive prosecution of criminal harassment and clear disciplinary action against individuals who target women leaders) are also evolving, though not quickly enough. Outright misogyny is an unfortunate reality women leaders may have to contend with in order to succeed. In addition, there are still lingering forms of less outright sexism that require calling out: despite decades of progress, in some fields, there may still be an 'old boys club' mentality or set of behaviours that has been driven underground and is out of plain sight, but still lurking and can still undermine women leaders. Building coalitions across organisations to ferret out these behaviours and swiftly addressing them should they actually emerge, is essential – and again a lesson that women mentors may be uniquely able to teach.

While the growing number of female politicians, judges, corporate leaders, professors, and entrepreneurs may make us think that sexism is dead and women are truly equal, the reality of course is that barriers still exist, differential harassment persists, and that women still have unique challenges in taking on leadership roles. This situation is improving, but not quickly enough. Building communities with like minded men and women who support and value women leaders, and finding mentors to inspire, can be effective ways of overcoming self-handicapping that may prevent smart, talented, and highly competent women from considering leadership roles.

BAME and BIPoC individuals

In Britain, the term 'BAME' is used to describe Black, Asian, and Minority Ethnic individuals; in North America the term 'BIPoC' is sometimes used to describe Black, Indigenous, and People of Colour; in Australia, the Australian Standard Classification of Cultural and Ethnic Groups (ASCCEG) may be used. In different jurisdictions, there are different ways of describing or discussing the unique issues faced by individuals who are not of the majority ethno-cultural group as they navigate life, careers, and systemic bias. While constitutional and legal protections have increased, and social awareness of historic inequities is growing, one's ethno-cultural heritage can sometimes serve as a barrier to considering leadership due to a variety of internalised personal reasons, and external systemic barriers.

The framing of one's ethno-cultural experience as an acronym such as BAME or BIPoC is inherently controversial, and reduces individuals to a demographic characteristic in a potentially unfair and unhelpful way. Though problematic, this framing permits the collection of data which could indicate there may be systemic reasons for the underrepresentation of certain groups in professions and in leadership roles. For example, in former British colonies such as Canada, Australia, and the United States, centuries of colonial practices have resulted in shocking disparities experienced by First Nations/Indigenous/Native American groups that persist to this day. In these same countries (and in the United Kingdom) members of visible minority groups and people of colour (who may or may not be recent immigrants) may also suffer disproportionately from social barriers and institutionalised racism. In the United States in particular, the historical experience and legacy of slavery continues to create racial divides that have led to the evolution of the Black Lives Matter movement.

Ethno-cultural and racial characteristics are realities that some may prefer to deny. It is tempting to believe we can all be 'colour blind' and – in the words of Martin Luther King – judge everyone not by the 'colour of their skin but by the content of their character'. The statistical under-representation of minority ethnic individuals in leadership roles across all sectors of society – including pharmacy and other professions – highlights the pervasiveness of colonial practices and systemic bias to this day. It also may produce an internalised response by some individuals that 'I'm not a leader...because I'm not white enough to fit in'. Particularly where ethno-cultural and racial characteristics are accompanied by certain behavioural norms (for example, around the consumption of alcohol, or clothing choices such as head-dresses), there may be a tendency to simply accept that others – but not me – are leaders.

As many scholars have highlighted, amongst the most pernicious and destructive legacies of the British empire globally has been the psychological privileging of whiteness at the expense of brown-ness and blackness.[10] To this day, in countries like India there is a social privilege that is placed on 'fair skinned' individuals of south Asian ancestry. In parts of Africa, skin-lightening products and hair straightening shampoos sell in astonishingly large quantities. In east Asian cultures such as Korea, large oval eyes are a sign of beauty and success. The internalised acceptance of 'whiteness' as better than everything is a distressing legacy that has long outlived the worst of the Empire.

Though challenging, it is an important journey for most individuals from these minority communities to reflect upon their internalised self-biases regarding privilege, status, and even what defines beauty, and to critically understand how their own perceptions of 'I'm not a leader' have emerged. The notion that one racial characteristic is 'better than' another, is intellectually repugnant and scientifically discredited...yet within some (perhaps many) individuals it persists at both a subconscious and conscious level and leads to self-handicapping. This is a difficult issue to overcome, one that is resistant to facile solutions like mentorship or diversity training, because it is so deeply engrained in the psyche of individuals and culture as a whole.

The success of many individuals who identify as members of racialised minority communities in countries like Britain, Canada, and the United States, highlights the reality that ethno-cultural and racial characteristics are not predictive of intelligence, success, or potential. Equally, the realities faced by many members of racialised minority groups indicate that system bias and discrimination continue to be a problem despite some advances. The fact that Barack Obama was once President of the United States does not mean discrimination no longer exists. There are no easy answers for individuals who have experienced discrimination personally – and for potential leaders who have internalised colonial and post-colonial messages that question their potential or value as leaders. Self-reflection, discussion, and community building are all helpful, but each individual will have their own struggle to overcome historical inequities and present realities. Hopefully, with time, inspiration, mentorship, self-reflection, and personal resilience, every individual will realise how much they have to contribute as a leader, and will do so in spite of an array of negative forces that may attempt to bring them down.

Members of the LGBTQ2S+ communities

In an era where television shows like 'Modern Family' and 'Will and Grace' exist, where corporate leaders at firms such as Apple and Qantas are openly and proudly gay, and when freedom to marry and live openly has never been greater in some countries, it is tempting to believe that the struggle for equality has been achieved. Indeed, the path from acknowledgement, tolerance, acceptance to fully embracing the lives of gay, lesbian, trans and queer people has been astonishing – and yet, there are still individuals who discriminate and systems that bias against these individuals in all parts of society. Unlike sex or racial identity, sexual orientations and gender identities may be more fluid, less overt, and more easily hidden, raising questions as to whether or not they are even real or matter with respect to career trajectory and leadership options.

It is essential to understand that orientations, preferences, and identities are integral to who we are as human beings. Who we love, how we live, and who we are and choose to be are as inherent to human existence as race and sex. Historically, there has been tremendous pressure for LGBTQ2S+ community members to 'hide' and 'stay in the closet' lest they bring unwanted attention to themselves and suffer reputational, psychological or physical harm. In the very recent past (and to this day), there are leaders who remain closeted, leading double lives or being desperately unhappy as a result. Fortunately, in most jurisdictions today, legislation exists to protect individuals from the most obvious forms of individual and system discrimination. This does not, however, cover the kinds of micro-aggressions that may cause some LGBTQ2S+ identifying people to think 'leadership is not for me'.

One key consideration for many is the notion that it is easier to stay hidden, out of the limelight, and to avoid stress and controversy if one opts to never take on a leadership role. The nature of leadership implies a kind of public profile and scrutiny that can be alarming to consider. While some people may feel comfortable being open and out with a carefully curated set of friends and colleagues, they fear they may lose control of this curated set if they assume a leadership role. Further, weaponising of sexual orientation or gender identity can undermine a leader's attempts to simply do a job well. Beyond name-calling and gossip/innuendo, there may be concerns that the charisma and inspiration that leaders are meant to instill may not resonate with a predominantly straight or intolerant group. In the corporate world, successful leaders who are open about their lives continue to be gay, white men – not racialised transgendered individuals. These gay white men often act and appear to be 'just like other leaders' even if they vigorously advocate for their communities.

Overcoming internalised homophobia and bias around what is possible if one is a member of the LGBTQ2S+ communities is amongst the first and most important steps in contemplating leadership. Considering one's own trajectory of coming out of the closet, living life honestly and openly, and being proud rather than ashamed requires significant introspection and psychological energy – but it is part of the whole leadership formation process. Even today, most members of these communities have experienced stigma, discrimination, name calling and bias, and that memory stings and persists...and may unfortunately discourage some from even thinking of themselves as leaders. While support groups, building networks of allies, and mentors can all be helpful, it seems that this still remains an intensely personal journey. Many leaders who find a way through these issues often say they found motivation and psychological energy to persist and resist by thinking of younger people in the next generation: being a trailblazer and opening doors for others helped them overcome the worst of the abuse they endured along the way.

It is absolutely clear that members of the LGBTQ2S+ have much to contribute as leaders in any organisation. First, they are members of a large and growing segment of society that has historically been under-represented. Second, the experience of growing up as a sexual minority provides unique insights and often results in development of unique skills related to observation, communication, and social interaction. Third, members of these communities often connect to social networks that bring new ideas and opportunities to organisations. Finally, as moves towards corporate and social responsibility increase, there are requirements for diversity in leadership roles.

Intersections

Women, BAME/BIPoC people, and members of the LGBTQ2S+ communities have been historically under-represented in all leadership spaces. Primarily, this may be due to internalised post-colonial structures and beliefs that negatively shape individual's thinking and beliefs with respect to the question 'can I be a leader?'. System bias and individual discrimination sadly continue to be a major issue, despite legislation and growing social awareness. The causes of this pattern are complex – and so too are potential solutions. Most importantly, each individual needs to find a path to come to the realisation that they belong, they matter, their voice is important – and they have much to offer as a leader...despite a mass of contradictory, insulting, and hurtful societal structures and individual behaviours that attempt to bring them down. The idea that a leader can succeed despite being a woman, and/or Asian, and/or gay must be transformed – the reality is leaders succeed precisely because they are a woman, and/or Asian, and/or gay.

There are so many other individuals and groups that have experienced historical marginalisation and exclusion: for example, those with physical disabilities, those from historically disadvantaged socio-economic backgrounds, or those with minority religious beliefs. While the specific experiences will of course be different, many of the general principles discussed in this chapter will apply. Further, in many cases, individuals will not simply self-identify as a monolithic member of one group. The concept of intersectionality highlights how each individual identifies with many different groups or collectives, and that the experience of a racialised gay religious cis-gendered man is very different than the experience of a racialised man, or a gay man, or a religious man. The complexities and realities of human life means there are no straightforward, simple solutions or checklists to follow. Instead, self-awareness, self-reflection, and self-understanding need to build self-confidence that allows anyone – regardless of their intersections – to say and believe, 'I am a leader'.

'So I'm a leader...what kind of leader do I want to be?'

The psychological process of becoming a leader is fascinating. Making the psychological shift to truly believing one can be a leader is only half the story. Becoming the leader one wants to become is just as complicated and fascinating, and involves even more reflection, introspection, and work. Each individual ultimately generates their own personal philosophy of leadership or leadership style. It is a rich amalgam of a person's history, their experiences, their interests, their strengths, their fears, and their hopes. Learning to shape one's own leadership philosophy – then working to find ways of actually articulating it and saying it out loud to others – is difficult, but it is essential to help reinforce and support one's own evolving leadership role.

Leadership literature is filled with models, ideals and typologies, and other individuals and organisations will frequently try to push or force-fit individuals into a mold or leadership role that may or may not be comfortable. One's personal philosophy of leadership can and should evolve over time and with more leadership experience, depending on specific circumstances and contexts. Some leaders are very comfortable adapting their leadership style to the immediate needs of the audience in front of them, while others will have a less flexible, more predictable style. Many different leadership typologies have been developed which purport to identify and describe leadership styles and the best contexts in which to be that kind of leader, but their value for individual leaders may be questionable. Similar to the concept of emotional intelligence, the idea of leadership style may be a useful starting point for reflection and building a vocabulary, but caution must be exercised in recognising it is not a diagnostic tool or definitive in any way.

One of the most widely used ways of describing leadership style was proposed by one of the leaders who studied and described emotional intelligence. Daniel Goleman has proposed a model of six different, sometimes competing leadership styles:[11]

- *Commanding leaders:* These leaders focus on compliance and obedience and expect those around them to listen and accept ideas or orders without question. They typically have a militaristic outlook, a strong drive to compete and win, and a high degree of self-control. When they themselves are led by others, they are generally compliant and obedient. For commanding leaders, there is usually a sense of urgency or crisis to their work, and in fact, commanding leaders may be most beneficial during such times. While a 'wartime' footing may be important for a leader on some occasions, it can be very difficult for others to work for a commanding leader all the time, and overall, this leadership style can be emotionally draining and create a negative climate in an organisation if it is overdone.

- *Visionary leaders:* These are individuals with creativity and ambition who are able to use self-confidence and charisma to inspire others. Rather than 'tell' people what to do, they create compelling pictures of the future that inspire others to want to follow them. They tend to use emotion effectively and positively, accentuating the positive while trying to eliminate the negative. Visionary leaders are most often successful in situations of social complexity where clear solutions are not obvious or perhaps even possible, and where individuals have a great degree of autonomy to decide for themselves independent of the leader. Such leaders may be less effective in a crisis situation or when urgent, immediate action is required.

- *Affiliative leaders:* These leaders focus strongly on the value of building harmonious and productive relationships with others, believing the strength of these relationships will be the fuel necessary to achieve leadership objectives. They are willing and able to invest considerable time and personal energy in conversations with individuals and actually draw strength from spending time with others. They usually have exceptional empathic communication skills and demonstrate superior interpersonal and non-verbal skills. Affiliative leadership works best in environments where leaders have limited clout or tools available to discipline or motivate others – for example, a health care environment populated by independent professionals. A particular strength for affiliative leaders is their ability to heal rifts and smooth disagreements that can arise during stressful situations – or from the efforts of overly commanding leaders. Affiliative leaders may be less capable in emergency or urgent situations and may be challenged by situations where 'happy endings' are simply not possible. Their need to create positive climates and workplaces can sometimes mean they are easily intimidated by others and can sometimes be overwhelmed by criticism.

- *Democratic leaders:* This type of leadership emphasises the involvement of everyone in making decisions: the democratic leader's job is not to make decisions but to ensure everyone gets involved and is heard. There is a strong focus on collaboration and communication – the leader's role is to simply keep the process going forward, organised, and on time. Democratic leaders emphasise the value of building buy-in and consensus and recognise that everyone has something valuable to contribute. They are willing to spend time and energy on consultation and recognise that this process is messy and does not yield quick, decisive answers or results. Many social service organisations rely on democratic leadership since the named leader may be too far away from clients to actually have a true grasp of a situation.

- *Pacesetting leaders:* These leaders are conscientious, have a strong drive to achieve and value initiative. These individuals focus on results in the short-term and sustainability in the long-term – they are less interested in people's feelings or democratic processes and more concerned about positive outcomes and success. They are often able to get 'quick wins' and find 'low-hanging-fruit' to get a group moving but may in the longer term exhaust and alienate individuals with their constant focus on productivity and outputs and their lack of attentiveness to individual's feelings and needs.

- *Coaching leaders:* They see their role as nurturing others and developing talent for the future. They are very empathic and self-aware but may be somewhat non-competitive and are not ego-driven. They take a hands-off role in dictating how a job is to be done and are more interested in people's feelings and experiences than the actual outcomes. Typically, coaching leaders are common towards the end of one's career, where there is little left to accomplish or prove and a greater interest in legacy.

The best and most successful leaders often find ways of balancing all six of these leadership styles with a sensitivity as to when each is most appropriate. Few successful leaders are only one style; learning how to adapt oneself to the context and situation at hand, then leveraging the most appropriate style to achieve the most positive outcome is difficult but generally seen as the best 'style'. This may require individuals to grow as leaders and to develop new strengths or propensities – and this too is the work of becoming a leader.

Arguably there is a seventh leadership style not explicitly described in Goleman's model: the title-less leader or an influencer. Increasingly, influencers are emerging as an important kind of leader. Influencers are individuals with no formal title, job description, or stated responsibilities, but they are able to exert influence over others because of who they are as individuals. Sometimes called 'thought leaders' these individuals are usually creative (like the visionary leader), but do not have formal rewards or punishments they can use to shape others' behaviours. Influencers are increasingly the kinds of leaders that actually (for good or for bad) produce outcomes. Title-less leadership has, for some individuals, significant value as a leadership style to pursue, particularly where ego perks associated with title, status, or salary aren't as significant to an individual. For title-less leaders, the value of not having a formal job description or responsibilities can be quite liberating, allowing them to focus their interests and energies on issues, rather than people or management problems.

Summary

The psychology of leadership and the answer to questions such as 'am I a leader' or 'what kind of a leader do I want to be' are complex but essential to reflect upon and articulate. Leadership is not a sterile technical activity: it is inherently psychological, interpersonal, and is rooted in a complex social context. As a result, there are no easy answers or checklists that allow individuals to 'solve' this problem or answer these questions without undertaking significant reflective and psychological work. The dividend of this will be a leader who is grounded in themselves, authentic, secure and therefore best positioned to be the best leader they can possibly be.

References

1. Hanbury G *et al*. Know yourself and take charge of your own destiny: the 'fit model' of leadership. *Public Administration Review* 2004; 64(5): 566–576.
2. Bracht E *et al*. Take a 'selfie': examining how leaders emerge from leader self-awareness, self-leadership, and self-efficacy. *Front Psychol* 2021; 12: 635085. https://doi.org/10.3389/fpsyg.2021.635085

3. Eurich T. What self-awareness really is (and how to cultivate it). *Harvard Business Review* [online] 2018. https://hbr.org/2018/01/what-self-awareness-really-is-and-how-to-cultivate-it

4. White S. Will there be a pharmacy leadership crisis? An ASHP foundation scholar-in-residence report. *Am J Health Syst Pharm* 2005; 62(8): 845–855. https://doi.org/10.1093/ajhp/62.8.845

5. Bachynsky J, Tindall W. It's time for more pharmacy leadership from within. *Can Pharm J* 2018; 151(6): 388–394. https://doi.org/10.1177/1715163518803875

6. Beales J, Austin Z. The pursuit of legitimacy and professionalism: the evolution of pharmacy in Ontario. *Pharm Hist* 2006; 36(2): 22–27.

7. Wang G *et al*. Does leader same-sex sexual orientation matter to leadership effectiveness? A four-study model-testing investigation. *J Bus Psychol* 2022; 37(3): 557–580. https://doi.org/10.1007/s10869-021-09767-y

8. Gundemir S *et al*. Think leader, think white? Capturing and weakening an implicit pro-white leadership bias. *PLoS One* [online] 2014; 9(1): e83915. https://doi.org/10.1371/journal.pone.0083915

9. Eagly A, Johnson B. Gender and leadership style: a meta-analysis. *Psychological Bulletin* 1990; 108(2): 233–256. https://doi.org/10.1037/0033-2909.108.2.233

10. McGibbon E. Truth and reconciliation: healthcare organizational leadership. *Healthcare Management Forum* 2018; 32(1): 20–24. https://doi.org/10.1177/0840470418803379

11. Saxena A *et al*. Goleman's leadership styles at different hierarchical levels in medical education. *BMC Medical Education* 2017; 17: 169. https://doi.org/10.1186/s12909-017-0995-z

CHAPTER 27

The psychology of entrepreneurship

Upon completion of this chapter you should be able to:

- outline what makes an entrepreneur
- understand the role of psychological safety in entrepreneurial psychology
- identify important characteristics of successful entrepreneurs
- examine the value of creativity and innovation in the context of execution
- understand the power of observation.

Who doesn't want to be an entrepreneur? In today's world, the popular view of entrepreneurs is that of super-human intellect, unbounded power and ego, and unimaginable wealth generated sheerly through the fruits of creative labour. Entrepreneurs such as Elon Musk, Mark Zuckerberg, or Jeff Bezos are household names who have fundamentally transformed the way people around the world live their day to day lives. There is even some small hope that entrepreneurship may unshackle the chains that have held back those from historically disadvantage groups: Peter Thiel (founder of PayPal and the first investor in Facebook) is a gay man, Oprah Winfrey is the most famous and wealthy media and entertainment entrepreneur in history and is an African–American woman, and Dhirubhai Ambani and Ratan Tata are successful Indian entrepreneurs whose businesses are global. While it may be optimistic that an increasingly entrepreneurial world is the ultimate way of addressing diversity, equity, and inclusivity, the reality is that more and more individuals from increasingly diverse backgrounds are finding ways of unleashing their talent and their potential to transform business and the world.

For many of us, however, entrepreneurship might seem like a step too far, well beyond our comfort zone and our own self-perception of strengths. Particularly for pharmacists, who (as Assimilators) may have greater confidence within well-defined workplaces structured around clear policies and procedures, the uncertainty and risk associated with entrepreneurship may seem unimaginable. Worse, the unbridled self-confidence, intellectual wizardry and passionate creativity entrepreneurs seem to possess in abundance might seem completely out of reach. While there is undeniably a personal element to successful entrepreneurship that is likely rooted in traits and psychology, it is also clear that there is a pressing need to mobilise more and more people from all backgrounds and psychological trait types to focus their interests and talents in solving the problems that face the world today. Entrepreneurship should be for everyone, not a select few, and is more about a way of thinking creatively and taking informed risks than about making money or garnering fame. Understanding the psychology of entrepreneurship can help all individuals self-reflect on how they can take full advantage of their personal gifts and talents to solve problems, build solutions, and be creative in ways that are impactful, rewarding, and simply fun.

What makes an entrepreneur?

The connection between creativity and personality has long been seen as the foundation of entrepreneurship. Innovations related to technology, entertainment, medicine and society have literally changed lives and the course of human history. Think about how we now take for granted the entrepreneurship behind the smart phone or social media, or the mRNA vaccines and the global mass vaccine rollout (that featured pharmacists front and centre) that transformed the trajectory of the COVID-19 pandemic.

What makes some people unusually productive, effective, and creative at problem-solving? Psychologists have noted that there are some characteristics that appear to be important, many of which are necessary for entrepreneurs. For example, MacKinnon's work has demonstrated that creativity and problem-solving in fields such as architecture appear to be connected to psychological preferences for asymmetry (rather than symmetry) and the capacity to maintain psychological equilibrium despite 'messiness' and unpredictability in the environment.[1] Kirby has identified a type of divergent problem-solving method, used by creative individuals, in which there is psychological comfort with the reality that there will be no single, pre-set solution, and that sometimes 'least worst alternatives' are all that is available.[2] Many psychologists have noted that creative innovators frequently demonstrate higher-than-average levels of internal motivation, comfort with environmental or situational ambiguity, and a type of non-conformity that allows them to be more self-accepting than many others.[3,4]

Does this mean that those who are more conventional, more conforming, and more troubled by environmental chaos or messiness are simply destined to be uncreative, uninspiring, office drones incapable of entrepreneurship? Of course not...

Finding psychological safety – the secret ingredient of entrepreneurship?

Recent pioneering work in innovation by Clark, has highlighted important insights into the psychology and process of innovation.[5] While in some cases, entrepreneurs are focused on an invention or product that is new and revolutionary, in many (if not most) cases, entrepreneurs are not really involved in or leading development of anything specific or novel. Instead, much of what is entrepreneurial is aimed at changing other people's behaviour – often using new or innovative tools, technologies, or products that have been simply lying idle and unused by the inventors themselves. Consider, for example, the case of Facebook and its founder/entrepreneur Mark Zuckerberg. Consider how social media has transformed the world and day to day lives of billions of individuals – including the ambiguous role social media may have played (and continues to play) in shaping thinking and behaviour in socio-political realms such as the rise of Brexit in the UK or the emergence of far-right ethno-nationalism in many parts of the world. Clearly, Mark Zuckerberg did not invent the internet itself, or the concept of algorithms or electronic messaging. Zuckerberg's entrepreneurial genius was in identifying how these pre-existing innovations could be repackaged in a creative way that would incentivise billions of individuals to change their social and communication behaviours with each other...and social media and Facebook were born.

Clark's work highlights that entrepreneurs often have a unique capacity to drive, cajole, or motivate other people to change pre-existing behaviours they haven't truly thought about or questioned in the past.[5] This often starts through the building of networks, alliances, or relationships with others in an informal way that allows otherwise change-resistant people to open their minds, let down their guard, relax a bit, form new or strengthen existing relationships...and in short find or reinforce psychological safety.

The role of creating and fostering psychological safety as part of entrepreneurial psychology is often overlooked, with disproportionate emphasis placed on the building of new products. Psychological safety is crucially important to encourage the spread of innovative ideas and products, but it is equally essential for the entrepreneur themselves. When individuals feel psychological safety rooted in trusting relationships with others, they don't fear failure or embarrassment at proposing new ideas or showing the fruits of their labours. Without these trusting relationships – and the psychological safety they generate – few individuals will manage the risk of behavioural change necessary to first showcase an innovation, then actually try another person's innovation for themselves.

Recent work by Haseltine has proposed there is a psychological formula for innovation at the core of entrepreneurship:[6]

$$\text{Innovation} = (\text{Talent} + \text{Relationships})/\text{Formality}$$

This formula suggests that the seed or starting point of entrepreneurship – innovation – is a function of one's talent, ideas and the relationships one has or can build. It is also enhanced by informalism: the denominator of this equation highlights the ways in which rigid structures and bureaucracies can inhibit innovation and reflects the notion that many (though definitely not all) entrepreneurs 'come from the outside'. Haseltine has said that the essence of entrepreneurship is to '...gather people with the requisite personality and cognitive traits for creativity, nurture trusting relationships among them, and do all of this with the bare minimum of process, procedure, and bureaucracy, while maximising informality...if possible over adult beverages and good food'.[6]

Purpose and gratitude

Jones has noted that successful entrepreneurs often have certain psychological characteristics in common.[7] His research comparing historically impactful entrepreneurs ranging from Walt Disney to Steve Jobs provides important insights for those interested in entrepreneurship to consider. In particular, he describes entrepreneurial characteristics of importance such as:

- *Purpose:* Few, if any, of the entrepreneurs Jones studied explicitly wanted to make money, have their own business, or generate fame for themselves. Self-interested 'purposes' for entrepreneurship are generally transparent and off-putting to others and are more likely to result in failure than success. For Jones, successful entrepreneurship often starts with an ambitious, wild-eyed, and completely unrealistic purpose or desire to do something that hasn't been done before. For example, Walt Disney's personal story involved being a teenager during the ravages of World War 1, being 'left out' during the roaring 1920s, then experiencing the worst of the Depression. As a result, he had an uncommon need to bring happiness – simple, pure joy – to humanity. In his work, in his thinking, and in his creativity that drive towards happiness, it is not only abundant...it was clearly realised through so many of the much beloved characters and stories who have lived on into the 20th century.

- *Simplification:* Few entrepreneurs consider themselves to be intellectuals, geniuses, or even much brighter than others. An important psychological characteristic that Jones identified is the psychological need – and the cognitive ability – to simplify and to clarify complexity. Innovators like Warren Buffet describe themselves in humble terms as 'simple men', but it is not the simplicity of themselves that is unique, it is their ability to take messy, ambiguous situations and find ways of distilling them into simple and straightforward problems to be solved. In part, this may be due to their ability (and willingness) to not let others' emotional states interfere with their drive to simplify; as a result, some entrepreneurs may appear strangely aloof or uninterested at times. At other times, it may come across as single-minded fixation on an issue, verging on rigidity. Importantly, Jones points out that this characteristic/trait of simplification yields dividends in terms of creativity and innovation, provided it does not tip over into over-simplification. Jones sites the example of the founder of Uber (Travis Kalanick) who was frustrated by the inefficiency and complexity (and accompanying unreliability and lack of consistent quality) of actually getting taxi cabs in large American cities he visited: his drive to simplify (coupled with his networks/connections to software engineers) allowed him to come up with the concept of Uber that has now revolutionised urban transportation.

- *High expectations:* Henry Ford is credited with having said, 'whether you think you can, or you think you can't – you are right'. This notion that belief in self, coupled with high expectations of what can be accomplished, differentiates entrepreneurs from many others. Jones points out that this combination of self-esteem and high hopes means that many entrepreneurs actually cognitively process environmental cues differently than most individuals: they tend to see outcomes first, then identify processes and potential barriers afterwards. In contrast, many other people cannot get to a vision of outcomes because they become mired in processes and barriers first. Jones questions whether the propensity to see outcomes first is simply a natural psychological trait or a behaviour that can be learned by everyone – in either case, it appears to be a necessary characteristic for most entrepreneurs who are successful.

- *Problem-solving:* For those who are currently not entrepreneurs, perhaps the most magical or mysterious element of entrepreneurial psychology is the ability of some people to solve problems we didn't even know we had: why worry about the expense and inconvenience of large anonymous hotel chains when there are millions of unused bedrooms and attic lofts homeowners would gladly rent out for a few nights in order to make a few extra dollars...and bingo, AirBnB was born. The entrepreneurial mind appears to be more flexible and able to parallel process inputs in a more efficient and rapid manner than for most individuals: harnessing this becomes the way entrepreneurs find, define, and solve problems that others overlook or simply give up on. At its worst, this can lead to a kind of hyperactive, hyperkinetic tendency towards distractibility and inattentiveness: at its best, this characteristic helps entrepreneurs put pieces together and synthesise ideas from seemingly disparate, incongruent parts that others may overlook.

- *Massive action:* The entrepreneurs Jones studied had more than simple good or novel ideas – they also had an ability and willingness to execute. The most successful of them invest in 'massive action', a term that describes the audacious, improbable, and risky things entrepreneurs do to see their ideas come to life. For less entrepreneurially oriented individuals, massive action frequently represents the most daunting piece of a puzzle: tales of successful individuals like Steve Jobs, Jeff Bezos, or Bill Gates quitting their jobs, re-mortgaging their houses, working tirelessly in their garages with no money and no recognition to pursue their dreams is the stuff of movies and television...but also reflects the kind of determined and confident actions that allow individuals to succeed. One lesson Jones draws from this is the notion that entrepreneurship can rarely succeed if it is safe, incremental, and measured: massive action implies risk, significant activity, and a scale that can be alarming. Imagine what those around Elon Musk or Jeff Bezos must have thought when they first started talking about their big ideas. 'Putting your money where your mouth is' describes the kind of massive action that can produce spectacular success – or horrendous failure – but the psychological ability to imagine oneself undertaking massive action is at the core of entrepreneurship.
- *Gratitude:* Jones states that 'when you are grateful...fear disappears, and abundance appears. Because you can't be angry or fearful while being grateful, that spark that prompts you to take action and achieve your full potential takes effect'. The role of gratitude in the psychology of innovation is interesting: it speaks to a tranquil emotional state in which raw feelings do not distort judgement or decision making, and where foundational elements of success – such as optimism, enthusiasm, energy, and determination – are more likely to flourish. Gratitude also makes it possible to build the kinds of networks and social relationships entrepreneurs need in order to allow innovations to flourish; no one likes being around negative, angry individuals, while positive gratitude is an infectious emotional state that generates its own positive outcomes. Of course, gratitude can rarely be faked or simply willed into existence; the psychological trait of optimism is likely an important element in this regard. Still, the finding that gratitude is part of the psychological makeup of most successful entrepreneurs – and that gratitude persists despite setbacks and failure – creates a picture of what entrepreneurs are like as individuals.

Other psychologists have identified additional important elements of the psyche of successful entrepreneurs that align with Jones' insights.[8] These include:

- *Proactive personality:* Procrastination appears to be antithetical to successful entrepreneurship. Simply, getting things done in good time and taking advantages of opportunities as they arrive appear to be important success factors.
- *Stress tolerance:* Successful entrepreneurs appear to have – or have developed – better coping and stress-management techniques than most individuals. In part, it may be because they do not procrastinate and ensure they put into place mechanisms to support them if the worst happens (e.g. put aside lots of savings first as a buffer in case of early failure). Much of the stress tolerance entrepreneurs appear to demonstrate is of a psychological/social nature and may reflect the 'social capital' theory. It is, perhaps, not a coincidence that most (if not the vast majority) of successful entrepreneurs are white, straight, cis-gendered men who may have self-confidence, self-efficacy, and historical privileges others do not, that can help them manage

entrepreneurial stress in ways that a single mother with four children simply cannot...because she is starting from a baseline of extraordinary stress.

- *Big five personality profile:* Studies have highlighted the ways in which entrepreneurs may be different than others (particularly managers in large organisations) using emotional intelligence theory and constructs described in Chapter 2. Across diverse studies and contexts, it appears as though entrepreneurs are more conscientious, less neurotic, more open to experience, less agreeable, and are no different in terms of introversion/extroversion than managers. The significance of these findings is not exactly clear.
- *Risk tolerance:* One of the most interesting psychological elements of entrepreneurs is their framing and tolerance of risks. (*See* Chapter 31 for further details.)

Understanding creativity and innovation – in the context of execution

Creativity and innovation are essential attributes of successful entrepreneurs, and many individuals may erroneously believe – 'you either are or you aren't'. The question as to whether innovators are born or made, or whether creativity is a foundational psychological trait or a behaviour/attitude that can be learned, is both important and provocative. Researchers have highlighted the ways in which innovation/creativity are necessary – but insufficient – for entrepreneurial success.[9] While some element of 'newness' is important, successful entrepreneurs need to ensure creativity and innovation are embedded within concrete and learned skills to allow ideas to come to life and actually be executed. Simply having a big idea, without the capacity to make it real, does not produce entrepreneurial success. In fact, focusing on the concrete and learned skills of entrepreneurship can help open doors, create networks, and ultimately generate the ideas that will fuel entrepreneurship...not the other way around. Thinking about creativity and innovation as the 'easy' part of the process – and execution of ideas as the 'harder' part – might seem counterintuitive, but the experience of most entrepreneurs suggests that the foundational elements of successful execution (such as network building and knowledge of market forces) are actually where the raw material for creative ideas often are to be found. Overemphasising the creative a-ha moment, or inspirational genius is commonplace. Key skills for successful execution that can help unleash creativity and innovation include:

- *Financial literacy:* All ideas need money to allow them to come to life, and entrepreneurs who are simply focused on 'big ideas' without a financial reality check, will be unlikely to succeed. Basic financial literacy around tools such as balance sheets and income statements are necessary for managers and leaders – but equally (if not more so) are essential for entrepreneurs. Ultimately, entrepreneurs are interested in converting big ideas into profitable businesses and knowing how a profitable business actually performs before daydreaming about big ideas is essential.
- *Understanding how markets work:* Entrepreneurs are generally outsiders who are trying to 'break into' established business markets or niches. The concept of a 'great idea' is directly tied to the needs, interests, and wants of markets and consumers, even if some (or many) times entrepreneurs generate ideas for things people don't even know they need. Understanding the

marketplace in which an innovation will need to compete and flourish to survive is essential. This means understanding competitors, understanding consumers, and understanding the supply and demand forces that govern current players in the field. Analysis of current market forces and conditions often helps trigger creativity and innovation: seeing how things currently work in a specific market can help entrepreneurs identify the gaps and opportunities that will ultimately translate into creative innovation.

- *Superior communication skills:* It is sometimes entertaining to listen to some of the most successful entrepreneurs (for example, Elon Musk) and ask, 'what planet did he come from'? The hyper-aggressive yet tone-deaf style of communication some entrepreneurs display may make it appear as though everyday skills such as active listening and rapport building aren't necessary for entrepreneurs. Of course, the exact opposite is true. Entrepreneurs need not just good or effective communication skills, but superior or exemplary skills to build the relationships with others that are needed to bring ideas to life. The process of leveraging these communication skills and building these relationships is often the way in which new opportunities are identified and ideas generated; rarely do entrepreneurs identify 'big ideas' in isolation or toiling way in obscurity. Innovative ideas almost always emerge through conversation and relationships – entrepreneurial creativity is a team sport or social activity, not an isolationist pursuit. Developing the communication and relationship building skills necessary to fully engage with others provides one of the most important pathways to innovation for entrepreneurs.

- *Networking:* Closely aligned with the importance of superior communication skills is the ability and willingness to develop and nurture social, professional, and cultural networks that are as diverse and broad as possible. Large and diverse networks provide important sources of information, data, and ideas for entrepreneurs and can help support the development and refining of creative innovations. Networking skills go beyond simple communicative competency. (*See* Chapter 32 for more details.)

- *Being a manager and leader:* Some individuals believe that 'entrepreneurship' is easier than being a manager or leader since you get to be your own boss and call your own shots. In fact, the most successful entrepreneurs are also incredibly effective managers and leaders, possessing the skills necessary to organise and motivate others, build high performing teams, and communicate with empathy, transparency, and clarity.

- *Time management:* Effective, sustainable, and consistent time management is essential for successful entrepreneurs, but is often overlooked as both a required skill and a conduit to innovation and creativity. Learning how to spend the right amount of time on the right tasks so that goals are achieved is essential: it is all too easy to indulge in the fantasy that 'creativity doesn't punch a clock' or that 'when a person is in an idea-generating mode, time stands still'. Wasting time is actually one of the greatest problems for unsuccessful entrepreneurs and is counterproductive to creativity and innovation. Disciplined management of time is essential for success.

Popular media depictions often distort the reality of the entrepreneurial mindset, by overemphasising 'creative genius' at the expense of other skills and competencies. Of course, entrepreneurs must be innovative, generate great ideas, and see the world differently than most other people. But those skills – in isolation – do not actually produce the kinds of outcomes and changes that entrepreneurs want, and rarely result in business success. It is sometimes said that 'a great idea and two dollars buys you a cup of coffee', meaning that everyone has great ideas from time to time...but not everyone is successful as an entrepreneur. Equally important is the insight that it is the actual process of building the skills of entrepreneurship – time management, network building, relationship management, understanding of markets, etc. – that will ultimately produce the fertile soil in which great ideas will germinate...not the other way around.

Entrepreneurship and the power of observation

Observation is simply the process of looking at things. For entrepreneurs, observation is often at the heart of their innovation and creativity and involves not simply looking at things in a blank or mindless way, but instead with a kind of consciousness and analytic filter that helps to explain or account for what is being observed. The term 'critical observation' is sometimes used to describe the unique human ability to take in information from the outside world while simultaneously prioritising, filtering, and analysing it. Critical observation focuses on generating ideas or theories about seen and unseen patterns, focusing on unspoken truths that drive behaviours, and even the realities that shape peoples' thinking and behaviours that are not even known to themselves. For entrepreneurs, the value of critical observation in shaping innovation and idea generation is essential. For those who do not see themselves (currently) as entrepreneurs, it is also a skill that can be developed. Critical observation can be enhanced by:

- *An open mindset:* Cognitive rigidity and a know-it-all belief system will inhibit the powers of observation. While some individuals are simply, by their nature and emotional intelligence, more open-minded than others, the importance of openness in the power of observation cannot be overstated. Learning to detect and suspend immediate judgements, biases, and assumptions, and intentionally rejecting one's knee-jerk reaction to assume understanding of a situation is important. While in some circumstances it may be appropriate to 'trust your instincts', for critical observation it is important to realise that instincts are frequently biased and tainted by our own experiences and wishes. A conscious effort to develop and maintain an open mindset in observation can be learned but requires constant vigilance to stay focused on the present and in the moment, rather than constantly being distracted by one's own impulsive assessments.
- *Use all your senses:* Critical observation requires us to not simply listen but also see, not only hear but also look. Frequently in human interactions, verbal and non-verbal messages will misfire or be at odds with one another. For example, in response to the question, 'how are you doing', a person may respond, [heavy sigh], 'fine'. The verbal message – fine – is at odds with the non-verbal heavy sigh. Most human beings will recognise this inconsistency but would prefer to avoid dealing with complexity and ambiguity, so in a case such as this most will simply ignore or de-prioritise the non-verbal heavy sigh, and instead think, 'great, you said fine, so everything must be good'. Critical observation requires us to train ourselves to avoid this instinct towards convenient oversimplification and instead engage all our senses appropriately. Where there are discrepancies between verbal and non-verbal messages,

or where something doesn't seem quite as it appears to be...critical observation means we continue to work to try to figure out why discrepancies exist, and where the truth lies.

- *Understand your filters:* The social complexity of human interactions is overwhelming and often leads us to take cognitive shortcuts to manage interactions more efficiently with others. This is the basis of stereotyping and bias: using convenient and obvious demographic or other characteristics to quickly categorise and pigeon-hole individuals, often unfairly. Critical observation requires us to think about and be able to articulate how certain filters can lead us to misinterpret situations and make assumptions. Misinterpretation and assuming will inhibit creativity, problem-solving, and innovation.

- *Memory and recall:* A central element to critical observation is the ability to infer patterns and build 'mind maps', models or mental representations that are based on observations but support some element of generalisation to other situations. This skill is supported by a strong memory and the ability to recall concepts, details, and states of mind. Memory and recall are often overlooked as an important entrepreneurial skill, but as a seedbed for creative innovation, they are essential. Strong memory facilitates the kind of pattern recognition that helps entrepreneurs identify opportunities and ideas; it is pattern recognition that helps generate creative solutions to commonly occurring problems and allows individuals to frame ideas amongst chaos. On a practical note, memory and recall are also instrumental in building networks and supporting interpersonal communication that is a necessary pre-requisite for idea generation.

- *Critical analysis/thinking:* Critical observation emphasises the importance of consistent and intentional attention to environmental cues and messages; by itself, however, critical observation is insufficient, if it is not accompanied by critical analysis or thinking. Critical analysis is a propensity and a skill that involves examination of observations and problems from multiple angles and multiple perspectives, in the hopes that this process will yield important insights and creative ideas. Critical thinking means not simply accepting at face value the observations being made, and not simply accepting that what has been observed is the complete truth of a situation. Questioning the veracity of claims, asking whether systems could be better, and simply not accepting that 'this is as good as it gets' are all essential attributes of critical thinking. Critical thinking is usually facilitated by the use of multi-stakeholder perspectives: imagining what different people who are affected by an issue might see, hear, or perceive can provide very important insights into a process or system. It takes imagination but also intentionality to systematically consider questions such as 'how would a patient see and experience this?', 'how would another health professional feel about this?', 'how would the media report on this?' and 'what would government think about this?'. Critical thinking is stymied when we assume that our perspective is the only true and meaningful filter through which observations can and should be considered. By consciously and deliberately asking questions from other stakeholder perspectives, creativity and innovation is more likely to flow.

- *Learning:* An important aspect of the entrepreneurial mindset is the expectation that learning is constant and life-long. A mindset that is rooted in acceptance of one's own certainty is rarely able to generate the creative insights necessary for innovation. Instead, when individuals adopt a learning mindset, in which each observation becomes a learning opportunity, there are greater opportunities for creativity to flourish. A conscious practice of simply asking oneself, 'what did I learn from this observation' in a routine and consistent way can help build an internal mindset that is more open and more likely to generate ideas. While it may sound contrived or hokey, the intentionality of reminding oneself to ask this question consistently and routinely is important, as it triggers the kind of reflection and analysis that can support creative insights.

Summary

We are often led to believe that the creativity and innovation demonstrated by successful entrepreneurs is almost magical: it is unique to a few individuals and not something the rest of us could even consider. Research has highlighted that entrepreneurs are not particularly gifted in any specific area of cognitive or emotional processing but instead have developed a series of practices or behaviours that are more likely to result in creative insight. By focusing on execution, creative insights are more likely to flourish. By thinking in terms of skills (like networking or effective listening), ideas are more likely to be generated. By realising that creativity and innovation are essentially social activities rooted in networks and relationships – not individual pursuits undertaken by loners in their parent's basements – entrepreneurship is more possible than many of us may initially imagine.

References

1. Mackinnon D *et al.* Networking, trust and embeddedness amongst SMEs in the Aberdeen oil complex. *Entrepreneurship & Regional Development* 2004; 16(2): 87–106. https://dx.doi.org/10.1080/0898562041000 1677826

2. Kirby D. Entrepreneurship policy: theory and practice. *Int Entrepreneurship and Management J* 2005; 1: 557–559. https://doi.org/10.1007/s11365-005-4778-3

3. Sondakh D, Rajah K. Developing an entrepreneurship culture: the Greenwich experience. *Int J Entrepreneurship and Innovation* 2006; 7(4): 231–241. https://doi.org/10.5367/000000006779111611

4. Frese M, Gielnik M. The psychology of entrepreneurship. *Annual Rev Organizational Psychology and Organizational Behaviour* 2014; 1(1): 413–438. https://doi.org/10.1146/annurev-orgpsych-031413-091326

5. Clark J, Lee D. Freedom, entrepreneurship, and economic progress. *J Entrepreneurship* 2006; 15(1): 1–17. https://doi.org/10.1177/097135570501500101

6. Haseltine E. The surprising psychology of innovation: it's less about creativity and problem solving than you may think. *Psychology Today* [online] 2021. https://www.psychologytoday.com/ca/blog/long-fuse-big-bang/202107/the-surprising-psychology-innovation

7. Jones K. The psychology of innovation: from purpose to gratitude. *Forbes Magazine* [online] 2016. https://www.forbes.com/sites/forbesagencycouncil/2016/04/06/the-psychology-of-innovation-from-purpose-to-gratitude/?sh=27ebf47b694a

8. Krueger N. The cognitive psychology of entrepreneurship. In: Acs Z, Audretsch D, eds. *Handbook of Entrepreneurship Research: An Interdisciplinary survey and introduction*, 1st edn. Manchester: Kluwer Law International, 2003: 105–140.

9. Davenport T. Entrepreneurial Execution: the future of strategy. *Harvard Business Review* [online] 2007. https://hbr.org/2007/12/entrepreneurial-execution-the

CHAPTER 28

Understanding your value proposition

Upon completion of this chapter you should be able to:

- explain what personal value propositions are
- understand the differences between value and money
- outline the difference between value creation for customers and for an entrepreneur in pharmacy
- describe how to develop a personal value proposition.

One of the challenges for many would-be entrepreneurs is recognising that they are not simply marketing or selling an idea or an innovation – they need to market and sell themselves. The connection between the individual entrepreneur and the idea, product, or service they have developed is very tight: in many cases, potential buyers will make no distinction between the entrepreneur themselves and the 'thing' they are working on.[1]

This is particularly true in the earliest stages of entrepreneurship when it is necessary to raise money, arrange bank loans, identify potential investors, and secure early clients for the product or service. While it is tempting to think that extroverted individuals may be better at this than introverted individuals, the reality is that that social skills associated with extroversion will only be marginally successful in convincing most people to part with their money. Relying solely upon glad-handing and communication skills will not produce entrepreneurial success.

The concept of the 'personal value proposition' (PVP) has been touted as an important tool for entrepreneurs to better understand themselves, their potential clients, and what they bring to a marketplace.[2] Many organisations are familiar with the traditional value proposition, usually associated with sales of a good or service. In that context, value propositions are statements that help companies more clearly define, specify, and prioritise their market segments, the unique benefits they can provide, and ultimately the cost-benefit of choosing their product/service over another. It is an essential marketing tool for external stakeholders, and a valuable educational tool for internal staff members, so their understanding of their organisation's work is better aligned.

For entrepreneurs who may be at different stages of having an actual product or service to sell, the personal value proposition is an important tool to help individuals develop a clear and concise vocabulary to explain who they are to other people who may be skeptical about what they are offering. Entrepreneurship usually involves some element of sales (whether it is selling an idea to a bank to secure a loan, selling an idea to a client to convince them to buy a product, or selling an idea to a regulatory body to gain approval). At the heart of this is faith in the entrepreneur themselves:

external stakeholders need to know the entrepreneur is trustworthy, honest, and is fairly representing themselves and their ideas. Since many 'pitches' that entrepreneurs make are speculative or future-oriented, they are asking external stakeholders to make a leap of faith and believe in them, their potential, and their integrity. A clear PVP can help make this case and provide a uniform vocabulary for introducing oneself and explaining one's unique strengths and value. It also serves as an aspirational goal post, reminding the entrepreneur of who they want to and intend to be. Finally, the PVP is also a useful mile-marker, an external document that can be used on a periodic basis by the entrepreneur to ensure that initial intentions and beliefs continue to be honoured.[3]

PVPs – what they are and what they are not

There are few standards for what PVPs are and are not. Importantly, PVPs are not resumes or curricula vitae stating accomplishments in chronological order. Equally, they are not slick marketing documents that bend the truth or gloss over inconvenient realities. One of the important elements of a PVP is its ability to help articulate difficult concepts. For example, many entrepreneurs pursue entrepreneurial pathways because they feel dissatisfied with or simply do not feel they 'fit' within traditionally defined job categories and hierarchically rigid organisations. Part of this sense of dissatisfaction and lack of fit is because most entrepreneurs have diverse skills and interests that sometimes defy easy, convenient, or even recognisable categorisation. This is part of the unique psychological profile of entrepreneurs: they tend to cross boundaries and silos, bringing diverse strengths and different experiences than would be expected in most situations. They may defy conventional expectations of individuals within certain professions: for example, while most pharmacists are expected to be rule-obeying, detail-oriented, collaborative non-risk takers, many of the most successful entrepreneurs in pharmacy are just the opposite; they often are big-picture people who wither in the face of excessive details, and they have a comfort with risk – and rule-bending – that may shock many of their professional colleagues. Not 'fitting' the mould of their profession may make these individuals more likely to pursue independent entrepreneurial opportunities, but this produces another problem: how can you sell yourself as trustworthy to a profession when you don't fit the mould of that profession? The main role of a PVP is to address this issue: clearly explain why you   as a convention-disrupting, rule-bending, innovative risk taker – should not only be trusted, but valued, for the unique contributions you can bring to your profession and your society.

Reflecting on value and money

For some, the connection between entrepreneurship and wealth is at the core of their drive to succeed. The perception that entrepreneurs are always wealthy and materially successful does not necessarily correspond to reality. While, of course, high-profile entrepreneurs like Elon Musk or Richard Branson have flashy lifestyles and untold billions of dollars in personal wealth, most entrepreneurs recognise that 'success' is about bringing ideas to life, not simply wealth. Importantly, where an individual brings value to a community or a society, some measure of material success will follow, even if it is not the jaw-dropping amounts enjoyed by high-profile celebrities.

'Value' and 'money' should never be confused. Entrepreneurs create value through the generation of new ideas and the implementation of innovations that are meaningful and impactful to others.[4] The personal value of an entrepreneur – and what needs to be showcased in a personal value proposition – is closely aligned with the value of the innovation and the idea itself. To some degree, entrepreneurs do need to sell themselves and their unique personalities, talents, and skills...but personality, talent, and skills that are devoid of ideas and innovation will not result in success. In crafting a personal value proposition, the connection between an idea that leads to an innovation that can be successfully executed to actually, truly, and believably be of value to others must be clearly represented.

From this perspective, 'value' has a double meaning that is both important and intentional. The first meaning of value for an entrepreneur is based on personal beliefs, behaviours, morals, and ethics – one's 'values' as a human being. Mindful reflection on one's values will help to clarify one's intentions as an entrepreneur: is it to simply make money and become famous, or is it to bring an idea to life? Does one crave material trappings of individual success or improvements for society that will benefit everyone? While there may be a tendency to want to avoid disclosing selfish motivations or materialistic ideals so as to appear to be 'noble', it is usually difficult to hide these personal values from others in the long-term. Honest self-appraisal of one's values – and how these are influencing thinking, decision making, and behaviour, is essential. Where material gain and self-interested materialism are truly at the core of one's values, entrepreneurial pathways will look different than where social benefit and translation of creative ideas into reality are at the core. Confusing or hiding personal values often leads to confusion for oneself and everyone else, and may undermine attempts to be successful.

The second meaning of value in this context is the creation or expansion of existing desirable benefits and gains. The term 'value creation' has been coined to describe the process by which an entrepreneur builds something valuable and provides it to others in exchange for something else that's more valuable to the entrepreneur. At its most basic, this might only be about profitability: an entrepreneur creates something new, sells it for money to others, and the money received is worth more to the entrepreneur than the thing that was created and sold. Monetary profit/gain and enlargement of personal wealth of the entrepreneur is, of course, important, but need not be the only consideration in value creation. Entrepreneurs may have the unique luxury of being able to define other forms of 'value' beyond simple monetary gain that are important: for example, producing a public benefit, becoming publicly recognised, or simply helping others live better lives. So called 'impact entrepreneurship' defines value creation in terms of non-financial gains that result in other people leading better lives, and this can be an even more powerful motivation to succeed as an entrepreneur than money. At times, financially motivated value creation may be at odds with, or simply incompatible with, impact entrepreneurship... but at other times the two can quite peacefully co-exist and mutually reinforce/support one another.

The key for entrepreneurs is to be mindful and intentional about reflecting upon the connection between 'money' and 'value', and be able to articulate one's own definition, clearly, honestly, and proudly, of 'value creation' that aligns personal values with the value being generated through entrepreneurial activities. Entrepreneurs are likely to fail when they cannot produce value for customers or themselves. Similarly, where entrepreneurs create value for their customers but in a soul-destroying and demoralising way which does not align with personal values, their success will be short-lived. Finally, where entrepreneurs create only value for themselves with alignment with their own interests but neglect to focus on value creation for customers, they may be engaging in time-wasting, self-indulgent but ultimately pointless endeavours.

Even the most altruistic of entrepreneurs, with strong commitments to social benefits, must recognise the practical realities of living life and running a business and the central role of money in success. Conversely, even the most self-interested and materialistic of entrepreneurs interested in maximising profitability, need to recognise that 'value' has important non-financial social benefits that must be considered. For successful entrepreneurs, the lesson is that where value is created and aligned with personal beliefs, sufficient money will flow to allow for a sustainable and rewarding life.

What is value creation for the customer?

At its simplest, value creation is the process of converting work and resources into something that meets the needs of others, in a way that the final output is more valuable to customers than the sum of the individual inputs.[5] For example, a farmer invests personal time and skill into their harvest, but also must invest up-front money into purchasing seeds, tractors, and storage facilities as well as renting land for growing. The ultimate harvest creates value if customers pay more for the crops than the sum of seeds + tractors + storage + personal time/skill invested.

For entrepreneurs, a similar value creation calculation formula will apply, but it can be somewhat trickier to work out as the intangible value of creative ideas is integral to the entrepreneurs work. Understanding value creation from a customer's perspective is essential to allowing entrepreneurs to critically evaluate their ideas as well as helping them to articulate their own personal value proposition.

Value creation for customers involves at least three distinct but connected elements: functional, positive emotional, and negative emotional components. The functional component of value for a customer is simply the job, activity, or task that the entrepreneur's innovation actually accomplishes. For example, a farmer's harvest generates food that sustains life. It has a clear function that is known and understood by both the customer and the farmer. While, clearly, not everyone will enjoy okra or aubergines, and some individuals may have gluten intolerance that precludes eating wheat, food that farmers produce will have an obvious market of some sort because of the function it fulfils. A more entrepreneurial farmer may consider: how can I convince people they actually do like okra and aubergines so I can grow the number of potential customers I have by fulfilling a function or need they didn't actually know they had? The functional component of value creation is focused on both known needs and unknown needs, and creating a pathway for customers to accept they have needs they didn't consciously know about as a way of expanding a marketplace.

Functional elements of value can sometimes be described in terms of different categories, including:[4,5] a) productivity (or the ability to do more with less and be more effective and efficient with respect to utilisation of resources); b) profitability (using an innovation to extract greater monetary returns than in the past, even after paying for the innovation itself); c) image (enhancing public perception, prestige, and customer awareness/appreciation in ways that may increase business, traffic, or loyalty); d) experience (enhancing the quality of interactions with customers as a way of building reputation, loyalty, and driving repeat customers); e) convenience (finding ways of making everyday activities/tasks easier, more reliable, less cumbersome and more enjoyable as a tool to enhance sustainability). Functional element value creation can be understood and described in terms of these five different categories as a way of more effectively communicating with diverse stakeholders.

The positive emotional component of value creation relates to an essential, but difficult to quantify, reaction customers have to an entrepreneur's innovation. Consider, for example, the value creation associated with organic farming. Organic produce is typically more expensive, rarer, and consequently should have fewer customers than 'regular' produce. The upsurge in organic produce consumption reflects a positive feel good emotional component of value creation: consumers of organic produce may feel more noble, or virtuous, and better about themselves for contributing positively by selecting (and paying more) for organic products. The value created here is not about function – organic and regular produce are more or less similar in terms of nutritive activity and biological function – but consumers are willing to pay more because of the positive emotional state that is triggered by the 'organic' label. This is the value that is added – and the value received by the entrepreneur who identifies the impact of positive emotions on consumer behaviours.

Similarly, negative emotional components can also contribute to value creation. In some cases, individuals may select organic produce not because they feel virtuous or noble, but because they are trying to avoid fear of chemical residues or pesticides. Providing these individuals with a pathway to reduce their negative emotional state (fear) is also a pathway to value creation for the entrepreneur.

Value creation from a customer perspective is an amalgam of function, amplification of positive emotional responses, and pathways to avoid negative emotional responses to an entrepreneur's product of service. In considering how to 'pitch' one's idea and oneself through a personal value proposition, it is important to consider all three of these elements in their totality and in a realistically calibrated manner. In some cases, entrepreneurs may overstate the importance of function at the expense of positive and negative emotion. In a pharmacy context, this can lead entrepreneurs to assume that dispensing fees alone drive customer loyalty and as a result cost containment to ruthlessly minimise dispensing costs are the way forward. In other cases, entrepreneurs may overstate the importance of emotions at the expense of function: over-investing in spa-like pharmacy settings and assuming 'if we build it, customers may come' may be unrealistic, especially for a relatively interchangeable and necessary commodity like a medication. Finding the most appropriate balance between function, positive emotion amplification, and negative emotion minimisation is an essential component of crafting a value creation strategy.

What is value creation for the entrepreneur?

Value creation from the entrepreneur's perspective is also important. Here, the emphasis focuses on alignment between personal values, beliefs, morals, ethics and entrepreneurial goals. Where an entrepreneur's success is built on a foundation that is fundamentally distasteful or contrary to personal beliefs and values, success will be short-lived and emotionally costly. Where it is simply not possible to align one's personal beliefs with the value creation needs of customers, the road to success will be difficult if not impossible.

For an entrepreneur, value creation involves both objective and subjective elements that need to be carefully understood and constantly monitored. Objective elements of value creation include the traditional markers of success in the business world, such as profitability, market share, market volume, etc. The higher one's profitability, market share, and market volume are, the more consumers are buying and using one's good or service – a direct and objective indication of success. Where these are sustainable over the longer term, true value creation for the entrepreneur has occurred.

However, the subjective or indirect elements of value creation for entrepreneurs often are the difference between long-term and sustainable success versus short-term profitability. Like value creation for customers, entrepreneurs need to think about value in terms of function, amplification of positive emotions, and minimisation of negative emotions. For entrepreneurs themselves, functional value can include the need to be gainfully employed and productive (even if in a non-traditional manner) and earning sufficient money to meet personal expenses and financial goals. Positive emotional value creation usually connects with the individuals core values or beliefs but can further extend towards subjective experiences related to being creative, fully engaged in their work, etc. Minimising negative emotional impacts may include not being constrained by a bureaucracy or 'boss', or feeling greater control over one's work and personal life.

The specifics of value creation for entrepreneurs will, of course, vary based on personality, personal circumstances, and personal characteristics. Each entrepreneur must determine for themselves what value they wish to and expect to create through their activities – and what is the 'bottom line' in terms of minimally acceptable value creation. Alignment of one's personal values and goals with the value creation work the entrepreneur is undertaking, is essential for long-term sustainability – and ultimately, personal happiness.

How to develop a PVP

There is no specific formula for developing a PVP. Much of the content of this chapter can help entrepreneurs reflect upon and learn more about themselves, their personal and entrepreneurial values and what value creation means to customers in the context of their work. This is the raw material from which an effective, honest, and impactful PVP will eventually flow.

One of the most significant challenges entrepreneurs may face with the PVP is the need to take time and pay dedicated attention to this self-reflection. Without it, clear articulation of 'value' can be difficult, and the PVP will likely fall flat. Remember, one's PVP is often the way that investors, customers, competitors, employees, and others will actually get to know the entrepreneur: a flat or less-than-effective PVP will inadvertently handicap the entrepreneur and require more work from them in the longer term to help others understand who they are – and why they should be trusted.

It is important to note that a PVP is not simply a cover letter that accompanies a CV or resume. A cover letter is a document that helps a hiring manager know whether a person is qualified and best suited for an employment role. While cover letters do try to focus on an individual's strengths, experiences, and skills, they serve a very different purpose and have a different format. Cover letters are usually 1–2 pages in length and written in a way that provide details on how previous experiences and education demonstrate suitability for a current role.

In contrast, a personal value proposition is typically much shorter, ranging from a single sentence to one or two paragraphs in length (but generally not exceeding 150 words in total). The power of a PVP is how concise, focused, and razor-sharp it is…PVPs should be memorable for the way in which they create a clear, accurate and highly positive image of the entrepreneur in a reader's mind. It does not speak to experience, education or skills demonstrated in the past but instead focuses precisely on defining and describing the value an entrepreneur brings to a community, a problem, or a customer.

A value proposition should not be overly jingoistic or filled with vapid, cheerleader-driven qualities. It is more than just a catchy slogan: it needs to convey clear information in a concise manner. It will often be the first thing that a potential investor or customer will see or learn about the entrepreneur, particularly in this era of internet-based connectivity and social media saturation; the PVP must speak for the entrepreneur when the entrepreneur is not able to speak directly to potential stakeholders.

There are three critical components to the PVP: relevancy, quantification, and differentiation.[1,2]

- *Relevancy:* The PVP must help readers understand why the entrepreneur – and by extension, the entrepreneur's ideas, vision, products, or services – are actually relevant. Relevancy is demonstrated by clear explanations of the problems or issues faced by stakeholders and how the innovation can address, solve, or in some way make things better. The distinction between the entrepreneur themselves and the idea being pitched is often blurred: no matter how great an idea, few customers will follow through if there is something untrustworthy or distasteful about the entrepreneur. Equally, no matter how wonderful an entrepreneur may be as a human being, there needs to be something meaningful and impactful by way of an idea, a product, or service. In focusing on relevancy in the PVP, the entrepreneur must satisfy the twin aims of showcasing themselves as a trustworthy individual and their idea as one that matters to consumers.

- *Quantification:* Lofty and idealistic statements of relevance can be inspirational and eye catching, but for them to be believable there also needs to be some concrete and quantifiable way of demonstrating and assuring the claims that are made. Quantification can include time saved, profits increased, productivity improved, or any other relevant measurement that is actually verifiable and reproducible. Relevancy claims made without quantification to verify will be quickly dismissed as empty rhetoric by most readers and may actually serve to reduce trustworthiness of the entrepreneur by suggesting they are 'all talk and no action'. Careful, evidence-based quantification of claims is one of the most important ways of reassuring investors, consumers, and other stakeholders of the seriousness of the entrepreneur and their capacity to actually deliver, not just talk.

- *Differentiation:* A personal value proposition needs to help readers understand why THIS entrepreneur and THIS idea are so truly unique; differentiation speaks to the ability to highlight and showcase specific features of the individual and the idea that warrants attention. In most cases – and most marketplaces – there are crowds of individuals who claim to have great ideas or purport to be uniquely qualified with desirable strengths. It is easy to make such statements but difficult to actually back them with fact. Differentiation means entrepreneurs need to have an in-depth and accurate understanding of their competitors, the marketplace, and the needs of consumers in order to explain clearly why they are better than the rest. Differentiation should focus on superiority, not simply meaningless differences; however, it is important to not overstate or become a vapid braggart in the process.

Examples of personal value propositions

There is no formula for developing a personal value proposition, nor is there a perfect PVP that serves as a gold standard. There are, however, better and worse examples that can be illustrative and helpful in supporting entrepreneurs in crafting their own PVP, based on principles discussed in this chapter.

Example 1: An entrepreneur with an idea to reduce the carbon footprint of community pharmacy

If health care were a country – it would be the 4th biggest polluter in the world. And community pharmacy would be the 3rd largest contributor to global warming. As a community pharmacist with 15 years experience, I have been part of the waste, the emissions, and the carbon footprint of our profession for too long and now, I want to be part of the solution. Join me in learning more about my innovative 3Rx program to Rxeduce, Rxuse, and Rxecycle in community pharmacy, that reduces waste by 35% in one year, to make a greener and more sustainable future for all of us – and help our profession lead the way forward.

What is good about this statement?
It is eye catching and memorable, leaning into an issue of global relevance. It quantifies the problem and the proposed solution, and clearly differentiates the entrepreneur as someone who is both a community pharmacist and an environmentalist. It has a jazzy tag line (3Rx program) that centres the innovation in community pharmacy, ensuring the audience/market/customer is clearly identified.

What could be improved?
The 3Rx program is dangled like a carrot without specific examples or descriptions of what this program is, forcing the reader to take an additional step to 'join'. Additional detail, or even a link to a website allowing a reader to learn more without committing to 'joining' might be preferable.

Example 2: An entrepreneur with an idea for an app that allows patients to 'carry' their personal medical health record (including pharmacy records) on a smartphone

I've been a community pharmacist for 15 years and know how frustrating it can be for patients like you to not have access to your medical records and details. It's frustrating for me too – how can I give you the best possible care and service for your health care needs without having the full picture about your health? Your frustration and mine led me to develop HealthCheck, a mobile phone based app that gives you full control over your medical records and allows you the choice to share with whatever professional you choose. It's flexible, it's secure, and it puts you in the driver's seat of your own health care.

What is good about this statement?
It builds a bond between the entrepreneur and the audience (patients) and establishes a common need and common problem to be solved. It highlights the entrepreneurs distinctive and unique background that builds credibility. It showcases an idea that seems to be simple and obvious enough and appeals to a relevant need expressed by patients – to control their own health care and records.

What could be improved?
A more critical reader may have many questions regarding integrity, safety, and confidentiality, and may be skeptical that a community pharmacist could solve these enormous issues; there is little in this statement to truly establish credibility and trustworthiness of the entrepreneur to actually 'deliver' the promises made in the statement. The terms 'full control' and 'driver's seat' might sound somewhat threatening to some stakeholders who are not the primary audience (e.g. physicians) which may produce longer term problems in the future. There are broad promises but little quantification or evidence provided that will give stakeholders assurance that these promises, can in fact, be delivered.

Summary

Entrepreneurs need to be able to clearly identify and articulate their value and the value of their idea, product, or service to diverse stakeholders. There are many dimensions to understanding value and this requires reflection, introspection, evidence, and ultimately a format for clearly describing and explaining this to diverse audiences. Taking the time to craft, test, revise, and refine a personal value proposition is essential and will form the foundation for success as an entrepreneur.

References

1. Indeed Career Guide (2021). *Personal Value Proposition: definition, template, and example*. Austin: Indeed. https://www.indeed.com/career-advice/finding-a-job/personal-value-proposition

2. Barnett B. Build your personal value proposition. *Harvard Business Review* [online] 2011. https://hbr.org/2011/11/a-value-proposition-for-your-c

3. Goldring D. Constructing brand value proposition statements: a systematic literature review. *J Market Anal* 2017; 5: 57–67. https://doi.org/10.1057/s41270-017-0014-6

4. van Praag C.M, Versloot P. What is the value of entrepreneurship? A review of recent research. *Small Business Economics* 2007; 29(4): 351–382. https://doi.org/10.1007/s11187-007-9074-x

5. Hitt M *et al*. Strategic entrepreneurship: creating value for individuals, organizations, and society. *Academy of Management Perspectives* 2011; 25(2): 57–75. https://doi.org/10.2139/ssm.1994491

CHAPTER 29

Business plans

Upon completion of this chapter you should be able to:

- explain the purpose of a business plan
- list the different types of business plans
- outline the sections that should be included in a business plan
- evaluate the success of a business plan.

Business planning is an essential component of success for entrepreneurs and provides a pathway or roadmap for bringing ideas to fruition. It is an ongoing and continuous process requiring constant monitoring and producing course corrections in response to evolving environmental and business changes. While some entrepreneurs may not think of themselves as being in 'business', the reality is that they are: business is a way for entrepreneurs to translate thoughts into action and innovations into reality. Businesses must be interested in, plan, and closely monitor their efficiency, cost-effectiveness, profitability, and other parameters to remain viable and sustainable. Entrepreneurs must therefore engage fully in business planning to succeed.

Principles of effective business planning are closely aligned with techniques of strategic thinking and planning (*see* Chapter 19). Business planning is not the same as strategic planning: strategic plans focus on how specific initiatives, goals and objectives will be achieved to grow and build a business, while business plans lay out in detail how a business will be run on a day to day basis in order to achieve the strategic plan. In most cases, entrepreneurs will want to start with strategic thinking and planning to gain the benefit of the big picture, 30 000 foot view of their environment, their market, and themselves before drilling down further into the details of running a business and generating a business plan. In this way, strategic and business planning can be better aligned and reinforced to one another. Every entrepreneur needs both a strategic plan and a business plan: in most cases entrepreneurs should strategically plan prior to business planning.

While business planning is an ongoing process, a business plan is an essential, written document that provides the entrepreneur and external stakeholders (including investors, banks, and regulators) with a formalised description and overview of the past, present, and future of the business. Typically, business plans serve three important purposes:[1]

1. To formulate and articulate an effective strategy to support the evolution and growth of the business.
2. To identify and justify expected financial resource and other needs to sustain and grow the business.
3. To attract and provide reassurance to potential investors (including banks and other lenders) that the business, the entrepreneur, and the ideas are indeed viable and sustainable.

Small or large, start-up or long-standing, every entrepreneur and business needs a coherent and solid business plan to form the foundation for growth and to inspire interest from external stakeholders.[2]

Types of business plans

Entrepreneurs must work in complex environments rife with ambiguity and with little certainty of success in either the short- or the long-term. As a result, there are different kinds of models of business plans that entrepreneurs may need to consider developing, based on their own needs and the interests of diverse audiences who will read the plan.[1,2,3]

- *The mini plan (or very short plan):* This type of business plan is often valuable to entrepreneurs to encapsulate their operational vision in a succinct and digestible way, both for the entrepreneur and for a potential new investor, shareholder, or banker. The mini plan typically has a short-term time horizon of less than one year, provides very clear timelines and measurements of success, and is best thought of as an appetiser rather than a main course: it is designed to build interest and awareness in the entrepreneur, and provide some initial reassurance that the entrepreneur is serious, and the innovation is viable. There is usually insufficient detail in a mini plan for an investor to make an informed decision, but its value is in introducing the innovation to a new audience and drawing their attention to the potential value creation...and thereby asking the entrepreneur for something more detailed, robust, and analytical. Mini plans are not simply fluffy, vapid marketing pitches: they must have sufficient substance and detail to allow a critical reader to conclude that there is some potential for sustainable value creation at the core of the idea, and that the entrepreneur themselves has the credibility and smarts to bring the idea to fruition. This means mini plans do need to have actual numbers, projections, quantitative data analysis, market shares, etc. in a condensed but defensible way, in addition to inspirational ways of highlighting the potential value of the innovation to specified market segments and customers. It is still a business plan, so many of the elements of a traditional business plan (such as sales forecasts, marketing plan, financial details, etc.) will need to be present, but in a summarised manner to generate an audience's interest to ask for more details.
- *The working plan:* The working plan is the more traditional business plan that provides sufficient detail to readers to truly understand the operational side of an entrepreneurial idea. In essence, a working plan is a roadmap that allows a potential investor to understand how the entrepreneur intends to run the business in a way that will be profitable, sustainable, and likely to create value. Of necessity, working plans are usually long on details and numbers, and short on presentation style and pizzazz. Working plans are usually judged based on the level of realistic detail they are able to present quantification rather than abstract projection. For example, rather than state, 'we anticipate being the dominant player in this market', the working plan should state, 'we anticipate having 35% of market share within three years because of these specific reasons/factors...'. Failure to include sufficient, realistic, believable quantified data in a working plan will undermine the entrepreneur's credibility. Working plans should also refer to industry norms/standards: for example, if the entrepreneur is expecting to

hire other people into the business, it is critical that this salary range be researched in advance and be comparable to what a person would expect to earn in another competitor's business. Further, working plans need to include details on how the entrepreneur is expecting to live and be paid, even in the initial start-up phase of a business: it is unrealistic and lacks believability for the entrepreneur to say, 'I will forego salary for three years while I'm building this business'. The working plan needs to provide reassurance to readers of sustainability, viability, and thinking that is grounded in reality.

- *The presentation plan:* Mini plans and working plans are typically written documents that must speak for themselves and provide details that are read and understood by others without the benefit of clarification from the entrepreneur. A third kind of business plan that entrepreneurs must develop is a presentation plan. Presentation plans include 'pitches', extraordinarily concise, targeted, and attractive ways of describing an innovation, its value, and the unique role of the entrepreneur themselves. Presentation plans typically start with a pitch but then must pivot quickly to provide the kind of quantitative data found in the working plan in a way that is both inspirational and believable. In most cases, presentation plans utilise software such as PowerPoint or Prezi, and are deliberately designed to be visually attractive and stimulating to an audience. They should encourage discussion and interactivity and should never be used in a way that the entrepreneur simply reads text off a slide to a bored audience. Care must be taken, however, to not over-invest in slick slides at the expense of substantive content. Finding ways of taking the 'boring' but essential details in the working plan and bringing them to life for an audience in a presentation plan is essential, with the goal of encouraging questions, interactions, and communication with the audience, not simply downloading information. A typical presentation plan should not exceed 20 minutes in length and cover key points that include the entrepreneur's personal story, the concept/idea, the strategic plan and mission statement, financial forecasts, and operational details.

- *The contingency plan:* The entrepreneurial journey can be exciting, but it is almost always laden with risks related to failure along the way. An essential part of business planning for entrepreneurs – especially at the start-up phase – involves contingency planning. A contingency plan provides the entrepreneur and potential investors with insights and ideas around how to manage 'known-unknowns' and 'unknown-unknowns'. Known-unknowns are those reasonably foreseeable risks and environmental circumstances that could arise during the life of the working plan, and what steps the entrepreneur will take to minimise these risks and manage them/deal with them, should they actually arise, in ways that will allow the business to continue. An example of a known-unknown in a contingency plan may be how the entrepreneur will manage an increase in inflation that affects prices of raw materials, or increases in interest rates on loans from banks due to economic uncertainty. Unknown-unknowns are those unpredictable events that still occur but cannot be reasonably expected: for example, what if a war breaks out in a part of the world where raw materials are sourced, or if a key member of the entrepreneur's team gets hit by a bus and can no longer work. Contingency planning allows the entrepreneur to start thinking about worst case scenarios and how the business will continue to survive – and thrive – despite these events. Developing a contingency plan alongside other forms of business plans is essential, and can help allay potential investors' or bankers' fears, by demonstrating the entrepreneur has actually considered a diverse array of potential scenarios in advance.

Elements of a business plan

While there is no required or single standard format for a business plan, most plans cover at minimum four key areas: a) profile; b) sales and marketing; c) operations; and d) financials. In addition, most plans will include an executive summary that provides a concise overview of these four elements in clear language. Historically, business plans have been prepared for – and have had as a primary audience – lenders, investors, or shareholders in a company. This is important because the historical function of a business plan was to allow an entrepreneur an opportunity to demonstrate the value creation and future potential associated with their work. Importantly, the interests and needs of these three groups can be quite different. As a result, entrepreneurs (particularly those just starting out) may need to have multiple, parallel forms of business plans based on specific audience needs. For example, bankers and other institutional lenders may be most interested in ensuring that their loans at fixed interest rates are likely to be paid back, while investors may be looking to maximise profits over a short time period then get out entirely, while shareholders may have a longer term perspective but are still interested in optimising profits, and creating value (including non-financial forms of value). The financial picture that will be painted for a banker may be different than for an investor: the profitability needed to repay a fixed interest loan in a reasonable time will likely be different (and significantly less) than what an investor expects to maximise in short-term gain.

Business plans are most effective and efficient when they not only address the needs of external funders but also help the entrepreneur develop a roadmap for actually building, managing and growing a new business, while providing all audiences with specific targets and benchmarks by which 'success' can be measured. The operational elements of the business plan are just as important to focus upon as the sales/marketing and financial elements, and all of these need to integrate effectively to demonstrate viability, sustainability, and the probability of value creation.

Most business plans should include the following sections or chapters:[4,5]

- *Business and marketplace overview:* Prior to developing this section, the entrepreneur needs to undertake focused and systematic research and mindful reflection. Research is needed to help the entrepreneur understand the context within which an innovation or idea is expected to flourish. What is this marketplace, who are the major players, and why and how is the entrepreneur's idea likely to change the dynamics of the marketplace? The business and marketplace overview provides an important point of connection between a strategic plan and a business plan; ideally, much of this research will have already been done as part of the strategic thinking and planning process and can be encapsulated in this section of the business plan. Particularly where entrepreneurs are working on their own, this section also needs to present the entrepreneur, their background/skills/ interests/passions in a way that is both compelling and credible, and tie this into the analysis of the marketplace itself. For example, a pharmacist who has entrepreneurial ideas related to optimising commuter train services may not be believable to some bankers and investors unless there is some reason to expect that professional background provides unique or transferable skills, knowledge, and networks. This section of the business plan also needs to clearly lay out the idea or innovation that is at the heart of the entrepreneur's business, in a way that is comprehensible to non-specialist audiences and in a way that makes it clear why the innovation matters, is important, and has the potential to create value for different stakeholder groups.

- *Operational plan:* It is often said that ideas are a 'dime a dozen' and what differentiates entrepreneurs from dreamers is the ability to actually execute ideas and bring them to real life. The operational plan section provides entrepreneurs with the opportunity to demonstrate they understand this, and they have thought through a cogent and credible plan that can actually turn an idea into a business. Particularly during the start-up phase of entrepreneurship, a viable operational plan needs to demonstrate how realistic, viable, effective, and efficient the business side of the idea will be. Key elements of an operational plan will include details related to space, equipment, processes, approvals, regulatory hurdles, etc. that need to be overcome to allow the idea to come to life. Operational plans should be written in a manner that is logical and makes sense to a reader; as a result, a chronological approach detailing steps, timelines/deadlines, and outcomes, and that demonstrates how each step of the operational process builds on previous steps and contributes to a specific outcome, is important. If the idea or innovation is more tangible in nature (e.g. producing a product rather than providing a service), it is essential to define clearly how raw materials are transformed into finished products and sent to the marketplace and customers. Where services are the focus of the innovation, the operational plan may focus more on supports related to information technology (IT), audio-visual (AV), and human resources (HR). Regardless of the nature of the innovation, the operational plan needs to outline how the entrepreneur plans on assembling and organising diverse raw materials and sources into a viable, sustainable, cost-effective, and efficient process to actually bring the idea to reality.
- *Human resources plan:* In virtually all cases, entrepreneurs will not work in splendid isolation but will need to find ways of building and managing high performance teams of skilled individuals to help them bring their strategic vision and their ideas to life. An important component of a business plan will be a human resources (HR) plan that provides details on staffing, policies, procedures, and an overarching philosophy that will guide team-building and development. Depending upon the nature of the innovation, highly skilled and professionally qualified staff may be required by the entrepreneur, and it can be difficult to identify, recruit, hire, and retain such individuals. The HR plan should clearly identify what personnel are needed, how they will be found, hired, onboarded, and retained, and what will be done to motivate them to perform to their greatest potential and stay with the entrepreneur in the longer term. A key element of a human resources plan involves contingency planning: what if key personnel leave suddenly, or an important type of skill is simply not available for hire? Describing ways of minimising and managing human resource risks such as this should be included in the plan. It may also be useful to consider how to manage the business should the entrepreneur themselves be suddenly incapacitated or worse: lenders like banks, in particular, are acutely aware that many entrepreneurs do not anticipate their own illnesses or even consider how their business can exist without them. Insurance or other risk mitigation instruments can be included in the human resources plan to indicate that contingency planning for human resource issues and risks has been undertaken.
- *Sales and marketing:* The business overview section of the business plan should provide readers with a clear understanding of the idea, the business itself, and the marketplace within which the entrepreneur will function. It is important to clearly outline how the entrepreneur plans on breaking into a crowded marketplace, generate awareness and interest

in their innovation, and manage and grow sales and marketing efforts. (*see* Chapter 30 for further details on entrepreneurial marketing.) Briefly, the sales and marketing plan needs to demonstrate how the entrepreneur will connect with potential customers, work with them to identify potential needs and opportunities for meeting these needs and build a customer/ client base that will focus on creating value for both the entrepreneur and the client. Part of this plan needs to be a systematic analysis of the marketplace itself – including competitors – to help readers understand both the potential for growth and risks that may exist within the environment. For many readers, the sales and marketing part of the business plan is the centrepiece as it represents the make-or-break activities that will define success. A key element of this section of the business plan will involve mechanisms to establish prices and values for goods and services produced and sold: a clear, coherent, and defensible mechanism for establishing a price for the entrepreneur's innovation is necessary to allow for the calculation of profits, losses, and other crucial financial information. Extra care and attention to this part of the plan is essential.

- *Financials:* The financials section of the business plan should clearly lay out how money will be spent, generated, and managed to ensure the business is viable and sustainable over the medium to long-term. Of necessity, financials will often involve assumptions and projections, not necessarily actual pounds and pence, especially for start-ups. While this is expected and acceptable, it is essential that assumptions and projections align with the marketplace and business overview sections, are grounded in reality and evidence, and that data and references are provided to back up whatever is stated or claimed. Particularly for certain kinds of lenders or investors, the financials section will be scrutinised closely, compared with competitors in the marketplace and will be used to make judgements regarding the fundability of an entrepreneur. Use of traditional financial reporting instruments like balance sheets, profit and loss statements, and cash flow statements should be used wherever possible: this is the language of finance and consistency with expectations is important to build credibility. (*see* Chapter 6 and Chapter 7) Credibility is strongly connected to financial literacy; using the terminology, techniques, and commonly understood tools of financial reporting and projecting are important. In many cases this may require external expertise, as few entrepreneurs have the accounting or financial management skills necessary to be truly credible. Particularly for start-up situations, it is imperative that entrepreneurs get the financial advice and support necessary to understand and articulate the financial needs and position of the business accurately and clearly. In many cases, an entrepreneurs' own personal financial safety and well-being will be important to consider: unrealistic, dishonest, or implausibly optimistic financial projections may not only compromise the success of a business but harm the entrepreneur personally. Seeking professional guidance in shaping the financials section of a business plan is an important investment and safeguard that is strongly recommended.

- *Timelines, outcomes, and actions:* A business plan is both a snapshot in time and a moving picture; while some of the elements above represent moment-in-time assessments, the business plan also needs to lay out, in some detail, a plan of action that will allow projections to come to life. A chronological timeline that highlights specific steps and tasks that will advance a strategic plan – accompanied by measurements or ways of assessing objectively how successful these steps or tasks were – should be part of the business plan. The time horizon for this section may vary; for a start-up, a 6 month to 1 year time frame may be appropriate, while for a more established business a 2–4 year time frame would be expected. In both cases however, a commitment to planning and attentiveness to details should be evident: readers of the business plan need to know that the entrepreneur can execute a complex implementation process by subdividing this complexity into smaller, meaningful, connected, and rational steps, all of which contribute to an overall strategic goal or objective. Connecting these steps to clear, measurable outcomes that provide feedback on success and allow for course corrections if success is not achieved, is also essential.

Measuring success of a business plan

Entrepreneurs recognise that business can be unpredictable, and the only constant is change. The best laid plans of entrepreneurs can easily become derailed by environmental or context changes outside of their control. Equally, these kinds of changes can also provide a springboard to unexpected and unplanned success. The reality of entrepreneurship means that it is essential to be constantly monitoring, measuring, and assessing the content of a business plan against the realities of day to day business life.

Measuring the success of a business plan can be complex and consists of both intangible and tangible elements. Most entrepreneurs have non-financial goals, objectives, and values that are important to them, and innovations that are not aligned with personal values are rarely sustainable or successful. Even before one considers objective measurement of entrepreneurial success, these values-based indicators need to be reflected upon, understood, and articulated clearly: no matter how much money an entrepreneur makes, it can rarely compensate for soul-destroying misalignment between a dream and reality.

Tangible measurements of entrepreneurial success are fortunately somewhat easier to conceptualise, though they can be difficult to implement and even more difficult to address once data is generated. Some of the most important metrics used to evaluate the success of a business plan include:

- *Financial statements:* The three main financial statements used in most businesses are the income statement, the balance sheet, and the cash flow statement. Income statements measure the profitability of a business over specified time periods and are useful for quantifying and highlighting profits and losses. In contrast, balance sheets demonstrate the overall financial health of the business, detailing how much is owned and how much is owed. Finally, cash flow statements help entrepreneurs to understand how liquid and flexible cash within the business really is. A business plan is a proposal and a projection for how to bring an entrepreneurial idea to life; it is essential to use financial statements on a regular basis to determine how accurate these proposals and projections were, and to determine what course corrections are needed in the event of a discrepancy.
- *Customer satisfaction:* In almost all cases, entrepreneurs seek to create value for their customers. While the specifics and details of value creation will vary based on the innovation itself, anyone in business must closely monitor customer satisfaction: if the target audience of an entrepreneur's work is not satisfied, they are likely to avoid buying goods and services in the future, and this will ultimately lead to the collapse of a business. There are many ways

of assessing customer satisfaction, and no single approach is usually sufficient. Widely used methods include: a) customer feedback through surveys (in apps, using telephone-based, or email-based methods); b) unsolicited/voluntary feedback from customers (usually in response to particularly good or particularly bad customer experiences); c) the CSAT (or customer satisfaction score, a widely used quantitative scale that asks customers to compare satisfaction with other competitors); d) the NPS (or net promoter score, a technique to determine customer satisfaction by assessing how likely a person is to recommend a product, good, or service to friends and family); e) the CES (or customer effort score, a measurement of how much time, effort, and energy was required by the customer to actually get the good, product, or service they wanted); f) web-analytics (an internet-based measurement that tracks online customer behaviours as evidence of satisfaction); g) social media metrics (a tool for determining how customers 'talk' about a good, product, or service on social media sites. While there are many ways of defining and measuring satisfaction (all of which are imperfect and incomplete), it is important for entrepreneurs to consider how they are going to build-in measurements of customer satisfaction into their practices as a way of assessing how successful their business plan actually is. In most cases, multiple forms of customer satisfaction data collection is most helpful in painting the most accurate picture of what customers think, but of course there are logistical and resource constraints that mean choices must be made amongst available methods.

- *Customer growth:* Most entrepreneurs expect their businesses to grow to thrive, and an important measurement of business plan success is simply tracking the number of new customers over time. Businesses that experience stagnant customer growth typically have difficulties in other areas of their operations as well and may over time not be sustainable or viable. The business plan should chart how the entrepreneur expects their business to grow and prosper; comparing these projections for customer growth to actual numbers experienced in defined time periods is an important metric of success.

- *Performance assessments:* While many of the ways of assessing the success of a business plan, understandably, are outward and customer focused, it is also important to consider a more introspective approach that involves performance assessment and review. Employees are essential to any business or entrepreneurial work: without them, businesses could not run or grow. Performance review and management (*see* Chapter 10) can provide entrepreneurs with invaluable information about the effectiveness and efficiency of operations which in turn will directly influence financial statements. Human resource challenges are amongst the most frequent reasons for the failure of entrepreneurial start-ups: effective performance assessment should be able to prevent small HR problems from becoming larger ones that can potentially destroy a business.

- *Constant marketplace vigilance:* A business plan is written at a moment in time and reflects that moment's assumptions regarding the present and future of the marketplace. An important component of evaluating success of a business plan is to constantly monitor the marketplace and compare those assumptions to the actual reality of marketplace conditions, including customer expectations and behaviours, competitors, changes in regulation, and technological evolution. Recalibrating initial business plan assumptions based on evolving marketplace realities is critical, as is understanding how and why initial assumptions were correct – or incorrect – to learn for future business plans.

- *Self-reflection and expectation management:* One of the most important ways of measuring success of a business plan is for the entrepreneur to mindfully self-reflect and recalibrate personal assumptions and expectations regarding their own business. Most entrepreneurs begin as optimistic and hopeful individuals who have faith in themselves and their ideas. The structure of the business plan is meant to channel this emotional optimism in a meaningful way that makes sense to external stakeholders, like investors, who may not be as optimistic, hopeful, or frankly interested in the emotional state of the entrepreneur. Evaluating the success of one's business plan is essential to help calibrate emotions and expectations in a way that still trends towards hopefulness and optimism, but is grounded in reality, data, and experience. It is a fine balance to navigate: pragmatic, realistic optimism is a difficult goal to achieve. Conversely, recognising that entrepreneurship is inherently risky, will involve failure along the way, and does not produce success in a linear, straight-line manner, is equally essential. Calibrating one's emotional response to the role of entrepreneur through self-reflection is an important way of better managing and controlling expectations in order to find that fine balance.

Summary

Business planning and business plans are essential tools for entrepreneurs and provide many different benefits. First, the process of generating a business plan will force entrepreneurs to think in pragmatic and objective terms and helps to ground them in reality. Second, business plans of different sorts help entrepreneurs communicate with different kinds of external stakeholders, including bankers/lenders, investors, and potential shareholders. Third, the business planning process forces a kind of discipline on entrepreneurs: the structure of the plan directs their activities around understanding the business environment and marketplace, connecting with customers, and developing operational, human resource, and financial plans that focus on sustainability and viability. Finally, the business plan provides a useful point of reference and check-in to determine and measure the entrepreneur's success – and to course correct along the way as necessary.

References

1. Haag A. Writing a successful business plan: an overview. *Workplace Health and Safety* 2013; 61(1): 19–29. https://doi.org/10.1177/216507991306100104

2. Abrams R. *The Successful Business Plan: Secrets and Strategies*, 5th edn. Palo Alto: The Planning Shop, 2010.

3. Greene F, Hopp C. Research: Writing a business plan makes your startup more likely to succeed. *Harvard Business Review* [online] 2017. https://hbr.org/2017/07/research-writing-a-business-plan-makes-your-startup-more-likely-to-succeed

4. Nunn L, McGuire B. The importance of a good business plan. *J Business and Economics Research* 2010; 8(2): 95–107. https://doi.org/10.19030/jber.v8i2.677

5. Corporate Finance Institute (CFI) (2022). *Business Plans*. New York: Corporate Finance Institute. https://corporatefinanceinstitute.com/resources/commercial-lending/business-plan/

CHAPTER 30

Entrepreneurial marketing

Upon completion of this chapter you should be able to:

- define the term marketing
- explain the alternative ways of successful marketing
- understand the value of promotion techniques
- consider the techniques for establishing a price for innovation.

The main function of marketing is to get other people – potential clients or customers – interested in the goods or services an entrepreneur has to offer.[1] Marketing is a complex intersection of finance, psychology, motivation, and strategy and requires a disciplined approach that is driven by data (not intuition) and that is constantly being recalibrated as the environment – and client needs – evolves.[2] Depending upon the nature of the innovation, good, or service being offered by the entrepreneur, an essential element of marketing involves price setting: establishing the correct and best possible price that the market will bear that will be acceptable for the entrepreneur in recognition of the time, creativity, and sacrifice required.[3]

What is marketing?

Marketing refers to a series of coordinated actions focused on the promotion and selling of products and services, and includes market research, advertising, and financial projections. Historically, marketing has been described in terms of the 4Ps or the 'marketing mix':[4]

1. *Product:* Developing the right product for the targeted audience is central to marketing. For entrepreneurs, a product can be an innovation, a good, or a service, but the key is to ensure the product being offered actually meets a need, is desired, and somehow improves the day to day life of the intended audience. For example, the original iPhone was a unique product that addressed a void in the market for a simple, easy to use device that paired the best features of an iPod with that of a phone, and later, with that of a camera and a web browser. For this innovation to succeed, it was essential to clearly define what the product did, and what unfilled needs or novel experiences it provided to customers. Since there was nothing like the iPhone prior to its development, this meant that potential customers did not actually know they needed or wanted such a thing, and so a key element involved highlighting how different the iPhone was from anything that preceded it...and how it would actually improve daily life for purchasers in ways they hadn't imagined previously but could actually relate to once it was clearly described to them.

2. *Place:* Historically, marketing has focused on tangible goods, so the place where these goods were purchased (e.g. a large department store versus a small corner store) was central to marketing. Today, in a world of social media and internet-based sales, 'place' simply refers to the way of ensuring the maximum number of potential customers are able to access and purchase the entrepreneur's products with minimal hassle. Attentiveness to the question of how potential purchasers will actually find, learn more about, and buy what is being offered is essential. Finding the right place to market and sell a product is key: if the product is offered in a place where target customers do not typically visit, it will not sell. For example, the initial target market for the iPhone was affluent, educated, busy professionals who were not likely to visit discount grocery stores. Placing iPhones in discount grocery stores would have been a failure as the demographic group who are most likely to shop there were not those most likely to value the innovation that was being sold. Placement also requires careful thinking of distribution channels to minimise risks of bottlenecks that can reduce accessibility, or potential 'funnel points' where it becomes impossible to overcome logistical barriers to providing as many customers as possible with access to all the product they wish to purchase.

3. *Price:* One of the most important decisions an entrepreneur makes is in establishing the initial price they expect for their innovation, good, or service. Accurate pricing is based on careful examination of data (costs for production, competitors in the market, etc.) as well as strategic and tactical thinking: initial over-pricing can result in market failure, while initial under-pricing can produce unsustainable financial pressure on the entrepreneur. Identifying a successful price requires careful research of the environment in order to assess: a) the price range of the product's competitors; b) the price range the target audience is willing to pay; c) clear definition of what price is considered 'too much' by the target audience; d) clear definition of what price is considered 'too low' for the entrepreneur to make it worthwhile; and e) what is the price range that best fits the needs of both the audience and the entrepreneur. For example, in establishing the initial price of an iPhone, it was important to recognise that the target audience was generally affluent and could afford to pay more than the price of a simple iPod or a single phone for the convenience of having both together in one convenient and portable unit...but that the cost to actually produce the iPhone and continuously update it was also higher than producing an iPod or phone. The 'value added' for the convenience and social attractiveness of the iPhone meant that the price that could be charged was greater than the sum of its constituent parts...within reason, based on a more affluent target market.

4. *Promotion:* Helping potential customers see the value creation and generation associated with the entrepreneur's work is essential: in some cases, potential customers may not even recognise they need or want the innovation, good or service that is being offered, and customised approaches help to build this awareness. A crucial element of promotion is to find ways of tipping simple awareness and recognition of value to an active decision to purchase what is being offered. Social media marketing has emerged as one of the most important ways for entrepreneurs to build awareness and to reach potential customers. Further, recognising that each target audience will respond in different ways to different kinds of persuasive techniques is essential. For example, in the initial promotion of the iPhone, it was clear that the target audience wanted to feel special, different, sexier, and cooler than other people and so much of the initial promotion for the iPhone concentrated less on functionality and technology and more on the 'look', the 'feel', and the jealousy purchasing an iPhone would trigger in other people.

The traditional approach to marketing has emphasised the notion of mixing different elements of these 4Ps in creative ways that are appropriate for the unique needs of individual entrepreneurs and what they are offering. There is rarely a one-size-fits-all approach to marketing as conditions will rapidly change, and innovation and surprise are key elements of success in capturing the interest and attention of audiences. As a result, since its inception, additional 'Ps' have been added to the 4Ps to highlight other important considerations in marketing:

5. *People:* Throughout the marketing process, the experience of customers and staff is important when considering the sustainability of any innovation and its ability to be executed effectively. Affluent individuals are likely to be willing to pay more – and to demonstrate greater loyalty – when the customer experience they receive is positive. For example, when the iPhone was launched as a consumer product, care and attention was paid to ensure those individuals selling the iPhone were not simply selling a product, but selling a lifestyle and an experience, making the customer feel valued, 'cool' and very chic for having made the purchase. This produced loyalty on the part of customers, but also helped build morale amongst the salesforce who felt they were doing something unique, not simply selling handsets.

6. *Processes:* Of growing importance in marketing is the recognition of the processes or systems in place that create the best quality customer experience. Customer experience is increasingly seen as absolutely essential to entrepreneurial success. Attempting to compete simply on the basis of price usually leads to a race to the bottom in terms of quality, while creating a process of caring and attentive customer service translates into greater sales and profitability. For example, when the iPhone was introduced, it was not simply sold as a phone, but as a lifestyle experience for the customer that was supported by all manner of helpers ranging from the salesperson to technical support to a worldwide community of users/other customers. A process for building a community around the purchaser provided for an enhanced experience that drove market interest and increased sales beyond a simple technological innovation.

7. *Physical evidence:* The 7th P of marketing is sometimes described as physical evidence, the ability of potential customers to 'see' or 'visualise' themselves as purchasers. For example, in conceptualising the iPhone as not simply a handset but a lifestyle experience, it was important to consider how that message would be transmitted and absorbed by the general population. Product placement in movies and television shows made it appear to the public that all 'cool', 'sexy', and well-heeled individuals had an iPhone, creating an impression that in order to become cool, sexy, and well-heeled, all that was needed was to purchase an iPhone. Physical evidence that reinforces the value-added message of the innovation, good, or service and creates a wide spread positive impression or image will drive interest, sales, and profitability.

The 5Cs – an alternative and complementary way of marketing

The 4 or 7Ps of marketing have been long understood by entrepreneurs but were originally developed in the context of tangible goods, products or certain kinds of services that were more pragmatic in their orientation. Particularly with the rise of innovations that are rooted in social media (for example, new apps), some of the principles of the 4 or 7Ps may not be as applicable, or may not fully reflect the reality of marketing needs entrepreneurs must consider. In addition to (or to complement) the 4 or 7Ps, the 5Cs have been proposed to help entrepreneurs more fully consider external factors of importance in promoting their work and ideas successfully:[5]

1. *Customer:* The audience, end-user, and target market for the innovation is the customer, and building goods, products, services and a marketing plan around the customer - rather than around the interest or quirks of the entrepreneur – is increasingly important. For example, when the iPhone was first introduced it represented a unique technological triumph...but the technology itself was actually peripheral to the marketing. Instead, there was a clear understanding of a marketplace gap for customers (even if customers themselves didn't identify or recognise such a gap) for a device that blended the best elements of an iPod, a phone, a camera, and a web browser. Anticipating customer interests, needs, and wants, even before the customer themselves is able to articulate them, helped drive the success of the iPhone.

2. *Company:* In the context of entrepreneurship, 'company' may be the entrepreneur themselves. A clear understanding of the entrepreneur's strengths, weaknesses, areas for improvement, and opportunities for growth will be essential for successful marketing. In particular, many entrepreneurs may overestimate the importance of their idea, and underestimate the importance of customer need in driving business growth. In focusing on company, the entrepreneur needs to honestly self-appraise gaps that should be filled by others: no matter how brilliant, no single individual or entrepreneur can possibly do everything needed for success, and as a result it is essential to be open to the idea that other people's expertise will be needed. For example, as brilliant as Steve Jobs may have been in conceptualising the iPhone, and as compelling a public figure he was in driving initial sales, he was not the most successful manager of a business and had reported difficulties in supervising and motivating his own staff. The iPhone would have collapsed as an idea had other professional and competent managers not been recruited and hired to address his gaps and weaknesses.

3. *Competition:* Entrepreneurial ideas do not evolve in a vacuum or miraculously appear out of nowhere. All goods, products, and services are part of a marketplace of competitors, and fully understanding the nature of one's competitors is essential for the entrepreneur. Careful and honest market research is necessary to understand the strengths and weaknesses the competitors have and the threats this may pose to the entrepreneur. Systematically addressing these strengths, weaknesses, and threats in a believable manner is essential. For example, when the iPhone was launched, its main competitor (Blackberry) was very successful. Blackberry was (arguably) technologically superior and had the advantage of being first to market with a unique product: but Blackberry was very much designed by and built for engineers, with a linear and functional look and feel that did not necessarily appeal to the iPhone's core market who were looking for 'cool', 'sexy', lifestyle experiences. In this gap, the seeming strength of Blackberry (its technology) was overshadowed by its weakness (lack of attentiveness to the lifestyle experience angle) ...and ultimately, Blackberry went bankrupt as iPhone became the go-to standard for the general public.

4. *Collaboration:* While the emphasis in this chapter has been on competition, building market share and presence, and crowding others out of one's target audience, there are times and circumstances where it may be both productive and profitable to avoid competition and instead collaborate. Rather than try to fight over a slice of pie...it can be to everyone's advantage to try to bake a bigger pie so everyone can have a larger slice. Such collaboration may at times seem counterintuitive

to the entrepreneur, but ultimately can lead to greater success. For example, the evolution of the iPhone and Android as separate and non-interoperable platforms resulted in a competitive stalemate when app developers were (at one time) only working in one universe or the other. At that time, it was thought that blocking the competitor's access to apps would actually improve or build a customer base, but in reality, this kind of competition simply produced a mass of frustrated customers who resented both iPhone and Android for creating such chaos. Collaboration does not necessarily mean compromised co-operation: now, as iPhone and Android apps are equally and seamlessly available it makes the customer experience for both kinds of users easier, and this has resulted in greater sales and profitability for both as the experience for all mobile phone users (regardless of platform) is simply easier and more pleasant.

5. *Climate:* One of the most important but challenging issues facing entrepreneurs today is the issue of climate. Climate refers to the general social, political, and economic context surrounding the market and the customer experience. For example, iPhone's interest in selling a lifestyle experience (not simply a technological innovation) raises significant questions around whose lifestyle is being promoted and privileged. This has led to the need for iPhone to take strong and clear stands in support of (for example) Black Lives Matter, LGBTQ2S+ issues, and reproductive rights for women. It is a complex balancing act: by clearly stating racists and homophobes are not the 'lifestyle' experience, there is of course the risk that racists and homophobes will not buy iPhones. However, by NOT being clear in terms of what lifestyle is being promoted, there is a greater risk that those whose political interests and allegiances are aligned in that direction will also not buy iPhones. As President of Apple (the manufacturer of iPhones), Tim Cook has made strong and public declarations regarding his personal experience as a gay man in corporate America – and this has triggered some backlash from some potential customers, while also creating greater general support from others. Importantly when considering climate, the reality is that neutrality or simply avoiding discussion of social, political or economic context issues is no longer possible or tenable: entrepreneurs (particularly those involved in the promotion of ideas that are pitched towards 'lifestyle') need to make difficult, principled choices and decisions as to how they wish to be perceived by their diverse audiences. Failure to take a stand on these difficult and divisive issues will be interpreted by many as a stand in itself, and leaves the entrepreneur vulnerable to being misinterpreted or worse, having others with a vested interest or agenda imposing their own views on the entrepreneur's image.

Promotion techniques

Promotion is crucial to success as it provides ways for the entrepreneur to communicate the value and value creation associated with the product or service, and a significant element of the marketing mix. Promotions should have a specific goal, budget, strategy, and a concrete outcome to measure to determine effectiveness, cost-efficiency, and success. It is essential to balance costs and benefits: being too stingy and under-investing in promotion can undermine entrepreneurial success by limiting exposure to key customer groups. Conversely, over-investment in promotion can be wasteful and divert precious resources away from other business functions. There is no specific formula or dollar amount that is prescribed for promotion activities, and it will depend entirely on the context, the innovation itself, and the entrepreneur's approach and strategy. A key consideration will be the form of promotion that will be primarily used to reach potential customers, each of which has costs, benefits, advantages, and disadvantages:

- *Advertising:* Mass communication allows a business to reach a broad, undifferentiated audience through television, radio, magazines, newspapers, and outdoor ads (like billboards). Mass advertising of this sort is typically expensive and then requires sacrifices in other areas of a business. The key advantage of mass advertising is the opportunity to reach the broadest and most diverse customer groups possible...which of course means that a target audience will be reached in addition to many, many additional 'non-target' audiences. As a result, mass advertising is sometimes deemed to be wasteful, or scattershot in its approach. It can be most useful in trying to build generalised public awareness, particularly at the launch of an innovation. For example, when the iPhone was first launched, considerable effort was spent on a variety of different print and television ads that resulted in millions of people who had no interest in – and no budget to afford – the iPhone learning about its existence, its features, and its value. On the downside, this represented wasted money as many people who would never have bought an iPhone in the first place saw ads that cost the company money. On the upside, however, it meant that the iPhone became a household name, a valued commodity, and a highly desirable purchase that drove the target audience to go out and actually buy them. For entrepreneurs, advertising is often a high-risk proposition given its cost and its inability to focus and target specific customer groups.
- *Social media:* By far the most common promotion technique for entrepreneurs is the use of social media platforms. The objective of using social media for promotion is to actually find a specific target market and provide a customised message to that target market based on their unique needs, interests, and wants. Unlike mass advertising, social media also permits two-way communication that can further support promotion activities. Platforms such as Facebook, Twitter, and TikTok, or Snapchat, Instagram, and Pinterest can be highly effective – and far less expensive in helping entrepreneurs find and connect with the actual customers they are most interested in finding. Importantly, not all social media are interchangeable; depending upon the specific profile of the target market, there may be a preference for one platform over another. It can be helpful to ask current customers about their social media preferences as a way of identifying priorities; alternatively, commercially available reports exist that help entrepreneurs better predict which social media platforms are likely to be preferred by the majority of potential customers. For example, younger and more technologically sophisticated customers are likely to gravitate to Instagram and TikTok, while older, less technologically sophisticated customers may prefer Facebook or even email. Using social media for promotion also requires consideration of the roles of 'influencers', high profile individuals who are followed by audiences and who may be valuable in introducing these potential customers to the entrepreneur and the product itself. It is very rare that the entrepreneur themselves will also be the best influencer on social media; managing one's own ego and recognising the way in which social media works should help entrepreneurs identify the best pathways forward for leveraging this important technique.
- *Government relations:* Government relations (or GR) is an important promotion method, particularly in highly regulated fields and professions such as pharmacy. Depending on

the nature of an innovation, an entrepreneur may be required to secure certain kinds of governmental or regulatory approvals before a product or service can actually be sold to a customer. In other cases, the target market for an innovation may actually be a government or a governmental agency (such as the National Health Service). Promotion to governmental and quasi-governmental agencies is qualitatively different than to other customers. First, the concept of 'value creation' will have a different meaning in a governmental context, and is rarely about profit maximisation or satiation of consumer needs. Second, governments must follow strict policies and guidelines with respect to purchases that limit discretion on the part of the actual purchaser. Third, government must also be attentive to political realities and the political nature of purchasing decisions. Fourth, transparency requirements means that all negotiations and contracts are generally conducted in complete openness which may alter the nature of promotion activities themselves. Government relations as a promotion technique often requires an expertise that is beyond what most entrepreneurs have experience with; fortunately, it is possible to hire GR experts to support the entrepreneur in this regard. Importantly, where the key or only customer for an innovation is government or governmental agencies, it is essential to tread carefully and recognise that 'second chances' may be rare. Investing in GR expertise to support this form of promotion is generally advisable rather than risk losing the largest – or only – potential customer for an innovation.

- *Public relations:* The goal of public relations (PR) is to highlight the ways in which the entrepreneur and their innovation are creating positive social change and contributing meaningfully to a community. Typical PR promotion activities include, for example, sponsorship of children's football teams in the community, hosting of events, and other ways of recognising that the business, the entrepreneur, and the innovation are all nested within a broader social context. The value of PR in promotion is considerable: for example, when Elon Musk first purchased Twitter in 2022, his profile as a rogue entrepreneur substantially damaged both the Twitter brand and his own personal standing in the community. Outrageous statements that at one point may have been dismissed as 'quirky' became more ominous, and Twitter users – and the advertisers that actually pay to be seen on Twitter – began leaving the platform in droves. At least initially, this would be seen as a PR disaster. The goal of PR is not necessarily to make immediate sales or to sign up new customers right away; instead, it is to create a positive impression of the entrepreneur and the innovation by positively impacting the community and creating goodwill that will eventually convert into sales and profitability.

- *Direct mail:* This promotion technique involves finding and targeting a desired customer sub-group through email, 'snail-mail' or other techniques. This individualised approach to contact allows for careful refinement of a promotional message to more effectively target an individual's interests, needs and wants, and can be particularly valuable in helping to build long-term relationships with customers. The main advantage of this approach is in building upon existing or latent interest in the innovation, in order to convert interest into actual sales. The disadvantage of this approach is the time and money that is required to find these individuals and to customise communication with them. Fortunately, with the rise of email-based communication or 'direct mail' using social media platforms like Facebook, the actual cost associated with the delivery of messages (e.g. what used to be called postage) is minimal. Direct mail approaches to potential customers can be very effective but usually require an enormous amount of time, energy, and resources to begin and may be difficult to sustain unless there is early success with this approach.

- *Personal promotion:* Most entrepreneurs are dedicated and believe passionately in their innovation, and consequently are often the most excited – and motivated – to share their story. In some cases, the entrepreneur-as-salesperson can be a highly effective technique for promotion as it can support the development of a highly personalised relationship with a potential customer. It can also be very difficult psychologically for the entrepreneur when a personal pitch fails – lack of success in a sales call can easily be misinterpreted as personal failure. Further, reliance on personal promotion can sometimes divert the time and attention of the entrepreneur away from the actual innovation itself. There is almost always a time and a place for personal promotion as part of the mix of techniques that will be used, but care must be taken by entrepreneurs to not overemphasise and not unrealistically distort the influence they may have on purchasing decisions.

- *Pricing and sales:* Depending on the innovation itself, one of the most important promotional techniques available is actually one of the other 'Ps' of the marketing mix: pricing. Classical economics theory suggests that price is a function of the interaction between demand and supply components within any market. Supply and demand represent the willingness and ability of customers and businesses to engage in buying and selling; where a supply curve intersects with a demand curve, customers and businesses will agree to sell a specified quantity of a product or service at a specific price. For entrepreneurs, this means that the higher the price, the lower the demand will likely be, or the lower the quantity of products or services sold. One of the most important – but difficult – decisions an entrepreneur must make is in establishing an initial price for the product or service they want to sell. Of course, there is an expectation that the price should cover all the 'costs' of production...but in an entrepreneurial context this can be very difficult to quantify. What is the 'cost' of creativity? Or the 'cost' of sacrificing personal time away from family? Looking to the market to determine how similar products and services are priced can be somewhat helpful in establishing a ballpark figure, but this too will be imperfect. Further, in many cases, entrepreneurs recognise that they must take losses in the early years of their business, simply to build widespread awareness of their product/service and to build market share, at which time increased sales will eventually lead to greater profitability. Entrepreneurs also need to recognise that unless their innovation is so truly unique they are actually irreplaceable – unrealistic pricing will simply result in competitors entering the market and undermining their existing markets.

There is no easy answer to the question of 'how much should I charge for this?'. Careful market analysis, including projections for costs, sales, revenues, etc. and constant monitoring of budgets is essential, but ultimately the process is often one of trial and error. Thinking of pricing as a promotional technique can be helpful, insofar as it helps the entrepreneur recognise that there are other measurements of success beyond simple profitability. For example, early in the entrepreneur's journey, it may be most important to simply build brand awareness and to get the name and the idea of the innovation into the public discourse. The financial value of this may translate into profitability in years to come...but may require some initial ability to absorb financial losses. In most cases, the unique and personal financial considerations of the entrepreneur themselves is the key determinant of pricing: if an entrepreneur's partner has a well-paying job with excellent benefits, perhaps the entrepreneur can afford to take losses for a few years as a way of building a business. If, on the other hand, the entrepreneur is the main breadwinner and has financial responsibilities to others, perhaps no short-term losses can actually be tolerated.

How to value an innovation – and market it

As discussed above, one of the most important but difficult elements of the marketing mix is pricing, which can, and often is, also used as part of promotion. Many entrepreneurs may be intimidated by balance sheets and financial statements and consequently may have difficulty in connecting the value of their innovation with a specific price. Ultimately, however, the objective pricing in the marketing mix is to enable a company to be simultaneously competitive within its market while also maximising (or at least optimising) profit potential. There are several different techniques for establishing the price for an innovation:

- *Cost-led pricing:* This is often the most straightforward method and simply involves careful accounting of all the costs required to produce the product or service and then adding an arbitrary and fixed profit margin over and above those costs. 'Costs' are typically defined in terms of direct costs for labour, materials, etc. and indirect costs associated with rent, utilities, salaries, etc. Typically, a 30% profit margin is applied but this may vary depending on the specific environmental context. For entrepreneurs, cost-led pricing has the advantage of being straightforward, but has a significant risk of underestimating intangible elements associated with creativity and sacrifice that are central to the entrepreneurial process. Cost-led pricing is usually most helpful when there is a tangible good produced, and may be less appropriate where services are provided. Still, as a first approximation – and especially to help prevent the risk of real financial losses associated with under-pricing – it is often helpful to include cost-led pricing as part of the process of determining the best price to set.
- *Premium pricing:* Sometimes referred to as 'perceived value pricing', this model recognises that costs alone are not the only way customers have of understanding the value of a good or service. Premium pricing requires the entrepreneur to quantify the actual value of the innovation to a customer, in terms of time saved, convenience, comfort, quality, or other intangible and difficult to monetise criteria. Premium pricing models are more speculative and require an ability to accurately assess the customer's willingness to pay for non-tangible qualities; when premium pricing misfires, it can be problematic as it means customers are walking away from an innovation and the entrepreneur has likely mis-calibrated the marketplace.
- *Penetration pricing:* At times, it may be important for an entrepreneur to consider pricing below competitors in the marketplace as a way of building awareness and gaining market shares. This may mean the business consciously prices in a way that they will lose money, but gain customers. Penetration pricing is a risky but effective short-term strategy that can sometimes lead to a 'price war' with competitors, resulting in everybody losing. In some cases, penetration pricing can be used as a way to drive less viable businesses out of the marketplace as they can not compete with nor sustain this kind of financial loss. Other terms for penetration pricing include 'loss leader pricing' or 'introductory offers'.
- *Customer-led pricing:* For services and particularly novel innovations, a model of customer-

led pricing can sometimes be used, in which customers will literally set the price based on what they perceive to be the value of the product or service being offered. Customer-led pricing is most typically accomplished through a survey or interviews with actual or potential customers and this is used to establish a price. This model is most popular and effective with technological innovations (like new apps) as other pricing models tend to underestimate the value customers place on unique features of an innovation.

- *Skimming:* This pricing model builds on the novelty or 'newness' of a product or service to justify charging the highest possible price of a product or service to 'make hay while the sun shines'. In many cases, an innovation will remain unique for a short period of time: if it is successful, competitors will quickly enter the market and drive prices down. Skimming means making the most profit as quickly as possible when the innovation is truly unique. This is why, for example, when new versions of iPhones are introduced, the price is quite high, but once the innovations of that new iPhone become more commonplace, the price quickly drops. Some customers value new and flashy innovations and are willing to pay a skimmed-price premium in order to be the first one to actually benefit from it. Over time, however, skimming must be reduced in order to maintain market share and be competitive.

- *Bundling:* This pricing strategy focuses on selling multiple units of products or services at a relatively reduced price to encourage customers to purchase more than once. For example, in the context of a service, a 5-year warranty on an iPhone is usually much cheaper on an annual basis than a 1-year warranty (i.e. than purchasing 5 lots of 1-year warranties). Bundling is applicable to both products and services. Its main benefit is in helping businesses gain more revenue per customer and to reduce the complexity of the order-taking process for both the business and the customer.

- *Odd numbers:* One of the most widely used pricing strategy involves the psychological value associated with making a price point appear visually attractive. Using odd numbers has a strangely powerful effect on purchasing psychology for many customers, even if by now this is a well-known pricing trick. The psychological difference between purchasing something for £50 versus £49.95 can be significant, even if profitability is not materially affected.

As part of the marketing mix, pricing has unique importance for entrepreneurs and must be carefully considered and constantly monitored. The models described above can provide ideas for entrepreneurs for how to best position their innovations to optimise uptake by potential customers.

Summary

Marketing is a complex but essential element of entrepreneurship and involves many different components. The variety of models described in this chapter (ranging from the 4Ps to the 7Ps, or the 5Cs, and the 7 pricing models) are not firm and fixed but merely illustrative, and can be useful guidance for entrepreneurs. Ultimately, the marketing decisions made by entrepreneurs will likely govern the success or failure of their innovation and their business, and considering many different perspectives, models, and approaches can help them make the most informed choices and decisions possible within the context of uncertainty and risk that is typical of entrepreneurial activities.

References

1. Alqahtani N *et al*. Entrepreneurial marketing and firm performance: scale development, validation and empirical test. *J Strategic Marketing* 2022; 22(1): 1–22. https://doi.org/10.1080/0965254X.2022.2059773

2. Collinson E, Shaw E. Entrepreneurial marketing – a historical perspective on development and practice. *Management Decision* 2001; 39(9): 761–766. https://doi.org/10.1108/EUM0000000006221

3. Morrish S *et al*. Entrepreneurial marketing: acknowledging the entrepreneur and customer-centric interrelationship. *J Strategic Marketing* 2010; 18(4): 303–316. https://doi.org/10.1080/09652541003768087

4. Morris M *et al*. Entrepreneurial marketing: a construct for integrating emerging entrepreneurship and marketing perspectives. *J Marketing Theory and Practice* 2002; 10(4): 1–19.

5. Bradt G (2017). *Consider 5Cs - Customers, collaborators, capabilities, competitors, conditions - in onboarding prep*. Jersey City: Forbes Magazine. https://www.forbes.com/sites/georgebradt/2017/11/22/consider-5cs-customers-collaborators-capabilities-competitors-conditions-in-onboarding-prep/?sh=383dc23c321c

CHAPTER 31

Risk management and mitigation

Upon completion of this chapter you should be able to:

- understand the benefits of risk management for entrepreneurs
- outline a risk management process
- list the risks an entrepreneur must manage
- explain how to evaluate and manage risk
- understand the importance of reputational risk management.

It is often said that 'no pain means no gain', or that 'high risks mean high rewards'. The notion that risks are central to entrepreneurship is generally accepted and most entrepreneurs recognise that they – like all business people – can expect to face risks that present threats to success. Risk is generally described in terms of probabilities of specified events causing negative impacts on outcomes; risk management is simply the act of using certain processes, methods, or tools to better manage, contain, prevent, and mitigate these risks.[1]

All businesspeople need to consider what might go wrong and evaluate which risks should be considered priorities for management. Thinking ahead about risks and risk management can better prepare – and insulate – businesses from the worst consequences in a more cost-effective and efficient manner. Entrepreneurs – particularly those just starting out – face unique vulnerabilities in both their business and personal lives, and consequently must be particularly well attuned to how to best manage and mitigate risks. At the centre of this process is the notion of organisation: 'hope for the best but plan for the worst' is a useful phrase to remember in the context of risk management.

Risk management is a process

While contemplating risks may seem like 'negative thinking' or pessimistic, it is actually one of the most important, constructive and strategic activities any entrepreneur should undertake. Risk management is part and parcel of strategic planning and helps to identify and address risks that can decrease the likelihood of success in achieving entrepreneurial objectives.[2] When undertaken in a coherent and systematic way, risk management should allow entrepreneurs to:[2,3]

- More effectively manage internal finances, and capital and resource allocations in ways to optimise the likelihood of success in the least risky way possible.

- Improve decision making through the use of projections and alternative what-if situational analyses.
- Better manage strong and spontaneous emotional responses to environmental events by anticipating and rehearsing alternative approaches to managing change.
- Reduce the need for 'firefighting' or ad-hoc responses to crises by having previously developed plans or frameworks to guide actions.
- Support strategic planning and prioritisation.

As a process, one of the most important reasons to undertake risk management is to help the entrepreneur think, in advance, through a diverse series of potential future scenarios. Having thought through such scenarios in advance can help reduce emotional tension should that specific scenario – or something like it – arise. Reducing emotional tension, in turn, will lead to better, calmer, and more reasoned decision making. Wishful thinking, unrealistic optimism, and wilful disregard for reality are no substitute for risk management, preparation, and planning. Of course, it is essential to temper the risk management process in ways that do not crush hopes and dreams: anticipating and planning for disasters should not lead the entrepreneur to conclude there's no point in proceeding and it is time to go back to bed, hide under the sheets and give up all ambition.

A risk management process should consist of a series of steps and activities, including:[4]

1. Systematically identifying potential and actual risks surrounding the business and the business's activities.
2. Finding a defensible mechanism for quantifying and assessing the likelihood of a specific risk event from occurring, then using this as a way of prioritising and planning.
3. Developing a mechanism, framework, or idea for how to respond to a risk event should it arise.
4. Putting systems into place to deal with a risk event and its consequences that reduces opportunities for emotion-led decision making and provides structure and reassurance for all who are involved.
5. Constant monitoring of the risk management approach and controls put into place.

Risk management is particularly important when entrepreneurs are just beginning: for example, when launching a new product or service, entering a new market, or targeting a new customer group.

Risks an entrepreneur must manage

There are several broad categories of risks that entrepreneurs need to consider in systematically identifying potential and actual threats to their business. These include:[2,3,4]

- *Strategic risks:* An innovation or breakthrough that drives an entrepreneur's passion is often the fuel that drives a business forward. It is the core of what the entrepreneur is interested in and at the heart of a business – and in most cases, if it is successful, will lead other competitors to quickly emulate, copy, or in some other manner, try to crowd the entrepreneur out. Strategic risks are essential to consider. How easy is it for a competitor to copy an idea and steal market share? What is to prevent others from simply replicating an innovation and claiming it as their own. Since ideas and innovations are at the heart of entrepreneurship, careful thinking about competitors and the risk they bring to a strategy is essential. Strategic risks are those that are associated with operation within a specific industry or context, and can arise from mergers/acquisitions, changes among customers or with general demand, changes in the industry itself, and evolution in research and development.

- *Compliance risks:* In a highly regulated field like pharmacy or health care, regulatory and legislative standards and rules are of central importance. Failure to comply fully with these will result in both legal and professional problems. At times, this compliance burden can be irritating for some entrepreneurs who may complain about 'policy wonks' or 'bureaucrats' interfering with innovation. At the end of the day, entrepreneurs must comply with all regulations and legislation, and in fact may face more scrutiny than established players in a market simply because they are new and may be a threat. Compliance risks are often more diffuse than one initially imagines; for example, an entrepreneur who develops a new cloud based app to allow for portability of an individual's medical record, may be surprised to learn how many different kinds and forms of legislation govern this activity, including privacy and other standards that may not be immediately or intuitively obvious. A systematic analysis of the regulatory and legal environment, and the relevant and even tangential legislation governing the innovation, is important in identifying potential and actual compliance risks that can undermine success. Consider, for example, the compliance risks faced by tobacco manufacturers a generation ago...and current compliance risks associated with the burgeoning medical cannabis business in many countries today.

- *Operational risks:* Whether a product, good, or service is the focus of an entrepreneur's innovation, there will always be some kind of operation in place that needs to translate an idea into reality. In some cases, this operation may involve an assembly line or a series of steps to produce a tangible product, while in other cases it may rely more on specialised personnel to deliver certain services or care. Operational risks refer to those kinds of events that may occur that threaten the processes that eventually result in the innovation reaching a customer. Examples of operational risks can include breakdown of equipment, power outages, or hackers interfering with websites. What-if scenarios that help the entrepreneur consider how will business carry on as close to normal as possible if X happens, are essential in contemplating how to manage operational risks.

- *Financial risks:* Few, if any, businesses operate without some kind of debt financing, including bank loans, loans from family or friends, or investments from others, including shareholders. Financial risks that need to be considered include how to manage changes in interest rates on money that is borrowed, or how to manage debt and equity positions in ways that advantage the business. In many cases, entrepreneurs must invest and spend considerable money in 'ramping up' or starting a business before it generates any revenue at all: managing that lag between spending and earning is a financial risk that must be considered carefully. In some cases, customers may go bankrupt, change their minds, or simply not pay the entrepreneur on time: considering how to manage non-payment is an important consideration for financial risk. One particularly important financial risk to plan for involves cash flow risk. If a business is too reliant upon a single few customers and they are delayed or unable to pay, this can have serious implications for success. The way in which credit is extended to customers, and the potential value of insurance to cover bad or doubtful debts should be considered.

- *Data risks:* As more and more entrepreneurs and innovations are based on the internet, the cloud, or other digitised formats, data hacks and breaches represent a particularly new and challenging form of risk management to consider. Even the largest governments and businesses have experienced hacking and compromise of their databases; considering how to minimise or prevent data risks is as important as contemplating how to manage them when they will (inevitably) occur.
- *Employee risks:* In many cases, entrepreneurs will work with others and will hire employees to help build their business. While a tremendous and irreplaceable asset, all employees introduce a different form of risk that must be considered. For example, a key employee may quit or become ill: how will this be managed? Potentially a key employee may decide to become an entrepreneur – and a competitor...how can this be prevented? As labour markets wax and wane, how will risks associated with not being able to hire enough of the right kind of skilled employees impact business success?
- *Environmental risks:* In the 21st century, all businesses must be mindful of the issue of climate breakdown and the environmental consequences and risks of global heating. Depending on the nature of an innovation, this may impact physical facilities (offices, production lines, etc.) or ability to maintain an online presence (due to power failures/disruptions). Considering and mitigating for environmental risks can be challenging but important, especially for longer term sustainability.
- *Political and economic instability:* In many countries, political polarisation has become the norm and formerly stable democracies have experienced once unimaginable threats. Entrepreneurs must function within a political and economic context that has become increasingly fragile and unpredictable. As centrist governments are replaced by right wing governments, this can introduce a variety of different risks for entrepreneurs, including changes in regulation, customer base, etc. Particularly where government or governmental agencies (like a National Health Service) are a large or only customer, this can be an important challenge. Further, economic instability caused by increasing societal disparities is a challenge that needs to be considered.
- *Health and safety risks:* In February 2020, few could have imagined what the COVID-19 pandemic would do in the months that followed. Global lockdowns, social isolation, and online pivots became the norm, all because of an infectious disease of unprecedented proportions and impacts. In the near future, infectious disease and other health and safety risks will likely become more commonplace and will directly influence entrepreneur's work and their success. These kinds of risks related to infectious disease, infrastructure breakdown (e.g. water or food shortages) and other similar problems are important to consider in risk management planning.

Evaluating risks

Listing and reflecting upon risks can be both daunting and instructive, and the list can appear to be never-ending. Risk evaluation is a process of trying to quantify and assess the significance of specific risks, as a prelude to deciding whether to simply accept a risk or actually develop a plan to manage or mitigate it.[2,5] Ultimately, ranking of risks that have been identified will help the entrepreneur to prioritise their time and energy more effectively.

Two key parameters that can help evaluate and rank risks include consequences and likelihoods. Examining a list of risks then applying a matrix such as the one below can help entrepreneurs make sense of and quantify them:

Table 1: *An example of applying a matrix to a list of risks*

	Very likely to occur in the next 3–6 months	May occur in the next 6–12 months	Unlikely to occur in the next 1–2 years
Will result in <80% reduction in market share and/or profitability	0.9	0.7	0.5
Will result in 30–80% reduction in market share and/or profitability	0.7	0.5	0.3
Will result in >30% reduction in market share and/or profitability	0.5	0.3	0.1

While the specific details regarding month ranges in terms of likelihoods or percentages of consequences will vary based on the specific business, this approach can provide a first approximation for risk evaluation. For example, if a competitor were to copy an innovation, it may decimate the business (high consequence) but it may take 18 months (according to the software engineer) for them to figure out how to do this (low likelihood). As a result, this strategic risk gets a quantitative rating of 0.5. In contrast, economists may project that rapid increases in interest rates due to inflation are likely to occur in the next 3–6 months (high likelihood) and the increased costs that flow from higher interest rates are projected to result in a 50% reduction in profitability (medium consequence). This financial risk gets a quantitative rating of 0.7. In terms of priorities, the entrepreneur should focus initial energy and attention on risk management and mitigation of that financial risk rather than the strategic risk.

As can be seen in the example above, quantification of risk for evaluation purposes means relying on data or evidence from outside sources (such as economists' projections of interest rate hikes or software engineers' predictions) as well as more internal reflections of impacts on the business. How 'consequences' are defined may also vary: in the example above, profitability and market share were the main consequences of interest, but other consequences (including effects on reputation or public awareness) could also be considered, depending on the innovation and the entrepreneur.

Alternative methods for evaluating risks also exist, including a simple 1–10 rating of risk with respect to 'importance' for the entrepreneur. Whatever method is used will depend on the particular nature of the innovation and the entrepreneur's preferences, but in all cases, some system of translating hypothetical risks into quantifiable evaluations for the purpose of prioritisation is essential, so the business can have a foundation for deciding how much time, energy, and resources must be dedicated to risk management and mitigation for that particular potential event.

Managing risks

In general, there are four ways in which identified and evaluated risks can be most effectively managed:[6]

- *Accept the risk:* In many cases, there are risks that are real and potentially important but are simply too complex or expensive to actually manage by a single entrepreneur. For example, the risk of geopolitical instability and nuclear war has (surprisingly?) increased in the 21st century – but few, if any, entrepreneurs can actually do anything to manage or mitigate this risk. Where risks are simply accepted, there is nothing really to be done other than to recognise the reality of a situation. Risk acceptance does not imply approval or acceptance of the source or perpetrators of the risk: however, risk acceptance does imply an informed and clear-eyed understanding that some events – regardless of likelihood or consequences – are simply out of the control of the entrepreneur.
- *Transfer the risk:* Risk transfer is one of the most important mitigation and management activities for entrepreneurs. It most typically is done through insurance. For example, a business that is built on an entrepreneur's personal expertise or reputation may take out life insurance on that entrepreneur so in the event of sudden death, there is money available to sustain the business, pay off debts, pay out employees, and wind down operations even after the founder/ entrepreneur has passed away. All manner of insurance for virtually any imaginable risk exists – however there is always a financial cost to risk transfer in the form of insurance premiums that must be paid. Calculating whether risk transfer is financially desirable or possible is important. For example, in managing environmental risk due to climate breakdown, certain forms of flood insurance are so prohibitively expensive that it may make more financial sense to simply accept the risk or eliminate it entirely by simply moving operations to a less flood-prone area.
- *Reduce the risk:* The most common form of risk management is risk reduction. Risk reduction involves implementation of policies, procedures, or practices that recognise and accept risks but use some kind of evidence-informed mechanism to reduce either likelihood, the consequence, or some combination of both should that risk event occur. For example, most organisations use workplace safety and health policies to protect employees who must handle potentially toxic substances as part of their jobs: these policies dictate how personal protective equipment must be used, what to do in the event of spills, etc. Such policies cannot completely eliminate risks associated with working with toxic substances but careful adherence can significantly reduce the risk of an event actually occurring. Further, documented attempts to follow scientifically valid risk reduction practices can further help insulate business and reduce monetary impact, particularly from the financial risks associated with legal actions taken by employees who may be harmed on the job by exposure to toxic substances.
- *Eliminate the risk:* The preferable way of managing risk is to eliminate it where able...but unfortunately this is rarely possible. Risk elimination might involve changes to the business itself (e.g. get out of any business that requires the use of toxic substances, or move locations to avoid building in a flood-prone area). It is always helpful to contemplate how risk elimination might be possible, but it is also realistic to expect that in many cases, it might not be entirely possible.

Insurance

Virtually every business will need to carefully consider insurance as one of the most practical ways of managing risk. Insurance can serve not only a risk-transfer function, but also a risk-reduction function: the existence of an insurance policy can help mitigate the worst potential financial damages associated with a risk event. Of course, insurance cannot eliminate or even reduce the probability of a risk event from actually occurring; it can however help cushion the blow and be a powerful financial tool to protect against certain kinds of losses. In some cases, for regulatory or legal purposes, certain kinds of insurance are mandatory and cannot be avoided. In other cases – for example, risks to reputation – there may not be any commercially available insurance that can be accessed by an entrepreneur.

In most cases however, some form of insurance from a third-party insurer can be purchased for a price. Where insurance is purchasable, insurers generally expect some kind of evidence that the business has put into place some form of risk reduction at the very least. Before even agreeing to sell an insurance policy, insurers may require proof that a business has policies, practices, and procedures in place that will minimise the likelihood of and consequences from a risk event. A coherent risk management plan, developed using the principles discussed in this chapter, is also often a requirement.

There are a variety of different insurance products that entrepreneurs might wish to consider, including:

- *Business interruption insurance:* This form of insurance is useful in protecting entrepreneurs from loss of income and profits that pay for a business to function, due to events such as weather-related damage, or breakdowns in machinery. In many cases, setbacks caused by these kinds of unexpected events are truly temporary; however, in the event that cashflow problems exist as a form of financial risk, then even a few weeks' delay caused by weather-related problems could literally bankrupt a company. Business interruption insurance provides some financial safeguards for continuity in these cases, but often require entrepreneurs to have a formulated risk management plan in place prior to being issued by the insurer.
- *Product liability insurance:* Depending on the nature of the innovation, product liability insurance may be mandatory or highly desirable. This form of insurance protects employers in case of damage or harm to customers of a business's products or goods. There are many different forms of product liability insurance and the specific version that is needed will depend on the product or innovation itself.
- *Professional malpractice insurance:* In regulated health professions, service and care are often the kind of innovation or 'product' that is being sold. Traditional product liability insurance cannot cover errors of omission or commission that cause harm in such situations, so professional malpractice insurance should be considered. Malpractice insurance is sometimes mandatory for some professionals; even when it is not a legislative requirement, it is often a useful risk transfer tool to consider for entrepreneurs, due to difficulties associated with defending oneself against claims of malpractice, negligence, or breach of duty. Even if one is completely innocent, the legal costs incurred to defend against such claims can be prohibitive and will often be covered by this form of insurance.
- *Key person insurance:* For many businesses – particularly new, entrepreneurial ones – there may be one of two key individuals upon whom the fate, prosperity, and viability of a business depends. Key person insurance provides a business with some protection in the event such a key individual leaves suddenly or dies. It is often used as a form of windup insurance, to allow a business that relies on a key person to wind down its operations in an orderly manner and pay off its debts.

Reputational risk management and mitigation

One of the most important but overlooked kinds of risk to entrepreneurs, is reputational risk. For entrepreneurs, their name and personal brand are often integral to success. Especially for start-ups, the reputation of the entrepreneur is often critical to secure funding, interest early customers, and to form the professional networks necessary to allow an idea to flourish and a business to succeed. Entrepreneurs with strong, positive reputations will be perceived as providing more value for employees and customers alike and will generate greater loyalty and willingness to accept risk. Particularly where an innovation or idea has an intangible element and it is difficult to quantify concepts such as 'brand equity', 'goodwill', or 'intellectual capital', reputation becomes a crucial way for entrepreneurs to monetise and convert concepts into reality.

Few entrepreneurs proactively consider the value of reputation management, and instead will simply respond to threats or crises associated with their reputation once a problem has actually surfaced. This kind of reactive approach aims to simply limit damage, rather than prevent damage from occurring in the first place. Reputational risk can be thought of in terms of three distinct dimensions:

1. *The gap between reputational rhetoric and reality:* Reputation is ultimately a socially constructed and psychologically oriented idea that other people have of an individual. While the construction of a person's reputation will be based on facts, events, and observations, reputation itself is simply a perception. An entrepreneur must interact with diverse stakeholders including bankers, customers, employees, suppliers, regulators, and the general community. Each stakeholder will develop its own perception of reputation, but equally these perceptions will intersect and interact to create a generalised reputation of the entrepreneur that will be different than any individual stakeholder's perception. Ultimately a reputation is built and evolves through multiple stakeholders across multiple types of individuals over multiple time periods. Of course, the reality may be different than the reputation (in either a positive or negative direction). Where a reputation is more positive than an underlying reality, there is the possibility of reputational risk, as the failure of an entrepreneur or business to actually live up to the reputation that has been generated can lead to difficulty in the future. It is important to do accurate self-appraisal: entrepreneurs must bridge reputation-reality gaps by either enhancing the reality of their real world performance (preferred) or somehow reducing public expectations (less preferred) to better align rhetoric with reality. Where gaps are large, this builds mistrust and suspicion about everything the entrepreneur says or does and will impact business success. Conversely, in some cases, entrepreneurs may suffer from an undeserved public reputation or may be unfairly labelled due to bias, discrimination, or stereotype, and this can be very personally difficult to manage.

2. *Evolution of beliefs and expectations of stakeholders:* It is important for entrepreneurs to recognise and respond appropriately to the reality that, over time, behavioural expectations will change. Certain practices or behaviours that were once deemed 'charming' or 'evidence of strong leadership' are now considered problematic and inappropriate. Reputational risk is heightened significantly when entrepreneurs do not remain aware of this evolution in expectations and respond accordingly. In some cases, this may mean expressing regret for previous behaviours or practices, or at least explaining the context in which they occurred. For example, today, most entrepreneurs will be expected to conform to broader societal norms related to climate

breakdown, or diversity/inclusion/equity. Importantly, this also means that simply because behaviours worked in the past to help build a positive reputation, they may not be appropriate today or in the future. Careful monitoring and self-assessment are essential to help manage and minimise reputational risk as beliefs and expectations of stakeholders evolve over time.

3. *The entrepreneur IS the business:* For many new start-ups, the distinction between the entrepreneur themselves and the business they run may be vanishingly indistinct. Even when an entrepreneur has employees, there is sometimes confusion on the part of stakeholders as to whose reputation is being generated. For example, an entrepreneur who is charismatic and makes bold promises to deliver a certain product, may have employees who know that such bold promises are completely unrealistic and cannot be achieved. The disconnect between a promise of an entrepreneur and the reality of delivery can have significant negative implications for the reputation of the entrepreneur, the employee, and the business itself. Where coordination between entrepreneurs and staff is weak and there is clear misalignment between promises and actions, the responsibility for addressing this belongs to the entrepreneur. More importantly, the responsibility for preventing this misalignment in the first place should also rest with the entrepreneur.

Reputational risks in entrepreneurial organisations is a significant concern; in general, risk management and mitigation will require the entrepreneur themselves to take control and responsibility of all aspects of reputation management, including assessing of reputation, evaluating the rhetoric versus reality gap, finding ways of closing or addressing gaps, and closely monitoring changes in beliefs and expectations. The entrepreneur's natural inclination towards being optimistic may need to be tempered somewhat, to ensure realistic appraisals are undertaken on a regular basis to ensure reputations remain strong, accurate, and supportive of the business's objectives.

Applications of risk management for pharmacist entrepreneurs

Arguably, the major risk concern that limits or prevents pharmacists in considering entrepreneurship is precisely the reason that many pharmacists selected the profession in the first place: the allure of a stable, secure, predictable job over the course of one's life. The psychological risks of instability and unpredictability can seem daunting to mitigate or manage. Applying concepts from this chapter, it may now be easier to see that the risk balancing of 'pharmacists' versus 'entrepreneur' has many dimensions to consider. From a mitigation perspective, the stability of the pharmacy profession should mean that no matter how poorly an entrepreneurial venture performs, it is likely that a pharmacist can usually find some work as a pharmacist in order to soften any financial blows. Thus, an important mitigation strategy for pharmacist entrepreneurs would be to continue to meet all registration/licensure requirements and continue to renew one's annual registration as a form of insurance against entrepreneurial loss. Further, maintaining some regular work as a pharmacist while building an entrepreneurial business can not only provide modest income, but help ensure the entrepreneur remains current and viable as a pharmacist should a full-time return to practice be required in the future.

Another significant risk concern involves imprecise calculations of 'opportunity costs' and 'sunk costs'. Some pharmacists are reluctant to consider entrepreneurship as they feel they have already 'sunk' so much time and money into completing a pharmacy degree and becoming a pharmacist and that this will somehow be lost if they do not actually and actively practice as a pharmacist. This view of sunk costs is incomplete: the financial 'cost' of entrepreneurship should not include the time and money required to become a pharmacist in the first place if being a pharmacist is actually the foundation of the entrepreneurial idea itself. Even if an individual's entrepreneurial idea has nothing to do with pharmacy or health care, there is cache and prestige associated with being a pharmacist that will confer benefit to the entrepreneur, so this time and money is neither wasted nor 'sunk'. The concept of opportunity costs as a risk factor to be mitigated should also be reconsidered. Opportunity costs usually refer to the financial loss suffered when an individual picks one mutually exclusive option or pathway over another: for example, a pharmacist who could be making money working as a pharmacist but ends up working for free while building up an entrepreneurial business may think they have actually 'lost' money along the way. Reframing opportunity costs as investments in one's own future and considering the rate of return of this investment over time, is an important way of understanding the actual magnitude of financial risk involved....and from this investment rather than cost perspective, it can frequently be positive when entrepreneurial ventures succeed.

One important risk calculation is often overlooked by those considering entrepreneurial options: the risk of personal unhappiness and unfulfillment, and the corrosive and potentially psychologically damaging impact of this over a person's career and life. How can one quantify unhappiness or ascribe a monetary value to professional malaise? The subjectivity of this experience means that traditional financial risk mitigation calculations are challenging to apply; however the experience of personal and professional malaise and unhappiness is real and has real world consequences that need to be balanced. Arguably for some individuals, it is far riskier (for one's happiness and mental health) to be stuck in an unfulfilling job squandering one's talents and life simply to receive a mediocre salary. No standard formulae or calculations exist to quantify this risk – but it is clearly an important risk factor to consider and take into account when determining whether to proceed with an entrepreneurial venture.

Summary

Risk is an inevitable reality of life and of entrepreneurship. Careful consideration and thoughtful analysis of risks can help entrepreneurs better manage and mitigate them to support successful business growth. Risk management planning is essential at all stages of business development and should be part of the general strategic planning processes used by businesses large and small.

References

1. Delmar F. The risk management of the entrepreneur: an economic-psychological perspective. *J Enterprising Culture* 1994; 2(2): 735–751. https://doi.org/10.1142/S0218495894000239

2. Clarke C, Varma S. Strategic risk management: the new competitive edge. *Long Range Planning* 1999; 32(4): 414–424. https://doi.org/10.1016/S0024-6301(99)00052-7

3. Ferreira A *et al*. Motivations, business planning, and risk management: entrepreneurship among university students. *RAI J of Administration and Innovation* 2017; 14(2): 140–150. https://doi.org/10.1016/j.rai.2017.03.003

4. Dvorsky J *et al*. Business risk management in the context of small and medium-sized enterprises. *Economic Research* 2021; 34(1): 1690–1708. https://doi.org/10.1080/1331677X.2020.1844588

5. Busenitz L. Entrepreneurial risk and strategic decision making: it's a matter of perspective. *J Applied Behavioural Science* 2016; 35(3): 325–340. https://doi.org/10.1177/0021886399353005

6. Info Entrepreneurs (2009). *Manage risk*. Info Entrepreneurs/The Chamber of Commerce of Metropolitan Montreal. https://www.infoentrepreneurs.org/en/guides/manage-risk/

CHAPTER 32

Networking

Upon completion of this chapter you should be able to:

- define the term networking
- list the types of networks
- outline the steps for successful networking
- understand the communication techniques for successful networking
- explain the general principles for networking for money.

Networking is usually defined as a process for establishing, building, and nurturing relationships with diverse stakeholders within a business, professional, or industry-specific context.[1] Its emphasis on fostering relationships that are mutually beneficial and reciprocal helps differentiate networking from mentoring or coaching.[2] Networking can occur in many ways and formats, and increasingly happens in both in-person and virtual/online ways. Entrepreneurs sometimes find networking difficult or may believe it is unnecessary and a waste of time. In reality, networking is one of the most important activities entrepreneurs need to undertake in order to connect with their peers, build their reputation, stay current in their field, understand their customers and markets, and observe their competitors. While some more extroverted individuals may find networking more natural or comfortable, even the most introverted of entrepreneurs will benefit significantly from developing their networking skills to build their networks.

What kinds of networks exist?

The term networking is widely used to describe a variety of different types of interpersonal connections, each of which may have unique and different characteristics. The three major types of professional networks entrepreneurs will form include operational, personal, and strategic.[2] While there are differences in each type of network, they often work synergistically together and consequently work best when simultaneously pursued.

Operational networks are those that form within an organisation, team, business, or workplace and that serve pragmatic organisational needs. In essence, these kinds of networks are positive working relationships with those the entrepreneur works with on a daily and regular basis (for example, employees or staff members). *Personal networks* refer to relationships outside a business or workplace setting, and even outside the industry category of the business itself. These kinds of networks are the ones that most individuals think of when the term 'networking' is used: it is about building strong and positive interpersonal connections with diverse arrays of individuals, within and outside one's own profession, for the purpose of ultimately enhancing professional prospects and business success. *Strategic networks* blend attributes of operational and personal networks, with the objective of helping individuals achieve a specific and focused objective. Strategic networks may or may not be enduring; once the objective is achieved the network may dissipate, or parts of the network may be folded into existing personal and operational networks.

How to get started with networking

It is sometimes said that it isn't what you know, it's who you know, that governs success and gets individuals to where they ultimately want to go. Reliance on interpersonal connections to build entrepreneurial success can seem daunting, especially for those who are not naturally gregarious or outgoing. A systematic approach to networking that builds relationships in an incremental way is important: ultimately the quality and value of a network is directly linked to the authenticity and positivity of the relationships that are built within that network.[3] Building a network too quickly or based on superficiality will minimise the value that network can have for the entrepreneur. Quality matters more than quantity...but quantity can be helpful in networking in certain situations.

Starting to build networks

Regardless of the type of network that is being developed, the first steps in networking are often the most difficult. An 'inner circle' approach is frequently helpful. For example, if trying to build a personal network, it can be most helpful to start with existing non-professional networks of family, friends, former classmates, or neighbours to identify where useful overlaps may exist. For example, a former classmate or neighbour may coincidentally be involved in some way in the profession or business the entrepreneur is interested in; while this individual may have been initially known in a completely different context, the fact that there is a pre-existing relationship can help form the nucleus of a new personal network in this space. The initial first steps in building networks can be tiring and awkward, and almost always requires a considerable investment of time and energy. Reaching out to existing relationships by email, text, phone, or other means and simply saying, 'hi, remember me? How've you been? Would you like to grab a coffee sometime?' is often all that is needed to rekindle a previous relationship and start to build a new network. Entrepreneurs may often feel awkward or overlook the potential benefit of family and extended family members, particularly reaching out to older relatives who may know or remember them as a child. In other cases, entrepreneurs may feel their extended family is too homogenous, representing 'only' a specific ethno-cultural or linguistic community. In both cases, careful consideration should be given to how family members will all have their own broad and diverse networks and how valuable these could be.

Leverage social media

The role of social media in everyday life has continued to evolve, and even the most technophobic of individuals is generally connected in some way via the internet. One of the particularly valuable attributes of social media (such as LinkedIn) is its ability to help visualise existing networks everyone may have...and providing a common point of reference in helping entrepreneurs start to reach out beyond their initial networks of friends, families and co-workers. An individual who is a 'friend of a friend' is much more likely to respond to an unsolicited message asking for information or an opportunity to meet than if the message came from someone who is a stranger with no connection whatsoever. Tools such as LinkedIn are particularly helpful for this as they facilitate access to geographically disbursed networks and help individuals map out the ways in which they are connected to one another, and through which individuals these connections occur.

Ask others to facilitate introductions

Networking is built on the premise that every human being is at the centre of their own, unique, and potentially powerful network...and that in accessing any person, there is the possibility of accessing that person's network. When the entrepreneur is aware that a person in their network has a contact within their own network that could be valuable or interesting, simply ask that person to facilitate an introduction via email or some other method. A short message such as 'hey, hope you're doing well - I'm writing today to introduce you to my friend/colleague/nephew who found your profile online and was interested in connecting directly to you' can open doors quickly. Facilitated introductions help people feel safer and more comfortable in speaking with a stranger, knowing that 'stranger' is actually a friend of a friend or a relative of a relative. This kind of accountability and connection heightens both interest in and comfort with this new person and is more likely to result in a response than if direct contact (without intermediation by the facilitator) occurred.

Attend events

Job fairs, professional association meetings, and other organised events can provide an outstanding opportunity for entrepreneurs to meet people who are not connected to their existing networks, but who are interested in similar things as they are. Organised networking events are commonplace in most professions. For relatively recent graduates, alumni meetings can also be a useful starting point. Organised events such as this can be intimidating at first: without the comfort and backing of a prior relationship or facilitator intermediary to make an introduction, it is necessary to be bold, professional, and confident. Importantly, these kinds of events help to remove one initial obstacle: commonality. The simple fact that an entrepreneur is attending the same specialised or professional event helps to establish comfort that they have at least some things in common...and this can form the foundation for further conversation. Where events are the starting point of networking, it is essential to take some care and pay attention to foundational issues related to how one dresses, one's appearance and hygiene, and general good manners. Dressing well, bringing business cards, and rehearsing opening lines when meeting new people is often helpful. It can be particularly helpful to research in advance who else will be attending the event (e.g. guest speakers/presenters, company sponsors, planning committee members, etc.) to help develop some initial ideas for how to introduce oneself and get a conversation going. Where possible and helpful – bring a friend along to help reduce social anxiety and to avoid looking lost or alone in the crowd. There is considerable value to being seen as part of an existing social group (even a group of two people) in such settings. Finally, a confident and well-rehearsed introductory sentence can enhance one's self-esteem in such an awkward and difficult situation: 'hi, my name is Quint Peters. I just graduated from the same school you went to and I heard your presentation tonight. It was so inspiring. I'm wondering if you have a few minutes for me to ask you about your career path so I can learn more.'

Collect – and organise! – business cards

In most professional and business circles, cards are an essential and expected requirement. When networking at live events, having one's own professionally produced, eye-catching and attractive business card is much preferred over scrawling an email address on a napkin. Professionally produced business cards are essential: it is an investment in one's future. Similarly, when networking online, a virtual business card can also be very helpful. Handing out business cards in a professional but not pushy manner is a useful network building technique. Importantly, when someone else hands you a business card, this usually demonstrates interest or openness to further communication and interaction, with the possibility of becoming part of a network. It is essential that all business cards are received with gratitude and professional politeness. Equally important is a system to organise and categorise business cards (paper and digital versions) to not forget who people were, their potential value to a network, and why they were of interest in the first place.

Networking communication: the pitch

These networking techniques can provide a starting point for supporting expansion of the diverse kinds of networks entrepreneurs need. These techniques do not, however, replace certain kinds of networking communication methods that are essential to develop. Simply being introduced to or exposed to potential new members of a network does not guarantee these individuals will elect to become part of that network. There is a complex and intricate interpersonal communication process that is necessary to inspire, motivate, and persuade individuals to join a network and to engage as fully as possible with it to help support an entrepreneur. Beyond initial meetings and facilitated introductions, an effective and professional communication style is necessary to help nurture and sustain networks. Central to this effort is a well crafted, authentic, cogent, and persuasive summary also known as 'the elevator pitch' or the 'hallway pitch'.

The essence of an elevator pitch is clarity and brevity. There is no formula or template to develop a pitch and where possible one's personal creativity should also shine through. The idea of the pitch is to provide a relative stranger with an encapsulation of who you are, what you want, and what your unique, value-added service could be to others. When someone at a networking event asks, 'what brings you here tonight?', it is important to have a clear, concise, interesting, authentic response that addresses all these issues – and takes no more than 30 seconds (the time of a typical elevator ride) to deliver in a relaxed and unhurried manner.

Box 1: Examples of elevator pitches from an entrepreneur

'My name is Rosie Macgruder. I've been working as a pharmacist for five years and have realised how important it is for me – and so many of my patients – to consider the environmental consequences of our behaviours. That's why I'm starting a new business to educate and help pharmacists practice climate conscious pharmacy in a profitable and sustainable way. If you have time to chat, I'd love to share more with you.'

Key attributes of a pitch such as this include: a) the full name of the individual; b) the background and qualifications necessary to confer legitimacy to attend the networking event and to actually spend time speaking with others; c) a personal reflection that explains motivation and interest; d) a 'hook' or interesting turn of phrase (like 'climate conscious pharmacy') that is memorable and intriguing; e) a clear statement of an idea that is unique and valuable to others; and f) an invitation to continue the conversation.

An example of a less successful elevator pitch may be:

'I'm here tonight because I've had it with all the waste and climate impact that exists in health care and pharmacy. We have to do something now, before it's too late for my generation and those that follow. I really think it is essential we re-examine all that we are doing and how we are directly contributing to climate breakdown in this profession. That's why I'm starting my own business to help pharmacies do better before it's too late. Can I give you my card in case you or someone you know is interested in working with me to make the world a better place?

'Key attributes of this pitch that make it problematic include: a) no name or introduction; b) no identification as a pharmacist, in order to establish legitimacy; c) a somewhat hectoring and demanding tone that could be off-putting for many individuals; d) a somewhat sanctimonious over-use of the word 'I', suggesting this person is the only person who truly understands this problem; e) a somewhat threatening closing statement that could come across as insulting to some.

Elevator pitches take time, rehearsal, and constant revision. As part of one's preparation of networking, it can be very helpful to video record oneself delivering a pitch to examine how it sounds and how it looks from an outside perspective. Care must be taken to not come across as being overly rehearsed or mannered, but practice is very helpful to build confidence, poise, and a delivery style that is fluid and relaxed.

Do not underestimate the value and importance of a strong elevator pitch as part of one's networking activities. The pitch is often the first and best chance to make a good impression on a potential customer or mentor. Importantly, many other entrepreneurs and people looking to set up new networks will most definitely have developed and rehearsed their own elevator pitches, so you will be competing for interest and attention with others in a similar situation. A poor, flat, or negative elevator pitch can shut doors quickly, firmly and will be remembered by others...so care must be taken to actually invest time and energy into putting one's best foot forward and crafting the punchiest, most interesting, and authentic pitch possible.

Communication techniques for successful networking

Networking – like so many other interpersonal situations – is both an art and a science. Part of the art of networking involves knowing how to communicate effectively with another person in ways that appear natural, relaxed, but engaging, and interested. In large part, success in networking will be a function of one's ability to accurately read another person and respond appropriately and proportionately. This is – in essence – emotional intelligence (*see* Chapter 2). Part of the science of networking involves a careful self examination of one's own emotional intelligence to identify opportunities to reinforce strengths and to address weaknesses, in order to optimise the likelihood of success in networking with individuals of all different emotional intelligence types. This requires a clear and grounded self-understanding of one's own emotional intelligence, honest acknowledgement of what this means in terms of communication style, interactions, conflict management, etc. and then focused efforts to align one's own communication style and preferred techniques with those of a network colleague of interest.

For some entrepreneurs who may be particularly enthusiastic to tell their own story and showcase their own accomplishments, this may require some careful calibration. Key mistakes some individuals make while networking include:[3,4]

- *Being overly enthusiastic to the point of pushy:* No one is ever going to be more interested in an entrepreneur and their work than the entrepreneur themselves. As a result, entrepreneurs should not feel disappointed, annoyed, or discouraged because someone they are speaking with isn't as excited (or excitable) as they may be. The reality is that in all business settings, it is essential to learn to be relaxed, measured, and dispassionate, especially in initial conversations and in informal meetings with new people. Learning to keep a conversation going just as though it were a regular chat is essential.
- *Not learning how to do 'small talk':* The social value of small talk is often overlooked by busy and motivated entrepreneurs. What seems like vapid conversation about the weather, local sports teams, or consumer purchases, serves an essential social function in networking: it signals to a stranger that you are a member of their 'tribe', that you speak the same language, and that you have the same cultural conventions and rules as they do, and this is essential in building familiarity, trust and rapport. While it can be tiring and irritating to complain about the weather (because no matter where you are, the weather is always wrong), it also serves a function in terms of indicating social ease and awareness of conventions. Learning to do small talk may not come easily or naturally for some entrepreneurs, but it is the 'price of admission' to many networking circles. Before chatting about business or financial matters, small talk provides an opportunity to build social bonds that will support better business-related conversations in the immediate future. Small talk means avoiding the use of all technical terminology, jargon, slogans – and even elevator pitches and resumes. Simply being an authentic human being who can demonstrate interests outside business and awareness of a world outside the entrepreneurial innovation itself, is necessary. In most cases, this means knowing when (and how) to deliver the elevator pitch or ask for a business card. Moving too quickly to these activities will appear selfish and obsessive, and will decrease the likelihood of networking success.
- *Telling too much:* Many entrepreneurs are understandably nervous, awkward, or shy when embarking upon a networking event. Depending on one's emotional intelligence, this may translate into a pattern of behaviour that appears socially awkward and off-putting: a tendency to 'show-off' and 'tell' rather than ask questions. In situations of social awkwardness, where connections with people may be difficult, questions are usually the best way to break tension and invite individuals to become more personal in their responses. A question like 'how did you get to the position you're currently in' invites an autobiographical response...and most individuals enjoy talking about themselves and relating their successes to strangers.

It is human nature to respond positively when other people seem interested in you; asking biographical questions is a powerful way of demonstrating interest...so long as these biographic questions do not become inappropriately personal or salacious. Even a simple question like, 'how are you enjoying tonight's networking event?' can be sufficient to move a conversation forward and indicate interest in another person's feelings and experience.

- *Asking questions the wrong way:* Much of the networking relationship involves individuals learning more about one another through questioning and listening. For some individuals, there is a general need to make overly quick and superficial judgements about others and whether they are suitable for further investment of time in building a networking relationship. This situation may result in the overuse of a certain type of questioning technique that relies too heavily on closed-ended questions. Closed-ended questions are those that have a 'yes' or 'no' answer; for example, 'does your company provide start-up funding for entrepreneurs in my field?' While it may be understandable that the entrepreneur simply wants to cut to the chase and get a quick answer to a practical question so as not to waste everyone's time, the use of closed-ended questions comes across as harsh, disinterested, and ultimately impersonal. A series of closed-ended questions asked in rapid fire sequence feels like a machine gun spitting out bullets, and is not likely to incline someone to be interested in you or your ideas. Learning to ask open-ended questions and genuinely listening to the responses is preferred, especially when first beginning to meet people in a network. Asking, 'what does your company look for when making start-up funding decisions for new entrepreneurs' is so much less aggressive and threatening, and allows the person being questioned far more latitude in responding....and this in turn makes the individual want to engage further and more fully in a conversation rather than a simple 'yes' or 'no'.

- *Not taking advantage of 'common ground':* It is human nature to feel more comfortable with, and be more supportive of, those with whom we share a commonality. That commonality could be a hobby or interest, an ethno-cultural background or language, or a religious or political affiliation. It could even be allegiance to the same football club, shared love of Italian food, or strong views on current TV shows. Networking is facilitated by common ground, and successful networking requires sophisticated communication techniques designed to find and nurture that common ground as a foundation for further interaction. It is essential to never 'fake' common ground simply for the purpose of building a connection: this is extremely transparent, insulting, and will ultimately be counterproductive to the goal of building a relationship. In most cases, individuals will find at least a few pieces of common ground they share, and this can be the foundation for building a networking relationship – even if there are many more differences they experience in other areas.

- *Determining what to do with differences:* In today's increasingly polarised political and social world, it is easy to imagine that everyone is everyone else's enemy and that we are all in a battle for survival of the fittest. It has long been understood that certain topics – for example, politics, religion, and sex – should be carefully avoided in professional and polite conversations, and for those attempting to build new networking relationships. This continues to be – in general – good advice. Still there may be circumstances where an entrepreneur wants to connect with an individual and is able to find some common ground – but also identifies a significant difference of beliefs or values with respect to an issue of personal importance. For example, a potentially valuable and influential network contact may have political or social views the entrepreneur finds odious or disagreeable: determining whether it is worth 'biting one's tongue' and continuing to focus on common ground while carefully avoiding this difference can be difficult. As in life, there is no easy answer for how to proceed in a situation such as this: the strength of one's personal convictions is an important determinant, as is the question of how opposite the other person's views really are. Ultimately, some differences cannot be papered over and ignored indefinitely, and in some cases no matter how 'valuable' a potential network contact might be to an entrepreneur, it is simply not worth engaging further for personal moral reasons as well as for business risk management reasons. Learning how to extricate oneself from a blossoming – but potentially negative – networking relationship is important. In almost all cases, it is essential to be both polite and grateful for the time already spent, and gracious in indicating no further contact is needed at this time, without diminishing or insulting the individual directly or obliquely.

- *Letting a potential relationship dangle:* One of the most irritating experiences for mentors and potential network colleagues is the experience of being ghosted. After having met a young entrepreneur, having an engaging conversation, offering a business card, and expressing openness to further conversation, it can be quite annoying if that young entrepreneur doesn't follow-up to say thank you and when can we meet again. Within a few days of meeting someone, it is important to follow-up – usually by email – with a polite, professional, and genuine thank you and sincere appreciation for the opportunity of getting to know them better. A short and easy to compose email such as this will make an enormous difference in impression management: an interaction with a stranger in an evening filled with interactions with strangers will become so much more memorable and remembered positively if it is wrapped up with a bow by such an email. If any promises or commitments were made in the initial networking conversation (e.g. 'I'll send over my CV to you straight away and would love your feedback') this needs to be followed-up as promised.

- *Overly-engineering network relationships:* The best and most valuable networks evolve naturally and organically, driven by spontaneity, humour, and shared experiences. 'Hanging out' rather than opportunistic networking is often a much more mutually satisfying experience and ultimately results in the kinds of interpersonal connections that yield solid and enduring business relationships. Only reaching out to individuals when there are problems to solve, jobs to fill, or money to make, creates a less-than-optimal interpersonal space. Like all relationships, building a network takes time – it cannot be rushed or pushed onto individuals without irritating or alienating them. Part of the process will involve rejection or less than hoped for outcomes, but this too is important for learning and development. Importantly, while this chapter has focused on the role of networks in entrepreneurship – networks are also not everything. They are only one component of some importance in the building of a business. Having realistic expectations regarding a network, its value and impact, and the roles of people within the network is essential. Ultimately, networks work best when the people in them actually and genuinely enjoy one another's time and company and are having some measure of fun beyond the utilitarian and business-related conversations they have.

Networking for money

One of the realities for most entrepreneurs is that a central function of networking is to support attempts to raise capital to fund new ideas and a new business. Asking for money is amongst the most awkward yet necessary activities of entrepreneurship. Even when 'initial investors' are family members or friends, using personal networks to raise funds for a business venture requires careful management of relationships, expectations, and communications. This can be amplified when the network being approached for financial support is composed of non-relatives or strangers who have no interest in the personal life of the entrepreneur.

There is more art than science to networking for money and for many entrepreneurs they will need to learn what works best for them, rather than reading general advice such as this. Still, experience suggests there are some general principles that are of importance when networks are being built and accessed for financial reasons.[5]

People invest in people they like

Despite Hollywood rhetoric that suggests 'business is never personal', the reality is that in most circumstances, interpersonal connections facilitate investor confidence. No matter how large or small an investor or funder may be, they are almost always more likely to want to work with an entrepreneur they like, they find charming or quirky, or that impresses them. Emotions and emotional investment are literally at the heart of finances and financial investments. An investors state of mind and emotional response to an entrepreneur will not only govern whether 'yes' or 'no' is the answer, but also the size of the investment and the terms under which it is offered. The interpersonal dimensions of financial decision making are essential to recognise. Of course, simply liking someone is not a guarantee that an investment will be made – many nice, funny, and charming people who ask for money won't receive it because, frankly, their ideas are not worth funding. Conversely, some entrepreneurs with great ideas will not be funded because an investor simply finds them unlikable.

One of the powers of networking is the ability to showcase the entrepreneur's personality, charms, and strengths in a context beyond business or the innovation itself. Using networking for this purpose will smooth the path towards the ultimate destination of asking for money – but it, of course, will never guarantee it. As a result, entrepreneurs must be constantly vigilant about the impression they are making and work towards the creation of a positive emotional state with each interaction. Building these kinds of bonds will be essential when the time comes to ask for and negotiate financial investments.

How you ask for money is as important as the money you ask for

While personal connections are a necessary precondition for most financial investments, the reality is that such relationships are only the first step. A key element of successful networking for money involves confidence on the part of the investor that their investment will be productive and profitable. There is a generally accepted way of presenting a confident 'ask' for funding from others that involves clear descriptions of the following:

1. This is what we've accomplished so far.
2. This is what we need more funding in order to finish.

3. This is what we will use the funding to do.
4. These are the results that we will measure and report on.
5. This is how long we expect it will take to see results.
6. This is what these results will do for the people who invest.
7. This is how much money we need – and how much I'm asking you for today.

Importantly, the actual 'ask' comes at the end of this sequence, after which no more really needs to be said. In fact, use of productive silence following the actual request can provide the entrepreneur with immediate feedback regarding the likelihood of success. The logical progression of information from item 1–7 should address most of the potential funder's questions and concerns, and allow them to process the information for their own decision making purposes. It is generally ill-advised to state up-front 'the ask': prematurely introducing financial details without providing the context of items 1–6 focuses the attention on money too soon, rather than an idea and its potential.

Find the people and networks that are right for you

Asking for money is never easy, but it is infinitely more complex if the entrepreneur fundamentally dislikes or disagrees with the individual being asked. In many cases, it is better to not get funding or an investment from an investor who will be problematic or worse. As much as the investor must carefully assess the 'fit' with the entrepreneur, so too must the entrepreneur assess the value of an investment from a particular individual or group. Networking is a two-way street: some money is simply not worth getting if it will compromise or adversely impact on the entrepreneur's reputation. The power of networking means that entrepreneurs have options – and opportunities to compare potential investors and supporters to determine the best possible fit, and not just simply jump at the first person who opens a wallet. What determines 'best possible fit' will of course vary from person to person and from idea to idea, but an alignment of values, interpersonal chemistry, and a track record of successfully supporting other new entrepreneurs are likely pre-requisites for a successful relationship.

Summary

Networking is an important, challenging, and frequently overlooked element of entrepreneurship. While there are many benefits to networking, it is usually a necessity when it comes to finding monetary support for entrepreneurs and asking for money. Networks have a unique power and ability to help entrepreneurs, but learning to build, nurture, sustain and benefit from networks takes time, energy, and attention. Even the most introverted of entrepreneurs will benefit from developing diverse professional networks – investing the time to do so effectively and to showcase one's potential to diverse audiences will yield impressive dividends.

References

1. Gino F *et al*. Learn to love networking. *Harvard Business Review* [online] 2016. https://hbr.org/2016/05/learn-to-love-networking

2. Jacobs S *et al*. 'Knowing me, knowing you': the importance of networking for freelancers' careers: Examining the mediating role of need for relatedness fulfillment and employability - enhancing competencies. *Front Psychol* 2019; 10: 2055. https://doi.org/10.3389/fpsyg.2019.02055

3. Goolsby M, Knestrick J. Effective professional networking. *J Am Assoc Nurse Practitioners* 2017; 29(8): 441–445. https://doi.org/10.1002/2327-6924.12484

4. De Janasz S, Forrett M. Learning the art of networking: a critical skill for enhancing social capital and career success. *J Management Education* 2008; 32(5): 629–650. https://doi.org/10.1177/1052562907307637

5. Cary A, Flynn R. The importance of professional networks. *J Archival Organization* 2019; 16(2-3): 144–150. https://doi.org/10.1080/15332748.2019.1680123

CHAPTER 33

Execution of entrepreneurial ideas

> **Upon completion of this chapter you should be able to:**
>
> - understand the importance of successful execution for entrepreneurs
> - list the three key elements of execution
> - explain the steps for successful execution
> - outline the tips for enhancing the likelihood of successful implementation.

Many – and probably most – of the best entrepreneurial ideas never become a reality.[1] It is sometimes said that great ideas are a 'dime a dozen' or that an entrepreneurial brainwave plus £2.50 buys you a cup of coffee...suggesting that ideas by themselves are in reality worthless. Of course, without an idea, without inspiration and creativity, entrepreneurship will not occur. Importantly, simply having an idea or a concept is equally unlikely to result in success. What is crucial is the concept of 'execution', the ability to convert ideas into reality. Execution is a rigorous, logical, and disciplined process of interconnected and purposeful activities, tasks and steps that enable an entrepreneur to take an idea, convert it into a strategy, then actually make it work through implementation.[2] Without a careful and planned approach to execution, ideas and strategies will rarely be successful.[3]

In the business world, there is a constant debate around which is most important: ideas or execution. Like the 'nature versus nurture' debate in psychology, the ideas versus execution debate in business is a false dichotomy. Both are essential, both are difficult, and each relies heavily on the other. Ideas and execution are inseparable. Execution helps to not only enrich and refine initially rough or vague ideas, but it also helps to test the potential of an idea at various stages to determine its viability, and the likelihood of success in the real world.

Ideas will typically fail to succeed for several reasons:[4]

- *Operational ineptness:* Basic business skills related to punctuality, reliability, organisation, and predictability are essential for entrepreneurs. The image of a wild-eyed, absent-minded entrepreneur who somehow manages to stumble into fame and fortune despite quirky interpersonal skills, is misleading and vanishingly rare. The reality is that most entrepreneurs are amongst the most organised and effective of individuals, with a disciplined work ethic, a strong sense of organisation, and superior interpersonal skills. Most entrepreneurs have skills that would be highly valued and rewarded in traditional large corporations and they would be likely to succeed in that environment; however, for personal reasons they choose a different path that allows them to leverage these important operational competencies in their own way.

- *Absence of a strategy:* An idea is not a strategy. A concept alone will almost never result in business success; however an idea that is used as the foundation for a systematic strategic planning process is more likely to be successful. Strategic planning is a foundational competency for managers, leaders and entrepreneurs, but is particularly important for entrepreneurs who need to understand and articulate their personal value proposition, their objectives, and their goals. While it may appear unnecessary or almost comical for a solo entrepreneur to initiate a strategic plan, it is both essential and practical. Having a reference point to constantly refer to as a business evolves and grows is the foundation for entrepreneurial success.
- *Accurately reading and understanding the marketplace:* In some cases, entrepreneurs may fall in love with their own ideas, and this can sometimes result in them making poor decisions or simply not accurately reading their environment or context. While the emotional and psychological energy that flows from falling in love with one's own idea is powerful and a significant driver for success, it must be tempered by a constant reading of the marketplace and the environment. In this context, this means understanding customers, understanding competitors, and understanding other players (such as regulatory bodies, or government agencies) that are part of this space. Understanding these marketplace players requires research that confirms assumptions and beliefs; it requires data from credible external sources, not simply the perception of the entrepreneur and their friends, and it requires close monitoring over time as trends are generally more important than a single snapshot. Aligning one's great idea with marketplace needs, realities and expectations is essential, and recognising that stubbornly clinging to a beloved idea is costly and likely to ultimately end in failure is important.

Entrepreneurs need not be creative geniuses or technological superstars; instead, a strong work ethic, a passionate belief, and business skills are essential. Three key elements of execution to consider – especially for a start-up – are feasibility, scalability, and passion.[5]

1. *Feasibility:*Almost everyone at some point has had a 'great idea' they were sure would convert into wealth and fame. Developing ideas is surprisingly easy – developing feasible ideas is actually difficult. Most entrepreneurs recognise that their initial concepts and ideas are simply not viable, and very quickly begin to incorporate feasibility constraints on their thinking before moving forward. Determining the feasibility of an idea will require external, objective scrutiny from others, and is not simply an internal calculation performed by the entrepreneur. Formal feasibility studies of ideas examine technical, economic, financial, legal, and environmental factors, even before considering marketplace or strategic issues. As part of a feasibility study, it is important to determine if the entrepreneur has – or has access to – the right people, the financial resources, and the technologies required to make an idea viable. It must also include some form of cash-flow analysis to determine the level of cash that can potentially be generated from revenues as compared to the operational costs of delivering the idea. A risk assessment should also be completed as part of a feasibility study to determine whether projected financial returns and gains are sufficient to offset the risk of undertaking the proposed idea. Importantly, simply because an idea is feasible does not necessarily mean it should be executed. Other considerations will impact on this decision. However, before even thinking of advancing with an idea, it is essential to demonstrate that it is, at bare minimum, feasible based on the parameters highlighted above.

2. *Scalability:* Most entrepreneurs with great ideas want businesses that will succeed – and a significant element of success in most businesses is the capacity to grow to some desired level. Scalability is an important element of execution to consider, as it requires the entrepreneur to consider factors beyond themselves that will accelerate or limit growth potential. In some cases, an entrepreneur's ideas are generalisable; other, similarly skilled individuals could have come up with a similar idea and could just as easily execute it if they wished. In other cases, there is something so unique about the entrepreneur and their idea that it is impossible for anyone else to ever really replicate it. Unscalable ideas such as this have a built-in limit to growth; if growth is an expectation of the entrepreneur (rather than a one-off delivery of the idea), an unscalable idea may not be suitable for execution. In contrast, an idea that is all-too easily scalable may be vulnerable to competition which may also influence decisions as to whether it should be executed. Midway, in an ideal situation, ideas are sufficiently scalable to allow for profitable, measured, and controlled growth but not so readily scalable that any competitor can quickly undercut the entrepreneur.

3. *Passion:* Despite the cautious tone of this chapter and the emphasis on execution, the reality, of course, is that virtually every entrepreneur needs to have a strong degree of passion for their idea to provide the psychological fuel necessary to sustain the expected and unexpected hardships associated with entrepreneurship. Entrepreneurship entails inherent risks and sacrifices; an entrepreneur needs to have faith in an idea and be sufficiently optimistic to endure these. Further, the passion of the entrepreneur can also be infectious and help customers, lenders, investors, and others 'see' the idea in fresh ways.

The pathway to successful execution

The following points should all be considered for successful execution:

- *Avoid choice overload:* Psychologists describe the process of choice overload as a situation where individuals have so many different options in front of them, they become cognitively paralysed and unable to actually make a decision.[5] Where decisions are made in a choice overload situation, they are often focused on immediate short-term gratification due to the mistaken belief that the abundance of choices will always be there – and the erroneous assumption that making a sub-optimal choice will not close doors or have other unwanted consequences. For many entrepreneurs, 'idea overload' is a similar problem: juggling too many great ideas – and indulging in the feel good satisfaction of being so clever as to come up with all these ideas! – is a cognitive trap that leads to an infinite loop of thinking and inaction. Idea overload can sometimes be managed by writing ideas down and then doing something – anything – with them to start the process of shifting from thinking to action. Ideas need to find a way out of the entrepreneur's head and into the world; simply writing it down on a piece of paper and showing it to someone else can often start a conversation that will be the first step in avoiding choice overload.
- *Understand and appreciate criticism as data:* The fairy tale of the single-minded entrepreneur who damns the torpedoes and slays the nay-sayers is an enduring Hollywood

fantasy. It suggests a kind of unrealistic optimism and faith that is more likely to be damaging than helpful for the entrepreneur. Negative thoughts can become paralysing and demoralising on their own but they should not be ignored or suppressed simply for this reason. One's own negative thoughts, or those of another person with whom an idea is being shared, are important pieces of data. Being open minded enough to recognise that an idea one loves can still benefit from review and comments from others is an essential part of execution. Do not discount and dismiss criticism as simply jealousy – actively solicit it and work to appreciate what it means for the refinement of an idea.

- *Think in terms of short, medium and long-term:* Entrepreneurs often find themselves in one of two camps: considering either immediate gratification and short-term wins, or being so long-term in their thinking that the here and now seems irrelevant. Assuming an unsustainable amount of debt in the name of 'long-term thinking' is as unhelpful as simply focusing on a fast buck today at the expense of established relationships tomorrow. While individuals may have their own personal tendencies towards long- or short-term thinking, entrepreneurs must be intentional in bracketing their planning around different time frames: shorter term (usually less than 1 year), medium-term (1–3 years) and long-term (3–5 years). Where ideas suggest longer time frames than five years, they are often best discounted at an early stage as environmental and societal changes occur so rapidly that five years from today will be utterly different than when a long-term plan was first conceived. Bracketing one's thinking and planning around three distinct time periods (each with their own unique issues) is very helpful for planning. For example, in the short-term, financial losses and extraordinary workload may be sustainable to launch an idea, build some initial market presence, and start up a new business. In the mid-term, unsustainable workload must stop, even if milder financial losses could be acceptable. If, however by the long-term (three years) financial losses continue, then there is a serious issue which must be managed. Carefully bucketing expectations, tasks, outcomes, and milestones into short-, medium- and long-term plans is an important way of executing ideas and bringing them to reality.
- *Descartes Squares as a tool for pros and cons:* Analysing one's ideas from multiple perspectives is an essential part of implementation. In many cases, the most straightforward and frequently used form of analysis is a 'pros and cons' list, in which reasons for proceeding with an idea (pros) are balanced against reasons for not proceeding (cons). A more sophisticated and helpful form of analysis for entrepreneurs is the use of Descartes Squares, as depicted below:

PROS of executing	PROS of NOT executing
• Market need • Desire for independence from work • Primary customer identified	• Less personal stress • More personal financial security • More time to refine idea
CONS of executing	CONS of NOT executing
• Personal financial burden • Increased workload and personal stress • What if no other customers identified?	• Someone else will steal the idea • Primary customer will go elsewhere • Market preferences might change in the future

As can be seen, the Descartes Squares approach to pros and cons analysis is somewhat more sophisticated and can help surface underlying issues that may undermine the entrepreneur's ability to execute an idea successfully. In particular, the pros of executing and the cons of not executing are often particularly relevant in this approach and can provide important data for the entrepreneur to consider enhancing implementation or support decision making.

- *Use your strategic plan effectively:* Every entrepreneur needs a strategic plan that has been generated through a methodical process of environmental and marketplace assessment. The use of SWOT (strengths, weaknesses, opportunities, threats) or similarly structured analysis is helpful in planning execution. Leveraging strengths and exploiting opportunities, while mitigating weaknesses and avoiding threats, is an important pathway to successful implementation. Explicitly addressing how each of these will be accomplished can help entrepreneurs avoid problems that will undermine successful execution.

- *360-degree feedback:* Entrepreneurs must function at the centre of complex business, social, and interpersonal networks. They must juggle customer needs, investor expectations, supplier requirements, and employee issues. To succeed, all stakeholders' needs must be carefully calibrated, understood, and eventually balanced in a way that is sustainable. 360-degree feedback is a tool to help entrepreneurs understand how they 'appear' to other stakeholders around, above, below, in front of, behind, and beside them. As the term implies, all stakeholders that surround the entrepreneur are consulted as part of the 360-degree feedback process. Traditionally, entrepreneurs have over-relied on only one or two sources of feedback, for example an investor, and a colleague. These important but limited slices of feedback will mean the entrepreneur does not get the full picture of where they are now and where they are going. While there are consultants and companies that will undertake formal (and expensive) 360-degree feedback sessions for clients, this is not always necessary. Simply being mindful of the value that everyone in the complex network around the entrepreneur can bring is the first step; the second step is to find ways to actively elicit their feedback, thoughts, and ideas in an anonymous way, through (for example) websites like SurveyMonkey which can provide invaluable data and information to support more effective execution of an idea.

- *Avoid procrastinating perfectionism:* Like new parents, many entrepreneurs have strong emotional attachments to their ideas, and may suffer from 'procrastinating perfectionism', the tendency to believe that a perfect answer/solution/time is possible and that by waiting long enough...that time will appear. Successful execution requires action, not perfection. There is no more 'the perfect time' to bring an idea to reality than there is a perfect time to have a new child; there will always be compromise and worry along the way. Successful execution starts simply with execution of some sort; the real work is to make execution successful given the conditions in place at the time. Rather than focusing on the perfect time to launch an idea, emphasise adaptability and responsiveness to rapidly changing and evolving environmental factors that are influencing success. Focusing on responding to those changes – rather than on finding the perfect moment to launch – is more likely to lead to action and success than procrastinating perfectionism.

- *Use the LEAN start-up philosophy:* The LEAN philosophy, popularised by Eric Ries, is another way of addressing perfectionist tendencies that may interfere with action and execution. This philosophy emphasises the 'minimum viable product' (MVP) or service. This MVP is '...that version of a new product which allows (the entrepreneur) to collect the maximum amount of validated learning about customers with the least effort'.[5] In essence, this means it is a product or service that barely meets the customer's needs...but that gives the entrepreneur sufficient data to know what to change, what to keep, and how to proceed next. By fully recognising that the MVP is not the perfect final product, service, or idea, it allows the entrepreneur to test drive different methods of production or service delivery, different kinds of marketing or sales techniques, and different kinds of audiences to target to see what works best. It is a form of prototyping that means the entrepreneur now has 'skin in the game' and is actively involved in the market, but is continuously reviewing data to keep improving performance, with the ultimate objective of reaching a point as close to the ideal or idea as possible.... eventually. While LEAN may not work for all entrepreneurial ideas, its emphasis on action, trial and error, and quality improvement can be applied to a variety of different products, services, and technologies.

- *Just do it:* Ill-advised, and half-baked attempts at execution are often as problematic as not proceeding until the perfect moment in time has arrived: both are likely to result in failure. At a certain point, every entrepreneur must simply gather their strength, take a deep breath and dive in. Avoiding execution of an idea today does not guarantee that it will be more successful tomorrow; indeed, endless avoidance often results in de-motivation and ideas dying before they can be realised. As the old saying goes...'if it were easy, everyone would have done it'.

- *Execution never ends:* Entrepreneurs quickly realise that execution is not a step or a process but an ongoing commitment and responsibility to helping an idea not simply come to life but to stay alive and thrive. It has been compared to childbirth and child rearing, a never ending process of constant evolution that brings great joy, heartache, stress, and pride, all at the same time. Like child rearing, there are different time horizons that must be constantly juggled; if parents indulged short-term tantrums to avoid going to school, children would never get educated. And similarly, if parents only fixated on long-term goals of every child becoming a concert pianist, many unhappy and unfulfilled adults would exist. Like parenthood, entrepreneurship is not just a description, it is a lifestyle choice.

Tips for enhancing the likelihood of successful implementation

The following tips all help to enhance the likelihood of successful implementation:

- *Know yourself – and the kind of entrepreneur you want to be:* A solid foundation for successful execution must begin with the entrepreneur themselves. Accurate and honest self appraisal allows for leveraging of one's strengths – and finding others to fill in potential weaknesses. Part of this is to understand and accept the kind of entrepreneur one is trying to be. In some cases, entrepreneurs literally invent and create new and revolutionary things and ideas...but this is surprisingly rare. Entrepreneurs who take other ideas and improve them, or entrepreneurs that plug into existing structures and systems are more commonplace. For example, in pharmacy, a common entrepreneurial pathway is independent ownership of a pharmacy, or perhaps a business that resembles a traditional pharmacy, like a specialty compounding centre. Fewer pharmacists will be entrepreneurs who invent something completely new – for example, an app to support patient care, or a new technology to enhance the quality of communication in teams. It is essential that entrepreneurs accurately categorise the kind of entrepreneur they are and not attempt to be something they are not...success depends upon it.

- *Create your own personal board of advisors:* Execution requires accountability and responsibility and one of the best tools for achieving both is the creation of a 'personal board of advisors'. A group of trusted individuals who will hold the entrepreneur to account, press them on details, and can question potentially flaky or ruinous decisions is an extremely useful tool for entrepreneurs. This group should not simply be cheerleaders who believe in the entrepreneur regardless of what occurs: like any board, a board of advisors needs to be able to hold the entrepreneur to account and push them to execute successfully – but also provide caution and guidance to prevent potential ruin. A personal board of advisors should not simply be family and friends, but needs to include some individuals with expertise, experience, and networks in the field itself.

- *Learn to manage emotional responses to risk:* One of the greatest threats to successful execution is the entrepreneur's inability to self-manage risks. Risk management and mitigation are an essential part of planning for success; equally essential is understanding how – as a human being who has sacrificed much – the entrepreneur themselves will manage the emotional roller coaster of the execution process. This is particularly important in situations where personal financial well-being is on the line: where entrepreneurs invest their own money and compromise their own financial security to build a business, emotional responses to risk can sometimes produce distorted responses. A personal advisory board can be very helpful in supporting the entrepreneur through this process, but ultimately the individual must learn to manage their own emotional responses in a calibrated manner.

- *Learn to be patient and proactive:* While the term 'execution' may imply action and a go-getting philosophy, in many cases successful execution is simply a balance of knowing when to wait and be patient and when to take proactive steps towards a defined objective. Many entrepreneurs are by nature impatient and action oriented, and this can sometimes interfere with successful execution. While some entrepreneurs may say, 'don't just sit there – do something!' in reality, in many cases, the reverse is true: 'don't just do something – sit there!'. Learning when patience is necessary and processes need to be followed – and when proactive interventions are best leveraged, is an art that takes time to develop but ultimately will enhance the likelihood of success.

- *Learn how to sell:* Ultimately, every entrepreneur is going to need to (at some level) be a salesperson. Learning to pitch, market, and create excitement about a new idea is the essence of successful entrepreneurship because entrepreneurs need customers, markets, and market shares to succeed. Learning to sell oneself and one's ideas may not come naturally to every entrepreneur, but successful execution of an idea requires an ability to sell in a way that resonates with primary markets and customers. Importantly, learning how to sell is not a generic activity or something that only cheerleaders indulge in. Learning to sell means understanding customers and markets, tailoring messages appropriately, calibrating delivery in a way that builds interest and respect, and ultimately ensuring professionalism and sustainability allow this to continue into the future.

- *Connect the dots – and the people you meet:* Entrepreneurs must interact with diverse arrays of individuals through the start-up process and into a more established business. Successful execution of ideas requires an ability to think in terms of big pictures, networks and the connections between individuals, organisations, and ideas. For example, a supplier can often end up being a customer, and a customer can perhaps become part of a marketing effort, and marketing can sometimes be used to build interest from investors – who may actually end up being customers eventually. The most successful entrepreneurs have an uncanny ability to actually see these connections in advance and find ways of building upon them effectively. While some individuals might prefer to compartmentalise and pigeon-hole people and organisations into single roles, this is a mistake: learning to connect the dots within and across one's environment and thinking in terms of networks not just individual relationships, can be instrumental in successful execution of an entrepreneurial idea.

- *Be and stay passionate:* The greatest asset any entrepreneur has is themselves: their ideas, their commitments, their dedication, and their passion. No one has as much to gain – or lose – as the entrepreneur themselves, so it makes sense that entrepreneurs have an 'invested passion' in what they do. Without passion, there may be little point in even considering entrepreneurship. While passion is essential, uncontrolled passion can be detrimental to success as it tends towards unreasoned, overly emotional decision making. Calibrating one's emotional state and passion – being 'just passionate enough' about the idea – is important. Equally important is the issue of sustainability: burning too brightly and too quickly can lead to flameouts. Learning to stay passionate for the long haul is important.

- *Be purposeful and intentional:* As important as passion is to successful execution, so to is organisation, purpose, and intentionality. Unbalanced emotion leads to poor decision making, but emotion balanced with purpose and intention is a recipe for success. Understanding the why and how behind one's decisions and actions leads to better and more sustainable decision making and more predictable outcomes. Not simply doing for the sake of doing but doing with purpose and for specific intention is a way to use precious resources and personal energy in a proportionate and sustainable way.

- *Momentum is important:* In physics, momentum refers to the impetus a body derives from moving forward – and in business, momentum refers to a positive virtuous cycle of success that builds when smaller triumphs accumulate upon one another. For entrepreneurs, momentum is often about small successes quickly accumulating to produce a forward trajectory that sustains itself. To achieve momentum, it means entrepreneurs recognise and value small successes, and not expect that the first customer they land will be a Fortune 500 company, or the first review they get will be in the New York Times. While ultimately, entrepreneurs can and should 'dream big', they should also value and appreciate momentum, and actively seek out small wins and 'low-hanging-fruit' that are the individual bricks upon which an impressive edifice of success will eventually be built.

- *Focus on always improving:* No idea – and no entrepreneur – is perfect. Everyone and everything can improve, and openness to feedback and suggestions, and treating criticism as data (and not as jealousy) can help entrepreneurs continuously improve themselves and their offerings. Expecting criticism and learning how to respond effectively to it is part of successful execution. Clinging tenaciously to one's initial ideas and beliefs with no capacity to accept feedback will undermine success.

- *Make work life balance and resilience a priority:* Execution is not a one-off process that is time limited and then completed. Entrepreneurs are constantly executing at all times they are entrepreneurs, and this reality can be exhausting. Overstressed and burned-out entrepreneurs cannot succeed in the long-term, so managing one's work-life balance and prioritising personal mental and physical health is an integral component of successful execution.

- *Take responsibility for your own legacy:* Many entrepreneurs compare the start-up process to parenting: giving 'birth' to an idea, seeing it through the difficult and cranky early years, managing the seemingly hopeless and unmanageable 'terrible twos', sacrificing sleep, finances and personal relationships to help nurture and grow the child...until, almost by magic, a child becomes more independent, delightful and (in an ideal world) independent and successful. For most parents, the idea that children are their legacy is both psychologically complex and fraught, but also an important part of the psychological fuel that allows exhausted and stressed parents to continue to survive and ultimately thrive. For entrepreneurs, the notion that their idea is 'their baby' and needs similar care, concern, nurturing and sacrifice in order to grow and thrive helps to highlight the notion of legacy. In taking responsibility for one's own legacy as an entrepreneur, many of the sacrifices and steps necessary for successful execution will fall into place and a greater meaning will be found.

Summary

Few, if any, entrepreneurs begin their journey thinking about execution, but no entrepreneur can succeed unless they think carefully about execution. Execution is a complex and nuanced process that is a function of the entrepreneur themselves, the idea being executed, the market and environment within which the entrepreneur is operating, and an uncountable number of other factors over which the entrepreneur has limited or no control. Yes – it is complicated. But as complicated as it is, execution is essential to success. There is no replacement for careful and systematic planning and constant self-reflection, reality checking, and course corrections along the way. While it is usually exciting to the point of self-indulgent to wallow in the glory of one's own genius and idea – it will never amount to anything without disciplined execution. The first and most important element of successful execution is self-discipline. Planning, organisation, methodical assessments, and evidence-based decision making should never squash passion and enthusiasm for one's ideas but needs to be seamlessly integrated into the entrepreneur's work in a sustainable and positive manner.

References

1. Davenport T. Entrepreneurial execution: the future of strategy. *Harvard Business Review* [online] 2007. https://hbr.org/2007/12/entrepreneurial-execution-the

2. Ching K *et al.* (2018). *Control versus execution: endogenous appropriability and entrepreneurial strategy.* Cambridge: National Bureau of Economic Research. https://doi.org/10.3386/w24448

3. Peterson A, Wu A. Entrepreneurial learning and strategic foresight. *Strategic Management J* 2021; 42(13): 2357–2388. https://doi.org/10.1002/smj.3327

4. Cote C (2020). *5 keys to successful strategy execution.* Boston: Harvard Business School Online. https://online.hbs.edu/blog/post/strategy-execution

5. Frigo M. Strategy, business execution, and performance measures. *Strategic Finance* 2002; 83(11): 6–8.

CHAPTER 34

Managing success and learning from failure to become the kind of entrepreneur you want to be

Upon completion of this chapter you should be able to:

- understand the importance of entrepreneurial self-reflection
- list the types of entrepreneurial style
- understand how to deal with failure
- recognise the importance of keeping your entrepreneurial sense of self separate from entrepreneurial ideas
- explain the psychological impact of rumination.

The Oxford dictionary defines an entrepreneur as '...a person who organises and operates a business or businesses, taking on greater than normal financial risks to do so.' From this description, it is clear that issues of risk are important, as is the notion of organising and operating a business. This may lead some to wonder what the distinction between an entrepreneur, a manager, or a leader is – managers and leaders also organise and operate different kinds of businesses, albeit without the same kinds of risks as entrepreneurs. The Merriam-Webster dictionary defines an entrepreneur as '...a person who starts a business and is willing to risk loss in order to make money'. Again, the issue of risk (especially financial risk) is front and centre in this definition, but so too is the concept of great reward...making money. Both dictionaries highlight the financial side of the entrepreneurial equation and while – of course – this is important and relevant, most entrepreneurs will describe something more nuanced and arguably less self-centred or tangible than mere profitability.

The term 'entrepreneurial mindset' has been coined to describe a set of skills and propensities common to most entrepreneurs, allowing them to make the most of opportunities, learn from and overcome setbacks, and ultimately achieve success.[1] The term 'mindset' highlights the important psychological facets of entrepreneurship, and, in particular, psychological relationships with issues such as risk, loss, creativity, and selling oneself to others. The entrepreneurial mindset is sometimes said to consist of five distinct characteristics: positivity, creativity, persuasive communication skills, intrinsic drive/motivation, and tenacity (the ability to bounce back and learn from failures).[2,3]

Some entrepreneurs bristle at being pigeon-holed or stereotyped with a single, all-encompassing definition. Initial reasons or drivers for individuals to consider entrepreneurship vary considerably from person to person. The idea of a 'mindset' might even be discomforting or appear unnecessarily intrusive. Regardless of one's perspectives, the psychology of entrepreneurship – and psychological self-awareness and grounding – appears to be an important element of success. While there is no one-size-fits-all mindset that encompasses all entrepreneurs, the concept of an individual entrepreneurial type or 'style' has increasingly been discussed as a way to promote self-reflection, and to better understand how one learns from both success and failure.

What's your style?

Increased interest in entrepreneurship in pharmacy has arisen since the start of the pandemic, as many pharmacists reflected upon their profession, their careers, their livelihood, and their lifestyle choices. Further, the pandemic helped illuminate the costs and consequences of inequalities in society – while some people got to retreat to the safety and sterility of their home office and work contentedly away from the ravages of coronavirus, others – like community pharmacists – continued to work in the front lines dealing with people every day under uncertain and potentially dangerous conditions. General surveys have found that interest in entrepreneurship across society has increased significantly since the start of the pandemic, with the top reasons being the opportunity to be one's own boss, freedom/flexibility to choose, and satisfaction in one's own work and success. The importance of entrepreneurship to the general economy and society is remarkable: for example, in the United States, virtually all net growth in jobs created over the last decade has come from entrepreneurial start-ups, while established firms and companies have reduced the size of their workforces significantly.[4]

Barlow has popularised the concept of entrepreneurial style to help individuals recognise their priorities, needs, and values as an entrepreneur, with the hope that this helps to better prepare them for the realities, the success and the inevitable failures associated with entrepreneurial start-ups.[5] Understanding one's entrepreneurial style can help to understand one's psychological responses to risk, the need to sell oneself to others, and many other aspects of entrepreneurship – including responses to successes and failures.

- *The innovator:* The 'classic' entrepreneur is the individual who has built a better mousetrap – or invented a new product or service that meets a marketplace need. Innovators are individuals who express their creativity in ways that aim to change the way other people think or live. Originality is the currency in which they deal: they identify gaps and work to fill them in ways that haven't been explored in the past. Innovators like Jeff Bezos (Amazon) or Steve Jobs (Apple) simply see opportunities where others see nothing. Within the pharmacy context, innovators will typically be individuals who, through their own professional experience, have identified gaps in products, services, or care for patients then leverage their creativity to find inventive ways to address these issues. In most cases, innovators are characterised by their high level of motivation to produce something new or different, their willingness to overcome nay-sayers or negative individuals in their family and networks, and perhaps a somewhat obsessive passion to do what they say they are going to do. Innovators may spend much time on their own, toying with and refining their ideas; this is often an advantage because until the idea is ready to debut, there is little financial or personal risk other than the loss of one's own time. At their worst, innovators may be too single-minded and self-confident that they have an idea where everyone else has failed, but at their best, innovators are creative, purpose driven, and passionate in their work.

- *The hustler:* Unlike innovators, hustlers rarely are involved in the invention or creation of something new or different; instead, they are entrepreneurs who have the capacity to see connections where others do not and bring individuals together for a greater (and more profitable) purpose. For the hustler, there is a great premium placed on the capacity to win over others, particularly skeptical audiences, and to change minds and hearts through the power of personality and persuasion. Hustlers like Donald Trump have made (and lost) fortunes through their ability to tell a story and inspire a vision, even if that story or vision is not of their own making. Hustlers may sometimes leverage the creativity and inventions of the innovators; they rarely have the time or inclination to create or invent things on their own but can quickly see and create opportunities for profit and growth from the work of others. Hustlers are generally comfortable with risk, understand the 'high risk, high reward' formula, and function most effectively in situations where there is some chaos, uncertainty, or ambiguity. At their worst, hustlers may come across as hucksters or scam artists making big and undeliverable promises leaving a trail of chaos and destruction behind (for which they take little responsibility). At their best, hustlers have unbridled energy and enthusiasm, an incredible capacity to make connections and build a following of fervent believers, and in the process can create tremendous outcomes. In the pharmacy context, hustlers are typical 'born salespeople' who can convince and captivate customers and an audience in ways that encourage them to buy products and services – and spend money in ways aligned with the hustler's ambitions.

- *The social entrepreneur:* These idealistic entrepreneurs are typically individuals who have a strong and altruistic need to make society a better place by solving social problems. They may be less interested in profit or personal fame. Social entrepreneurs may emphasise both products and services. For example, Bernard Kouchner is widely credited with being amongst the first volunteers to found the humanitarian organisation Médicins Sans Frontières (Doctors without Borders). His story reflects the power and potential of the social entrepreneur, a person who identifies a desperate social need not connected to profitability, works collaboratively with other like-minded individuals, and ultimately builds an organisation that literally has saved tens of thousands of lives. Also, consider the story of Greta Thunberg and her entrepreneurial spirit in addressing climate breakdown. The desire to drive positive change in the world and create value through their hands-on efforts is particularly strong for social entrepreneurs. Equally, they have the capacity to inspire others through their own stories and actions, to build networks, to advocate fiercely for causes that are important to them, and to be creative in solving social problems. Importantly, social entrepreneurs face all the same risks, need all the same skills in sales, marketing, advocacy, and strategic planning that other kinds of entrepreneurs require. Their efforts, however, are in service of something greater than themselves and are deployed in the context of a cause that is of significant personal importance and value. At their worst, social entrepreneurs can appear hectoring and may overleverage guilt in a holier-than-though manner and despite their best intentions, can make situations worse through an almost selfish need to help others. At their best, social entrepreneurs literally change the world and save lives with only limited self-interest and concern for their own profitability or well-being. Within the pharmacy context, social entrepreneurs are frequently individuals who express their creativity and innovation by working with medical missions or organisations like Médicins Sans Frontières, cleverly findings ways of bringing high quality pharmacy services to places that may be experiencing significant social turmoil.

- *The imitator:* It is sometimes said that imitation is the sincerest form of flattery. Imitators are entrepreneurs who build on existing ideas with the objective of simply doing it better, more efficiently, more effectively and ultimately more profitably. Rather than 'reinvent the wheel', imitators emphasise process refinements and improvements as a way of executing existing ideas in creative and new ways. While some may dismiss imitators as a poor facsimile of a 'real' entrepreneur, in reality, the majority of the most successful entrepreneurs are actually those who have never invented anything new but instead have found ways of using existing ideas in better and more strategic ways. The great strength of the imitator is their ability to focus on strategy and execution, and not be bound too tightly to a single idea or creative impulse. They can 'shop around' for the best ideas without feeling personally invested in their own innovation. They see themselves as being able to refine existing ideas and solve problems with prototypes that already exist – their role is to simply improve rather than innovate. At their worst, imitators may seem too opportunistic and not sufficiently invested in their work, only seeking self-gain and profitability. At their best, imitators are self-confident, able to learn from other's mistakes, and get things done. In the pharmacy context, most pharmacy owners are imitators, refining existing ideas for how to run a pharmacy and imprinting their own unique interests and skills in the process.

- *Intrapreneurs:* Perhaps the largest number of entrepreneurs are not individuals who ultimately have their own business or assume their own financial risks...instead they are intrapreneurs who have stable and secure jobs with large, well-known organisations and apply their creativity, skills, and passions to innovate and lead improvements within a company structure that ultimately increase profitability and bring good ideas to life. For example, some of the most entrepreneurial individuals in pharmacy are hospital pharmacists who must navigate complex bureaucratic and political structures, manage difficult workplace conditions, and experience great pharmacotherapy challenges daily. With the safety and security of a salary with benefits and the backing of a large institution, these individuals do not assume personal financial risks in the way more traditionally defined entrepreneurs may, but they still express creativity and solve complex problems in highly meaningful ways. In fact, for many pharmacists, the 'freedom' associated with a full time job provides them with the peace of mind necessary to truly be innovative, creative, and entrepreneurial – and their employers benefit significantly from this. To these individuals, personal financial gain or fame is less important than the innovation itself and solving meaningful problems in ways aligned with personal needs and values.

The notion of an entrepreneurial 'style' can be helpful to consider as it provides a structure for explaining motivations, hoped for outcomes, and underlying psychological needs that will be satisfied through entrepreneurial expression. It is essential to be honest and accurate in self-appraisal: while it may be more ennobling to self-define as a 'social entrepreneur', this type of individual is clearly different to a hustler. Trying to fool oneself is rarely successful in this regard: if profit maximisation is one's goal, then social entrepreneurship is not the best vehicle to achieve this. Similarly, there is no shame in recognising that one's need for safety, security and stability is crucial to psychological well-being – and that an intrapreneur route is a more satisfying option that minimises personal financial risk while still allowing for opportunities to express creativity and innovation (albeit with someone else making the profit and taking on the risks).

What you call yourself helps you to understand success

Hollywood movies and business fiction are replete with examples of risk-taking entrepreneurial swashbucklers who said 'damn the torpedoes, full speed ahead!' in order to achieve their dreams. Of course, there are some very high profile cases of extremely successful entrepreneurs who were innovators and hustlers and succeeded beyond their – or anyone's – wildest dreams. Less well publicised are the imitators who quietly go about improving ideas and running businesses that are the cornerstones of their communities, in a less flashy or well-known way. Even less well publicised are the intrapreneurs who – by the tens of thousands – work in corporations big and small and allow those companies to grow, prosper, and innovate, without the need for a spotlight or personal financial gains.

It is estimated that close to 90% of start-ups – and even 75% of investor-backed businesses – will likely fail within the first three years of operation.[6] This sobering reality is frequently overlooked in movies and biographies that showcase the breathless opportunities that afforded the risk-taking entrepreneur. When the default state of entrepreneurship is failure, it may raise questions as to why anyone would want to bother at all.

The reasons for entrepreneurial failure vary considerably, including overinvestment in the wrong idea or product, improvident depletion of capital, bad choices with respect to partnerships/employees/investors, or miscalculating risks. Especially in the early days of a venture, small problems can lead to existential threats because few entrepreneurs have the financial backing to withstand years of losses. Most 'successful' entrepreneurs (and remember, successful entrepreneurs are the vast minority of all those starting out in this enterprise) highlight their own experiences with failure as crucial to supporting their ultimate success. Several common themes in terms of dealing with failure emerge, regardless of the entrepreneur's individual style:[7,8]

- *Failure is feedback:* The term 'failure' has a strongly negative emotional connotation, particularly for an entrepreneur who may have invested the best part of themselves in an idea. One cannot help but interpret the failure of an idea as a personal shortcoming, and this in turn can't help but trigger strong defensive and negative emotions. While this all-too-human response is understandable, it is unfortunately catastrophic for entrepreneurs. Most successful entrepreneurs will say they have unusually strong comfort with failure, even if they interpret failure in a personal way. The key is to think of failure as feedback, not an insult. Analysing failure and learning from it is essential. Dwelling on failure, railing against it, and blaming others for it is neither productive nor a way of dealing with it. Instead, trying to overcome a strong initial negative emotional response, then methodically analysing the failure to identify underlying causes and reasons can help prepare for the next time around.
- *Solutions to actual problems:* A significant cause for entrepreneurial failure may be the entrepreneur's unwillingness to acknowledge the absolute need for their innovation to solve an actual, real world problem. A clever idea or brilliant innovation that doesn't solve a problem may be a cocktail party conversation starter but will rarely translate into success. Accepting that one's idea

– no matter how imaginative or creative it is – actually doesn't solve anyone else's problem can be difficult, but failure to do so will likely lead to entrepreneurial failure. Innovators and hustlers are at highest risk of this, as they may overinvest personally in ideas. Social entrepreneurs may also overestimate the significance of their personal social crusade for other people.

- *Entrepreneurship is a team sport:* While many entrepreneurs opt for this route as a way of 'breaking free' from organisations, bureaucracies, and (most of all) 'bosses', the reality is that entrepreneurship is a team sport that involves organisations, bureaucracies, and bosses. In any business, large or small, success depends heavily on teamwork and collaboration, and entrepreneurial failure is most likely when entrepreneurs choose not to believe this reality. Entrepreneurship should never be an option for an individual who doesn't like working with other people or feels uncomfortable being part of a team; these are unavoidable realities of entrepreneurship and actually determinants of success.

- *Learning to hire:* One of the most important lessons from failed entrepreneurs is the reality that hiring decisions are amongst the most important – and impactful – ones that will govern success. In some cases, entrepreneurs may be too resistant to hire others for fear of losing control. In other cases, they may hire people too quickly without adequate screening, training, and onboarding to support success. The managerial functions of entrepreneurship are rarely showcased but they are pivotal to success. It is often said that the only thing worse than not being able to hire someone is hiring the wrong someone: learning how to hire properly – with sufficient diligence, support, clarity of purpose, and commitments to onboarding – is essential for success.

- *Learning to manage personal energy in a sustainable way:* The stereotype of an entrepreneur is of a highly energised and extraverted individual who is always thinking, always doing, and is always 'on'. While entrepreneurship does require a certain kind – and amount – of personal energy, it is also important to recognise that all human beings have limits. In some cases, alarming dedication to entrepreneurship may signify a deeper mental health issue that just happens to express itself in this way. In most cases, entrepreneurs will need to learn lessons regarding how to balance energy expenditures, ensuring there is sufficient energy remaining to manage day to day personal life. Burn-out and emotional/physical exhaustion can occur and will undermine attempts to create successful business ventures. While each person has a different baseline capacity for energy expenditure, even the most highly energetic of individuals must find ways of slowing down, stopping, and resting.

- *The limits of perseverance:* In popular culture, entrepreneurs are seen to have a 'never take no for an answer' attitude. No doubt, perseverance and tenacity in the face of negativity is essential for entrepreneurs. Successful entrepreneurs recognise that mindless perseverance is counterproductive and will hinder their development. It is a fine balancing act: sufficient perseverance to overcome reasonable obstacles is necessary, but single-minded obsession can be both emotionally and physically damaging to the entrepreneur and contribute to failure.

You are not your failures – or your successes

The connection between one's ideas, one's business, and one's personality are incredibly tight for most entrepreneurs. The time, energy and sacrifice required to be an entrepreneur means that in most cases, entrepreneurs have a difficult time disassociating their situation from themselves. Where entrepreneurial ideas are successful, this can be an enormous ego-boost. Some of the highest profile (and badly behaved) entrepreneurs in the public eye are often wildly successful as business people, and this leads them to believe that somehow they are more than, or better than, the average person.

Learning to be justifiably proud of one's accomplishments while still maintaining basic civility and human decency can be surprisingly tricky, particularly in a media and societal context where roguish and outrageous entrepreneurs are admired. Entrepreneurs like Elon Musk and Donald Trump appear to cultivate their personae to be larger-than-life figures who act as masters of the universe. Such ego-driven behaviour may be transiently gratifying or even lead to election as President, but in the longer term there is a corrosive and psychologically damaging element to 'believing one's own press'.

Success as an entrepreneur produces as many psychological complications as failure. In reality, it is not clear why some entrepreneurs succeed, and others do not. Seemingly random factors beyond the control of the entrepreneur clearly have a significant influence on both success and failure. Unfortunately, human beings tend to believe that their successes are entirely or predominantly due to their own hard work, intelligence, and creativity, while failures are due to external factors. Both success and failure are highly reliant on uncontrollable external factors; the objectives of business planning, risk management, and marketing are actually to better manage these external factors while still recognising they can never be controlled entirely by the entrepreneur. Where entrepreneurs start to believe they have super-human or magical powers that other human beings do not, simply because their business has succeeded, this will set the stage for a subsequent and spectacular failure in the future. Consider the sobering example of Donald Trump: while his success as a businessman and entrepreneur was always questionable from a financial perspective, he was able to parlay the manufactured impression of himself into being elected as the 45th President of the United States. When disagreements arose that led to failures, it was (almost) always other people's faults – not his own. A spectacularly public unwinding of his carefully manufactured persona occurred during the final years of his presidency and in the years that followed. His 'success' as an entrepreneur led to an overconfidence bias of Shakespearean proportions.

On the other hand, failure can also be challenging to manage. Where an entrepreneur has become too personally invested in their idea, failure can be particularly bitter and psychologically damaging. In situations where entrepreneurs have not only invested personal time, hope, and energy into a business, but have also mortgaged their house, borrowed from family members, and have enormous financial liabilities, the personal and the entrepreneurial are completely intertwined. In such cases, 'failure' will be felt in a highly personal way: it is not just the idea that has failed, but the entrepreneur as a human being has failed as well. In many cases, there will be early warning signals of this risk: where entrepreneurs are unable to accept valid criticism or helpful suggestions from others, it may be a sign that the personal and the entrepreneurial are too tightly attached to one another. Recognising this issue and preventing it from becoming bigger is vitally important to ensure the worst psychological outcomes of failure do not occur.

Regardless of one's entrepreneurial style or mindset, it is essential that entrepreneurs remain mindful and vigilant to keep themselves, their personalities, and their psychological health ringfenced and separate from their entrepreneurial ideas. Passion, excitement, and strong belief in one's ideas is essential for success and, of course, do entail some measure of intertwining of the personal and the entrepreneurial. Finding a way of maintaining a healthy and sustainable balance, and always ensuring there is a psychological off-ramp available to ensure neither failure nor success fundamentally changes one's personality, is essential.

Rumination: the curse of the entrepreneur?

Psychologists describe rumination as an unhealthy fixation or the inability to shift one's thinking away from a topic despite conscious attempts to do so.[9] The cognitive work of entrepreneurship is significant, time-consuming, and exhausting. Entrepreneurs will often spend almost all waking hours – and some sleeping hours – refining their ideas, developing what-if and hypothetical scenarios, and rehearsing elevator pitches or business plan deliveries. This is part of being an entrepreneur and for many individuals, part of the fun and excitement of the process. Where productive idea generation becomes problematic is when fixation and rumination emerge. Worse, when considering failure, some entrepreneurs may find themselves incapable of overcoming post-hoc rumination and analysis, always looking for who to blame and what went wrong.

Everyone who has ever accomplished anything significant has also failed along the way. J.K. Rowling had her Harry Potter books turned down by many publishers. Albert Einstein was unsuccessful in being hired as a professor. Even Donald Trump declared bankruptcy on several occasions. The emotional intelligence of most pharmacists (Assimilators) may actually leave them particularly prone to rumination because of their tendency towards 'procrastinating perfectionism'. Rumination can be dangerous to mental and physical health as it can prolong or intensify depression, as well as interfere with one's ability to think clearly, process emotions, and interact appropriately with others in social situations.[9] It can lead to feelings of isolation because it causes individuals to push other people away from them. In the context of entrepreneurial failure, rumination might be understandable, but one must be vigilant to ensure it does not reach dangerous or unhealthy levels.

There is no magical cure-all for rumination. Entrepreneurs who have experienced failure and rumination often highlight how important a supportive social network can be in helping them overcome the tendency to ruminate. Family, friends, colleagues – and even competitors who truly understand the experience of entrepreneurial failure – can all be important sources of comfort. Importantly, social connectedness is probably the most helpful way of overcoming rumination as it forces individuals to look outside themselves, grounds them in an objective external reality, and opens the possibility of social interactions that are distracting and fun. More internalised techniques such as meditation, mindfulness, yoga, or journalling may also be helpful.

Activity and action are thought to be particularly powerful antidotes to the more cerebral activity of rumination. Making a list of what to do and actively ticking off items as they are accomplished gives individuals a sense of control, mastery, and success – and disrupts the cognitive spiral of rumination. Finding trusted individuals in one's social and professional networks who can 'call out' rumination and ruminating behaviours is important; often, in failure, entrepreneurs are incapable of seeing how they appear to others. Psychotherapy or counselling should not be considered a last resort but instead simply one more activity to help the entrepreneur process and manage failure in a productive and healthy way. For those who are less psychologically oriented, career or life-coaches may serve a similar function in being a sounding board and reflector of one's thinking and experiences. Finally, learning to identify one's triggers for rumination is important: when rumination emerges, it is important to take mental note of the situation and reasons why it started (for example, the presence of another person, the time of day, a particular location). Learning to avoid or manage these triggers to prevent the rumination cycle from even beginning is important.

Not all entrepreneurs will ruminate in light of failure, but many will. The toxic effects of rumination are significant and must be managed vigorously and proactively. Entrepreneurs recognise and accept many risks when they embark upon this path but may underappreciate the psychological risks they may face should failure occur. Being clear-eyed and realistic about this is important – and will allow entrepreneurs to ultimately learn from failure to set themselves up for success in the future.

So how do I start?

Most of us have what we believe to be a great idea – something new, innovative, important, and unique that is a reflection of both our experiences and our personalities. It is exciting to daydream and speculate about what could possibly be...if only we plucked up the courage to get started. Entrepreneurship seems to be something that is hard-wired into most human beings – it taps into our creativity, our desire to solve problems, our hope to make our mark on the world, and our need for autonomy and being our own boss. Despite this, few of us actually become entrepreneurs.

There is no roadmap or magical formula for how to get started as an entrepreneur. The experience of successful – and unsuccessful – entrepreneurs suggests that introspection, reflection, and honest self-awareness are the foundation. Knowing oneself and accepting one's deficiencies makes it easier to know where to concentrate one's attention. There is no substitute for planning, forethought, and being organised. Entrepreneurs can control very little in the universe around them...so the things they can control need to be controlled as best as possible. Entrepreneurship is, in many ways, a job like any other. There will be times where it is a slog, times when it is a pleasure, times when it is frustrating, and times when it is rewarding beyond words. The amplitude of this rollercoaster ride may be larger than in more traditional jobs, but the experiences are broadly similar. Entrepreneurship will never solve all one's personal problems or be a magical pill that transports us to a world of wonders and delights.... but it can open new possibilities, provide exciting opportunities, and allow individuals to explore parts of themselves they never knew even existed.

Part of this process of reflection and introspection means figuring out for oneself how best to get started on this voyage. For some individuals, it might mean bringing on a partner or colleague immediately, because they know they need the social reinforcement and support of another human being to help them along the way. For others, it might mean jumping in with both feet and going through cycles of failure and success to get it just right....and that's okay because they are perfectly fine with failing occasionally. For some, it might mean finding a regular job in a big company that provides salary, stability, and security...but ensuring that big company lets them be intra-preneurial in ways that are meaningful.

There is no one-size-fits-all solution for how to get started as an entrepreneur...but there are clearly steps along the path that everyone will need to take. Developing a personal value proposition, a business plan, thinking about risk management and entrepreneurial marketing, and building networks will be relevant to all entrepreneurs. Perhaps most importantly, doing the work of learning about oneself and answering the question, 'what kind of entrepreneur do I want to be?' is essential.

What are you waiting for?

References

1. Lynch M, Corbett A. Entrepreneurial mindset shift and the role of cycles of learning. *J Small Business Management* 2023; 61(1): 80–101. https://doi.org/10.1080/00472778.2021.1924381

2. Jiatong W *et al*. Impact of entrepreneurial education, mindset, and creativity on entrepreneurial intention: mediating role of entrepreneurial self-efficacy. *Front Psychol* 2021; 12: 724440. https://doi.org/10.3389/fpsyg.2021.724440

3. Wiklund J *et al*. Entrepreneurship and well-being: Past, present, and future. *J Business Venturing* 2019; 34(4): 579–588. https://doi.org/10.1016/j.jbusvent.2019.01.002

4. Abraham L, Master B (2021). *Entrepreneurship in America: challenges and opportunities*. Santa Monica: Rand Corporation. https://www.rand.org/content/dam/rand/pubs/perspectives/PEA1100/PEA1141-1/RAND_PEA1141-1.pdf

5. Barlow S. *Unprepared to Entrepreneur: A Method to the Madness of Starting Your Own Business*. New York City: Kogan Page, 2021.

6. Klimas P *et al*. Entrepreneurial failure: a synthesis and conceptual framework of its effects. *Euro Management Rev* 2021; 18(1): 167–182. https://doi.org/10.1111/emre.12426

7. Jenkins A, McKelvie A. What is entrepreneurial failure? Implications for future research. *Int Small Business J* 2016; 34(2): 176–188. https://doi.org/10.1177/0266242615574011

8. Pan L-Y *et al*. Entrepreneurial business start-ups and entrepreneurial failure: how to stand up after a fall? *Front Psychol* 2022; 13: 943328. https://doi.org/10.3389/fpsyg.2022.943328

9. Smith J, Alloy L. A roadmap to rumination: a review of the definition, assessment, and conceptualization of this multifaceted construct. *Clin Psychol Rev* 2009; 29(2): 116–128. https://doi.org/10.1016/j.cpr.2008.10.003

Index